ADVANCED
ORAL SURGERY

Andreas Filippi | Fabio Saccardin | Sebastian Kühl (eds)

ADVANCED
ORAL SURGERY

With contributions by:
Stephan Acham, Daniel Baumhoer, Michael M. Bornstein, Thomas Connert,
Dorothea Dagassan-Berndt, Henrik Dommisch, Tobias Fretwurst, Mathieu Gass,
Norbert Jakse, Ronald E. Jung, Georgios Kanavakis, Adrian Kasaj, Khaled Mukaddam,
Katja Nelson, Puria Parvini, Michael Payer, Martina Schriber, Michael Schwaiger,
Frank Schwarz, Bernd Stadlinger, Frank Peter Strietzel, Silvio Valdec, Carlalberta Verna,
Jürgen Wallner, Wolfgang Zemann

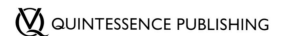 QUINTESSENCE PUBLISHING

Berlin | Chicago | Tokyo
Barcelona | London | Milan | Mexico City | Paris | Prague | Seoul | Warsaw
Beijing | Istanbul | Sao Paulo | Zagreb

One book, one tree: In support of reforestation worldwide and to address the climate crisis, for every book sold Quintessence Publishing will plant a tree (https://onetreeplanted.org/).

A video shows more than a series of photographs

Numerous videos are included in this book to illustrate the content and enrich the reading experience. These can easily be played on a smartphone or tablet using the QR code.

Alternatively, the videos can also be accessed via this link: https://video.qvnet.de/b23530/.

A CIP record for this book is available from the British Library.
ISBN: 978-1-78698-133-2

Title of original issue: Das große 1 x 1 der Oralchirurgie
Copyright © 2022 Quintessenz Verlags-GmbH, Berlin, Germany

QUINTESSENCE PUBLISHING DEUTSCHLAND

Quintessenz Verlags-GmbH
Ifenpfad 2–4
12107 Berlin, Germany
www.quintessence-publishing.com

Quintessence Publishing Co Ltd
Grafton Road, New Malden
Surrey KT3 3AB, United Kingdom
www.quintessence-publishing.com

Translation: Susan Holmes, Brighton, UK
Editing, layout, and production: Quintessenz Verlags-GmbH, Berlin, Germany

ISBN: 978-1-78698-133-2
Printed and bound in Croatia

Preface

Our book *Basic Oral Surgery* was published in late 2022. It became clear even during the creation of that first volume that if that book was about "basic" oral surgery, there would need to be a successor. And so we set about creating this book, *Advanced Oral Surgery*, the content and scope of which is based on advanced training programs and the range of clinical advanced training in oral surgery provided by university departments. The book is aimed at our advanced oral surgery colleagues who frequently perform oral surgery procedures in their practices and want to update or develop their skills as well as current and prospective specialists in oral and maxillofacial surgery.

Like the first volume, *Advanced Oral Surgery* is not designed as a textbook but as an atlas. Particularly in the clinical chapters, the theoretical content is outlined in short passages of text that all follow a similar structure: indications, contraindications, step-by-step clinical procedures, and postoperative course, together with just a few relevant literature references. These chapters come to life in the series of photographs in the book and the videos linked via QR codes, which can be viewed very easily and almost instantaneously on any up-to-date smartphone or tablet. This significantly expands the scope and value of the book beyond mere static images. We hope that as a result our book

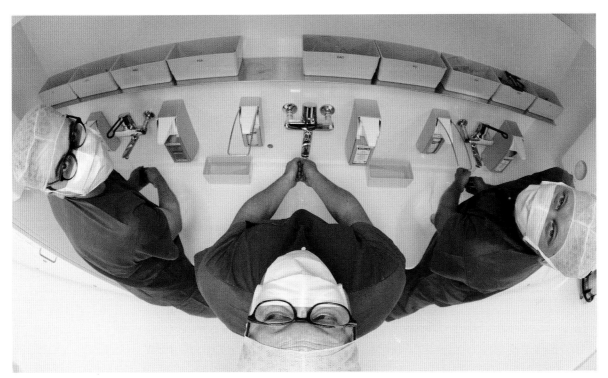

The editors in the operating room at the dental clinic in Basel before surgery (from left to right): Fabio Saccardin, Andreas Filippi, and Sebastian Kühl.

Preface

will give practitioners more confidence before, during, and after oral surgery interventions. Some redundancies in the content as well as a few contradictory statements by the team of authors drawn from three nations are intentional on the part of the editors.

Our special thanks again go to everyone who has been involved in the creation of this second volume: our co-authors Stephan Acham, Daniel Baumhoer, Michael M. Bornstein, Thomas Connert, Dorothea Dagassan-Berndt, Henrik Dommisch, Tobias Fretwurst, Mathieu Gass, Norbert Jakse, Ronald E. Jung, Georgios Kanavakis, Adrian Kasaj, Khaled Mukaddam, Katja Nelson, Puria Parvini, Michael Payer, Martina Schriber, Michael Schwaiger, Frank Schwarz, Bernd Stadlinger, Frank Strietzel, Silvio Valdec, Carlalberta Verna, Jürgen Wallner, and Wolfgang Zemann.

Our thanks also go to Sabrina Peterer for the cover image, which continues the style of the iconic covers of books by Andreas Filippi; Anita Hattenbach from Quintessence Publishing, Andreas Filippi's favorite editor for her ever-reliable, incredibly pleasant, and highly professional editing (and that is compared with all the other publishers with whom Andreas Filippi has previously worked); and to all the staff involved at Quintessence Publishing in Berlin.

Finally, thank you to all our colleagues at our really fantastic Department of Oral Surgery at UZB in Basel for your support, your motivation, and your dedication. It is tremendously enjoyable to work with all of you every day.

Andreas Filippi, Fabio Saccardin,
and Sebastian Kühl

Editors' contact details

Prof Dr Andreas Filippi
Dr Fabio Saccardin
Prof Dr Sebastian Kühl
Department of Oral Surgery
University Center for Dental Medicine Basel UZB
University of Basel
Mattenstr. 40
CH – 4058 Basel, Switzerland

Authors' contact details

Priv-Doz Dr Stephan Acham
Clinical Department of Oral Surgery and Ortho-
dontics
Department of Dental Medicine and Oral Health
Medical University of Graz
Billrothgasse 4
A – 8010 Graz, Austria

Prof Dr Daniel Baumhoer
Bone Tumor Reference Center and DOESAK
Reference Registry
Department of Medical Genetics and Pathology
University Hospital Basel
Schönbeinstr. 40
CH – 4031 Basel, Switzerland

Prof Dr Michael M. Bornstein
Department of Oral Health & Medicine
University Center for Dental Medicine Basel UZB
University of Basel
Mattenstr. 40
CH – 4058 Basel, Switzerland

Priv-Doz Dr Thomas Connert
Department of Periodontology, Endodontology
and Cariology
University Center for Dental Medicine Basel UZB
University of Basel
Mattenstr. 40
CH – 4058 Basel, Switzerland

Dr Dorothea Dagassan-Berndt
Center for Dental Imaging
University Center for Dental Medicine Basel UZB
University of Basel
Mattenstr. 40
CH – 4058 Basel, Switzerland

Prof Dr Henrik Dommisch
Department of Periodontology, Oral Medicine
and Oral Surgery
CharitéCenter 3 for Oral Health Sciences
Charité – Universitätsmedizin Berlin
Aßmannshauserstr. 4–6
D – 14197 Berlin, Germany

Prof Dr Tobias Fretwurst
Department of Oral and Maxillofacial Surgery/
Translational Implantology
University of Freiburg
Hugstetterstr. 55
D – 79106 Freiburg, Germany

Dr Dr Mathieu Gass
University Clinic for Caniomaxillofacial Surgery
Inselspital, University Hospital Bern
Freiburgstrasse 20
CH – 3010 Bern, Switzerland

Contact details

Prof Dr Dr Norbert Jakse
Clinical Department of Oral Surgery and Ortho-
dontics
Department of Dental Medicine and Oral Health
Medical University of Graz
Billrothgasse 4
A – 8010 Graz, Austria

Prof Dr Ronald E. Jung, PhD
Department of Reconstructive Dentistry
Center of Dental Medicine UZH
University of Zürich
Plattenstr. 11
CH – 8032 Zürich, Switzerland

Dr Georgios Kanavakis
Department of Pediatric Oral Health and Ortho-
dontics
University Center for Dental Medicine Basel UZB
University of Basel
Mattenstr. 40
CH – 4058 Basel, Switzerland

Prof Dr Dr h c Adrian Kasaj, MSc
Department of Periodontology and
Operative Dentistry
University Medical Center
Augustusplatz 2
D – 55131 Mainz, Germany

Dr Khaled Mukaddam
Department of Oral Surgery
University Center for Dental Medicine Basel UZB
University of Basel
Mattenstr. 40
CH – 4058 Basel, Switzerland

Prof Dr Katja Nelson
Department of Oral and Maxillofacial Surgery/
Translational Implantology
University of Freiburg
Hugstetterstr. 55
D – 79106 Freiburg, Germany

Priv-Doz Dr Puria Parvini, MSc MSc
Outpatient Department of Oral Surgery and
Implantology
Center of Oral Health (Carolinum)
Johann Wolfgang Goethe University Frankfurt
am Main
Theodor-Stern-Kai 7
D – 60596 Frankfurt am Main, Germany

Prof Dr Dr Michael Payer
Clinical Department of Oral Surgery and Ortho-
dontics
University Department of Dental Medicine and
Oral Health
Medical University of Graz
Billrothgasse 4
A – 8010 Graz, Austria

Dr Martina Schriber
Department of Oral Health & Medicine
University Center for Dental Medicine Basel UZB
University of Basel
Mattenstr. 40
CH – 4058 Basel, Switzerland

Priv-Doz Dr Dr Dr Michael Schwaiger
Clinical Department of Oral and Maxillofacial
Surgery
University Department of Dental Medicine and
Oral Health
Medical University of Graz
Auenbruggerplatz 5
A – 8010 Graz, Austria

Prof Dr Frank Schwarz
Outpatient Department of Oral Surgery and
Implantology
Center of Oral Health (Carolinum)
Johann Wolfgang Goethe University Frankfurt
am Main
Theodor-Stern-Kai 7
D – 60596 Frankfurt am Main, Germany

Prof Dr Dr Bernd Stadlinger

Clinic of Oral Surgery –
Clinic of Cranio-Maxillofacial Surgery
Center of Dental Medicine
University of Zürich
Plattenstr. 11
CH – 8032 Zürich, Switzerland

Priv-Doz Dr Frank Peter Strietzel

Department of Periodontology, Oral Medicine
and Oral Surgery
CharitéCenter 3 for Oral Health Sciences
Charité – Universitätsmedizin Berlin
Aßmannshauserstr. 4–6
D – 14197 Berlin, Germany

Priv-Doz Dr Silvio Valdec

Clinic of Oral Surgery –
Clinic of Cranio-Maxillofacial Surgery
Center of Dental Medicine
University of Zürich
Plattenstr. 11
CH – 8032 Zürich, Switzerland

Prof Dr Carlalberta Verna

Department of Pediatric Oral Health and Ortho-
dontics
University Center for Dental Medicine Basel UZB
University of Basel
Mattenstr. 40
CH – 4058 Basel, Switzerland

Priv-Doz Dr Dr Dr Jürgen Wallner

Clinical Department of Oral and Maxillofacial
Surgery
University Department of Dental Medicine and
Oral Health
Medical University of Graz
Auenbruggerplatz 5
A – 8010 Graz, Austria

Prof Dr Dr Wolfgang Zemann

Clinical Department of Oral and Maxillofacial
Surgery
University Department of Dental Medicine and
Oral Health
Medical University of Graz
Auenbruggerplatz 5
A – 8010 Graz, Austria

Contents

SOFT TISSUE SURGERY

HARD TISSUE SURGERY

Contents

Complex patient profile in oral surgery

1

Martina Schriber, Michael M. Bornstein

There is often very little separating success from failure in oral surgery, and several factors influence the outcome. Firstly, the skills and experience of the surgeon play a key role. Studies have shown that surgical skills improve with the number of procedures performed, and hence the risk of complications also decreases. Correct patient selection is an equally important factor in the success of oral surgery. In the process, it is crucial to take a thorough general medical history, which helps to avoid local and systemic complications resulting from a surgical procedure. It is the surgeon's responsibility to give patients a thorough explanation prior to surgery and to gather any general medical information that may be missing. Furthermore, the surgeon needs to assess whether the patient is able to tolerate the procedure under local anesthesia or whether treatment under sedation or general anesthesia is required because of a dental phobia, for example. An oral surgery procedure is successful if attention is paid to patient-specific factors as well as the actual intervention and if medical complications can be avoided.

Importance of history taking

History taking forms the basis on which a diagnosis is made at the start of any medical or dental treatment and is an integral part of the work of medical and dental practitioners. The purpose of history taking is to record all existing or previous illnesses and diagnoses of the cardiovascular system, gastrointestinal tract, metabolic and nervous systems, blood and coagulation system, and musculoskeletal system as well as infectious diseases. Furthermore, patients should specifically be asked whether they have ever experienced intraoperative or postoperative complications such as difficulties during procedures, allergies, bleeding or failure of anesthesia.

Age itself brings with it physiologic changes that have an influence on patient positioning and resilience. In addition, elderly patients frequently have several concomitant diseases and an extensive list of medications. A characteristic of multimorbidity is the simultaneous presence of two or more systemic diseases such as metabolic, cardiovascular, psychosomatic, mental, neuropsychiatric, and gerontopsychiatric conditions as well as combinations of diseases (known as a "cluster"). These illnesses are usually treated or kept under control by patients regularly taking medication. This means they are simultaneously taking many different medications. When a patient is taking five or more prescription medications per day, it is referred to as polypharmacy[38]. Overprescribing is not uncommon, especially among elderly people who have been taking medication for a long time[51]. Inappropriate polypharmacy is a relevant problem, particularly for older people, and is associated with negative health consequences[46]. In 2010, 13% of the population in the USA were aged 65 and older and were receiving 39% of all prescribed medications[16,51]. In this population group, 68% suffered from two or more chronic illnesses (i.e. multimorbidity). These typically involved high blood pressure (61%), heart disease (32%), arthritis (31%), and diabetes (28%)[15].

History taking enables complex patient profiles with multimorbidity and associated polypharmacy to be properly recognized. This can also help to categorize patients into high- and low-risk groups for outpatient oral surgery measures. For polypharmacy and multimorbidity patients, it is therefore advisable to obtain a list of medications and diagnoses routinely from their attending physician. Possible drug interactions can thus be checked and avoided.

Relevant problem areas from general medicine

Increased bleeding tendency

Intraoperative or postoperative bleeding can pose a serious problem in the course of oral surgery procedures (Fig 1-1). When patients have an increased bleeding tendency, a distinction must be made between congenital, acquired, and drug-induced hemorrhagic diatheses.

Congenital hemorrhagic diathesis

Patients with congenital hemophilia A or B or a deficiency or faulty formation of von Willebrand factor have an increased risk of bleeding. In such cases, it is imperative to consult with the attending hematologist before oral surgery procedures and ideally perform the procedure at a specialist clinic.

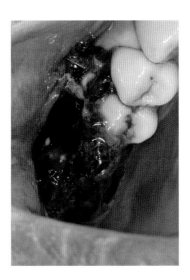

Fig 1-1 Bleeding 1 day after implant placement with horizontal bone augmentation in the region of the maxillary right first molar in a 55-year-old healthy patient not taking anticoagulants.

Acquired hemorrhagic diathesis

Acquired hemorrhagic diathesis occurs in patients with hepatic, renal, and autoimmune diseases; infectious diseases; and leukemia. Disturbances of liver function such as cirrhosis of the liver can arise in the context of alcohol addiction or as a result of autoimmune and drug-induced hepatitis. In cirrhosis of the liver, the function of the liver is impaired to the extent that clotting factors are no longer formed. It is therefore advisable to obtain preoperative laboratory blood values for clotting factors.

Thrombocytopenia or thrombocyte dysfunction occurs in the context of kidney diseases and malignant bone marrow diseases (leukemias) where the healthy thrombocyte-forming bone marrow is suppressed by the growth of malignant cells.

Thrombocytopenia and thrombocyte dysfunction also occur in association with HIV, hepatitis B and C and Epstein-Barr virus infections, and autoimmune diseases (e.g. systemic lupus erythematosus or rheumatoid arthritis). Prior to oral surgery, the platelet count is particularly significant because in some circumstances the administration of platelet concentrate may be required before the procedure.

Drug-induced hemorrhagic diathesis

Drug-induced hemorrhagic diathesis occurs in patients receiving oral anticoagulants or platelet aggregation inhibitors. More and more patients are taking these drugs, in some cases for life, in order to prevent thromboembolic events. There is still a lack of clarity among physicians and dentists with regard to the preoperative, intraoperative, and postoperative management of these patients, together with a degree of uncertainty on the part of patients. The various groups of anticoagulants (vitamin K antagonists, novel oral anticoagulants, platelet aggregation inhibitors) should be correctly recorded during history taking, and their effects also need to be understood (Table 1-1). In the case of patients taking anticoagulants, potential bleeding risks during the course of oral surgery if anticoagulation is continued must be weighed against possible thromboembolic complications if the medication is suspended, altered or reduced. Patients under oral anticoagulation/platelet aggregation inhibition usually have a very low risk of bleeding complications that cannot be managed with a topical hemostatic agent. No fatality due to blood loss during or as a direct consequence of an oral surgery procedure has been reported in the literature to date. This contrasts with a similarly low but highly significant risk of serious thromboembolic complications with the resulting persistent morbidity or even death in patients with reduced or discontinued anticoagulation therapy in the context of dental procedures[62].

Typical representatives of indirect anticoagulants are the orally administered vitamin K antagonists (VKAs) (e.g. Marcoumar [phenprocoumon]), coumarin derivatives, and heparins (low molecular weight/fractionated, e.g. Clexane [enoxaparin]; high molecular weight/unfractionated, e.g. Fraxiforte [nadroparin], Fragmin [dalteparin]). The group of VKAs is used for long-term blood dilution primarily in tablet form and inhibits enzymes that are required in vitamin K metabolism for the formation of certain clotting factors. Orally administered VKAs have an onset of action of 48 to 72 hours and a long plasma half-life of approximately 160 hours (Table 1-1). Their action is highly effective but subject to fluctuations due to, for example, certain foods (e.g. cabbage, spinach, parsley), stress, other medications, and sports. The prothrombin time is determined by the international normalized ratio (INR), which is a laboratory value to measure the functional capacity of the extrinsic blood clotting system. Depending on the therapeutic indication, the INR lies between 2 and 3.5. In the case of vitamin K antagonists, therapeutic levels (INR < 4) are possible for oral surgery measures because the risk of postoperative, uncontrollable,

life-threatening bleeding is negligible[34]. As a precaution, however, the INR should be measured on the day of surgery or, if not possible, one day beforehand. From the dentist's perspective, a target INR below 2.5 would be desirable, provided this is considered possible after consultation with the attending physician.

Heparin anticoagulation is usually only carried out in an in-patient setting, which means a dentist in private practice will hardly ever encounter a patient with heparin in their system. The rapid onset of action and short half-life of 5 to 7 hours are advantages of heparin.

Nowadays, it is accepted that VKAs should not be discontinued or reduced for oral surgery or even bridged with heparin products. One important reason is that adjustment to the appropriate target INR takes several days and is relatively complex and time consuming. Suspension or reduction would carry a considerable risk of a thromboembolic complication[6,47]. Despite strict hemostatic measures being followed, easily controllable bleeding should nevertheless be anticipated[22,34].

The novel direct oral anticoagulants (NOACs) exert their effect by direct interaction with individual clotting factors. Important active ingredients in this group of drugs are dabigatran (e.g. Pradaxa) as a direct thrombin inhibitor as well as edoxaban (e.g. Lixiana), apixaban (e.g. Eliquis), and rivaroxaban (e.g. Xarelto) as factor Xa inhibitors (Table 1-1). Their action is reliable, starts or decreases rapidly, and is rarely subject to fluctuations. The anticoagulant effect cannot be determined routinely in clinical practice but can only be measured by special laboratory tests. For this reason, it is important to ask about the individual bleeding tendency during history taking prior to surgery. What matters is when the last tablet was taken and at what dose as well as identifying the active ingredient[28]. Antagonization with an antidote is possible for all NOACs. Based on data from general surgery, dabigatran

Table 1-1 Group of oral anticoagulants modified from the German S3 Guideline on Oral Surgery under oral anticoagulation/platelet aggregation inhibition (as at August 2017) and adapted to the products available in Switzerland.

Group of oral anticoagulants (active ingredients)	Product name in Switzerland	Indications	Plasma half-life
Vitamin K antagonists			
Phenprocoumon	Marcoumar	1. To prevent recurrence of thromboses 2. Atrial fibrillation 3. Artificial heart valves and vascular prostheses 4. Coronary heart disease (CHD)	Marcoumar 50 h
NOACs			
Dabigatran Rivaroxaban Apixaban Edoxaban	Pradaxa Xarelto Eliquis Lixiana	1. Primary prevention of venous thromboembolic events after an elective surgical procedure (e.g. artificial knee or hip joint) 2. Prevention of stroke and systemic embolism in non-valvular atrial fibrillation 3. Treatment and prevention of (recurrent) deep vein thromboses (DVTs) and pulmonary embolisms (PEs)	Pradaxa 12–17 h Xarelto 7–11 h Eliquis 8–14 h Lixiana 10–14 h
Oral platelet aggregation inhibitors			
Acetylsalicylic acid (ASA/aspirin)	Aspirin Cardio	1. CHD 2. Prevention of transient ischemic attacks (TIAs) and strokes after TIA or stroke 3. In peripheral arterial occlusive disease (PAOD) after procedures and to prevent secondary vascular complications such as myocardial infarction, stroke, and vascular death	Aspirin Cardio 15–20 min
Thienopyridines	Clopidogrel Prasugrel	1. Dual therapy with aspirin in the context of coronary interventions and in acute coronary syndrome 2. Secondary prevention after ischemic stroke and myocardial infarction 3. Secondary prevention in cardiovascular diseases as an alternative to aspirin	Clopidogrel 6 h Prasugrel 15 h

h, hours; min, minutes

should be discontinued 2 to 3 days prior to surgery with bleeding risks if creatinine clearance is > 50 mL/minute. Early preoperative discontinuation may be advisable if renal function is impaired. The general advice for rivaroxaban is to stop the drug 1 or 2 days prior to invasive procedures, although this approach is disputed[28,54,55]. Again, based on general surgery data, apixaban should be discontinued more than 2 days and edoxaban 1 to 2 days preoperatively. It is true for all NOACs that they can be resumed after procedures once complete hemostasis has been achieved[28]. NOACs have not been as thoroughly researched to date as VKAs and most of the recommendations, especially regarding dentistry issues, are therefore based on expert opinions. Even so, it does not seem necessary to suspend NOACs for oral surgery procedures[35].

Platelet aggregation inhibitors (PAIs) achieve their effect by an inhibition of platelet function that is induced by various mechanisms, which distinguishes them from other anticoagulants. The best-known active substance in this group is acetylsalicylic acid (aspirin). Thienopyridines (Clopidogrel, Prasugrel) belong to the novel, orally administered active ingredients in this group (Table 1-1). Only specific laboratory tests are able to determine the exact bleeding tendency in a patient taking PAIs. If PAIs are taken in combination with certain nonsteroidal anti-inflammatory drugs (NSAIDs) (e.g. ibuprofen, diclofenac), an increased bleeding tendency is to be expected because these NSAIDs lead to reduced platelet production and hence to thrombocytopenia[28,35,54,55].

Mono-, bi- or triple therapy

For monotherapy with PAIs there is only a weak correlation, if any, with prolonged bleeding tendencies[4,26]. However, if acetylsalicylic acid is stopped 7 to 10 days before a procedure, the risk of a cardiovascular event increases threefold[61]. Therefore, it is not advisable to discontinue acetylsalicylic acid prior to oral surgery procedures, although discontinuation might theoretically take place if the risk of thrombosis is low[2,4].

Patients who have had stents implanted are commonly given combined therapy with PAIs (known as bitherapy) for several months postoperatively in order to avoid stent thrombosis, but this can result in relevant postoperative bleeding after oral surgery[26]. Minor oral surgery procedures can take place while bitherapy is continued[40]. However, elective dental procedures should be postponed, if possible[27]. In an emergency procedure, antiaggregatory drugs are not suspended, but platelet concentrates, desmopressin, and/or antifibrinolytics are used, if required[55]. In this situation, topical hemostatic measures yield good results in terms of preventing and managing bleeding complications[52].

If a patient is receiving long-term anticoagulation due to atrial fibrillation and needs a stent because of coronary heart disease, triple therapy is used, which means a combination of oral anticoagulation and two PAIs[53]. The procedure for these patients is identical to that adopted for patients on bitherapy with PAIs.

Oral surgery procedure in patients with increased bleeding tendency

A patient's hemorrhagic diathesis or risk of bleeding is dependent on the severity of the systemic disease, the nature of the oral surgery procedure (high or low bleeding risk), wound care, and postoperative compliance as well as the life circumstances of the patient. Oral surgery procedures are generally classified as having a low bleeding risk[29]. Oral surgery procedures with a higher bleeding risk include the treatment of infected wounds and abscesses as well as interventions in the floor of the mouth, the maxillary sinus, and the retromaxillary space[34]. These factors dictate the choice of oral surgery approach and whether in-patient admission to a specialist clinic is required[12]. Bridging is currently

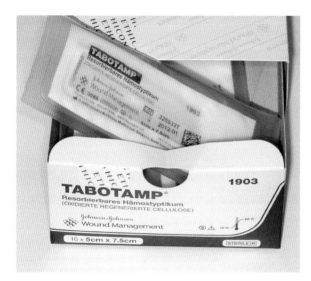

Fig 1-2 Classic hemostat made of absorbable, regenerated cellulose, which can be placed in the socket after a simple tooth extraction, for instance. However, packing the socket should be avoided as it may impair wound healing.

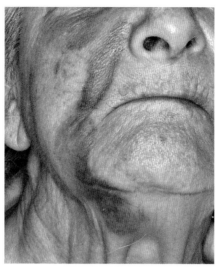

Fig 1-3 A healthy 94-year-old patient with an extensive hematoma on the right sight of her face and neck after surgical extraction of the maxillary right canine.

controversial even for major procedures and can be carried out with heparin in the case of VKAs and NOACs, if need be, but not in the case of PAIs[20].

A minimally invasive approach is important for congenital, acquired or drug-induced hemorrhagic diathesis. Oral surgery procedures should ideally be scheduled for early mornings or on weekends. Large wound areas should be avoided, which means the treatment should be planned on a phased basis, if need be. Local anesthetics with vasoconstrictors are subject to the usual contraindications in this group of patients, while increased bleeding (rebound effect) may be expected if the adrenaline effect is diminished. Complete removal of granulation tissue is important when treating sockets in order to prevent postoperative bleeding. The placement of hemostatic agents such as absorbable sponges or cellulose and collagen cones is advisable (Fig 1-2). The overlying suture

fixes the material and further reduces the risk of bleeding[8,18,26]. Physical compression where the patient bites on gauze[5] or the provision of pre-operatively prepared gingival shields[21] are very simple and effective measures. Postoperatively, tranexamic acid is also helpful as an antifibrinolytic mouthwash, which significantly reduces the frequency of bleeding after oral surgery[25,58]. It is not uncommon for patients taking anticoagulants to develop hematomas, so prophylactic antibiotic administration may be considered (Fig 1-3). It is advisable to consult the attending internal medicine physician or cardiologist when prescribing antibiotics and analgesics in order to avoid drug interactions.

Cardiovascular diseases

Patients with very poorly controlled high blood pressure have an increased bleeding tendency and a higher risk of myocardial infarction and stroke. For this group of patients, especially those over the age of 60, it is advisable to monitor blood pressure, pulse, and oxygen saturation during the procedure. The appropriate medications (e.g. Nitroglycerin Streuli, oxygen) should be kept ready during surgery on patients known to have angina pectoris. After a recent myocardial infarction, the attending cardiologist should be contacted in the event of imminent treatment. A period of at least 3 months after myocardial infarction is required before elective surgeries are performed. If there is a risk of endocarditis (e.g. patients with heart valve replacement or congenital valve defects), prophylactic antibiotic administration is required before oral surgery or periodontal procedures in accordance with the endocarditis prevention identification card. Local anesthetics containing adrenaline are not contraindicated for patients with cardiovascular diseases, but the dose should be adjusted depending on the disease and medication (e.g. beta blockers). Patients with heart failure should not be treated in the supine position in order to avoid dyspnea[49].

Liver diseases

Impairment of liver function occurs in autoimmune or drug-induced hepatitis and alcohol abuse with cirrhosis of the liver and can cause acquired hemorrhagic diathesis, as described above. In liver disease, it is important to bear in mind the increased bleeding tendency as well as the resultant impaired drug metabolism. Therefore, if liver function is impaired, alternative drugs should be chosen that are not broken down in the liver. It is advisable to discuss the drugs being prescribed beforehand with the patient's attending internal medicine physician.

Kidney diseases

Chronic renal failure, caused for instance by diabetes mellitus, hypertension, pyelonephritis or polycystic kidney disease, leads to an increased bleeding tendency because of

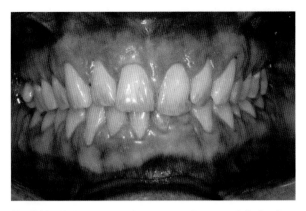

Fig 1-4   Subtle gingival overgrowth, especially in the papillary area, in a 47-year-old patient who is taking a nifedipine drug (calcium channel blocker) daily for hypertension.

thrombocytopenia or thrombocyte dysfunction, increased susceptibility to infection, and altered drug metabolism. Patients with terminal renal failure require hemodialysis, for which they are anticoagulated. Surgery in patients with renal impairment, renal failure or with a history of kidney transplant surgery should routinely be discussed preoperatively with the patient's general practitioner or nephrologist. Appropriate hemostatic measures should be taken intraoperatively. Postoperatively, infection prophylaxis by means of antibiotic treatment should be considered.

Diabetes mellitus

Type 1 and 2 diabetes are autoimmune diseases. Patients with type 1 diabetes are reliant on taking insulin for their entire lives because the beta cells in the islets of Langerhans of the pancreas are no longer functioning. Patients with type 2 diabetes primarily show a reduced response of the body's cells to insulin and have beta cells that are limited in their function. Type 2 diabetes is treated by lifestyle changes, weight reduction, insulin administration, and oral antidiabetic drugs. If a patient is known to have type 1 or 2 diabetes, whether this is well controlled should

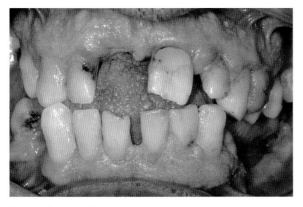 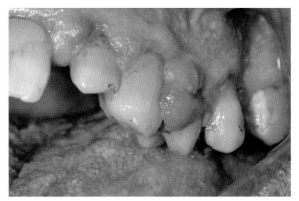

Figs 1-5 and 1-6 Generalized gingival overgrowth in the area of the residual dentition in a 56-year-old patient who is taking a nifedipine drug (calcium channel blocker) daily for hypertension. A pronounced increase in substance is very noticeable, especially in the papillary area between the maxillary left canine and first premolar.

be checked before any oral surgery treatment. The long-term glucose level (HbA_{1c}) is a reliable benchmark and should ideally be below 7%. Patients usually know what their HbA_{1c} value is. If the diabetes is poorly controlled, delayed wound healing and infections are likely. Appointments should be planned for early morning to enable patients with diabetes who are on insulin therapy to stick to their usual mealtimes and insulin doses. The blood sugar level should ideally be measured prior to an oral surgery procedure. During treatment, it is important to watch out for symptoms of hypoglycemia (e.g. agitation, sweating, pale skin, tachycardia, palpitations, tremor, ravenous appetite, vomiting) and react to them promptly. Antibiotic administration should be considered for patients with poorly controlled diabetes or after major oral surgery procedures in order to aid wound healing and avoid infection.

Epilepsy

The increased stress caused by surgery can trigger a seizure in patients with epilepsy. Patients should be asked about the frequency and intensity of their seizures and the date of their last seizure. If seizures are frequent and poorly controlled by medication, referral to a specialist clinic is advisable, and treatment under sedation or general anesthesia is indicated. In addition, certain antiepileptic drugs belonging to the group of "old antiepileptics" such as those containing the active substance phenytoin cause gingival overgrowth as a side effect. Such changes, previously known as gingival hyperplasia, are nowadays mainly diagnosed in patients with hypertension who are taking calcium channel blockers (e.g. nifedipine-class drugs such as amlodipine) as an antihypertensive active substance (Figs 1-4 to 1-6).

Antiresorptive agent-related osteonecrosis of the jaw

A considerable number of adults worldwide are treated with antiresorptive (AR) drugs as a result of various benign and malignant bone metabolism disorders and hypercalcemia. Bisphosphonates (BPs) and monoclonal antibodies such as denosumab (DNO) belong to the group of ARs (Table 1-2). The main indications for AR treatment include multiple myeloma, bone metastases of solid tumors (e.g. breast, prostate or lung

Table 1-2 Antiresorptive drugs from the group of bisphosphonates (BPs) and denosumab (DNO), commonly administered in Switzerland, and novel substances: mammalian target of rapamycin (mTOR) inhibitors, vascular endothelial growth factor (VEGF) inhibitors, tyrosine kinase (TK) inhibitors, multikinase inhibitors.

	Active substances	Product name in Switzerland (excluding generics)
Bisphosphonates (BPs)	Alendronic acid Alendronic acid and cholecalciferol	Fosamax Fosavance
	Ibandronic acid Risedronic acid Zoledronic acid	Bonviva Actonel Aclasta Zometa
Denosumab (DNO)	Denosumab	Prolia Xgeva
mTOR inhibitors	Everolimus Sirolimus Temsirolimus	Afinitor Rapamune Torisel
VEGF inhibitors	Aflibercept Bevacizumab Brolucizumab Ranibizumab	Eylea Avastin Beovu Lucentis
TK inhibitors	Erlotinib Gefitinib	Tarceva Iressa
Multikinase inhibitors	Sorafenib Sunitinib	Nexavar Sutent

carcinomas), osteoporosis (primary and secondary), and Paget's disease (Table 1-3).

Numerous clinical trials have shown that ARs lead to a reduced frequency of bone fractures and pain in patients with nononcologic diseases (e.g. osteoporosis). In patients with cancer, AR drugs help to prevent pathologic fractures and to improve quality of life. On the other hand, the side effect of AR agent-related osteonecrosis of the jaw (ARONJ) is relevant (Figs 1-7 and 1-8). ARONJ is a potentially serious disease because it is associated with relevant functional impairments. Event rates of 0.001% to 0.01% are reported in patients with osteoporosis who are taking AR agents (BP and DNO), and 1% to 15% in patients with cancer who are taking AR agents[36]. As the individual risk profile for ARONJ differs and is dependent on various factors, prophylaxis and prevention should be adapted to the patient's particular risk profile (Table 1-3). Patients are assigned an individual risk profile (low, medium, high) based on pharmacologic properties, indications, doses administered, frequency, and duration of AR treatment. The patient's general medical condition as well as existing nicotine use and comedication with agents such as glucocorticosteroids or immunomodulators also play a role. Patients with malignancies receive a much higher AR dose than osteoporosis patients and therefore belong to the high-risk group.

Approximately 1% of BPs are taken orally and 99% are administered intravenously. Long half-lives of 10 to 12 years are reported. The pharmacokinetics of BPs cause a cumulative effect, thereby explaining why the observed event rates increase with the duration of treatment. Unlike BP, DNO is not deposited in the bone. Half-lives of 24 to 26 days and efficacy for up to 5 months are reported for DNO. Therefore, it is assumed that there is no longer a risk of ARONJ after a break of half a year from DNO treatment.

Table 1-3 Risk profiles modified from the S3 Guideline on ARONJ (as at December 2018).

	Low risk profile (range: 0% to 0.5%)	Medium risk profile (range: > 0.5% to < 1%)	High risk profile (range: 1% to 21%)
Indication/ Patient group	Primary osteoporosis	In treatment-induced osteoporosis In secondary osteoporosis Avoidance of skeletal-related events Comedication with immuno-modulators (antirheumatic drugs, including methotrexate) Underlying diseases, treatments or status with impaired wound healing and/or influence on the immune system: diabetes mellitus, anemia, hyperparathyroidism, dialysis, chemotherapy, glucocorticoid therapy, anti-angiogenic therapies, advanced age	For BP: Bone metastases Multiple myeloma combined with novel substances (mTOR, VEGF, TK inhibitors)
Medication	BP: Oral: including alendronate, ibandronate or risedronate IV: zoledronate 5 mg every 12 months, ibandronate 3 mg/3 mL every 3 months DNO: SC: DNO medication 60 mg every 6 months	BP: IV: e.g. zoledronate 4 mg every 6 months IV: zoledronate once a year or oral BP with comedication with immunomodulators and/ or with underlying disease that modifies wound healing or modulates the immune system	BP: IV: e.g. zoledronate 4 mg every 4 weeks DNO: SC: DNO medication 120 mg every 4 weeks
Prevalence with BP medication	0.0%–0.5% BP medication < 4 years: 0.04% BP medication > 4 years: 0.21%	1%	1%–21%
Prevalence with DNO medication	0.13%–0.21%		2%–5%
Prevalence with BP medication and novel substances*			BP combined with TK inhibitor (Nexavar, Sutent): 17% BP combined with VEGF inhibitor (Avastin): 0.9%–2.4%

IV, intravenous; SC, subcutaneous. *Novel substances: mammalian target of rapamycin (mTOR) inhibitors, tyrosine kinase (TK) inhibitors, vascular endothelial growth factor (VEGF) inhibitors.

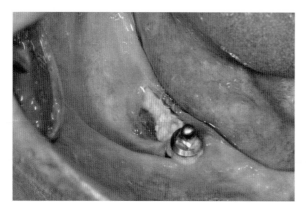

Fig 1-7 A 74-year-old patient with prostate cancer and bone metastases receiving treatment with denosumab (Xgeva). ARONJ in the right mandible in the second premolar to second molar region crestal and distal to the implant in the first premolar region.

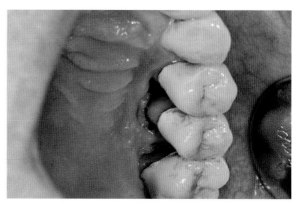

Fig 1-8 A 62-year-old patient with breast cancer and bone metastases receiving treatment with denosumab (Xgeva) showing exposed bone areas palatally and marginally in the maxillary left first premolar to first molar region after a dental hygiene session, which corresponds to the clinical picture of ARONJ.

There are some other substances worth mentioning that also pose a risk of osteonecrosis of the jaw (ONJ) or can worsen existing ONJ. These include radium-223 dichloride, which is used in the treatment of prostate carcinoma, and novel substances/small molecules (mTOR, VEGF, and TK inhibitors) that are used in cancer chemotherapy, for instance (Table 1-3). Patients should always be told about their risk profile for ARONJ. Any AR therapy should be preceded by a search for foci of infection, and prophylactic measures should be carried out as well as the eradication of infection and bacterial portals of entry. It is important that the start of osteoporosis therapy is not delayed by dental ONJ prevention because a low ARONJ event rate is present. This applies particularly to osteoporosis patients being treated with oral BP. When DNO is administered, however, it should be borne in mind that an increased risk of ARONJ exists from the first injection due to a rapid onset of action and short half-life. The aim is to complete the prophylactic measures before therapy starts. In oncology patient groups, eradication of infections and bacterial portals of entry in the oral cavity before the start of BP therapy can lower the ARONJ event rate.

If oral surgery is indicated for a patient who has an AR history or is currently receiving AR therapy, an individual risk profile is drawn up on the basis of how long the medication has been taken, the active substance group, and the current dose. The efficacy of a treatment break (drug holiday) with high-dose AR medications remains uncertain[41]. It is impossible to make any conclusive recommendation for or against a drug holiday prior to oral surgery procedures in patients receiving ongoing AR medication. The decision to suspend the AR therapy is always made in an interdisciplinary manner in consultation with the relevant attending specialists. For oral surgery procedures, perioperative systemic antibiotic administration usually takes place from the day of surgery until follow-up or suture removal and until there are no signs of infection.

Osteoradionecrosis

Osteoradionecrosis (ORN), especially of the mandible, is a serious complication following curative radiotherapy of oropharyngeal and oral

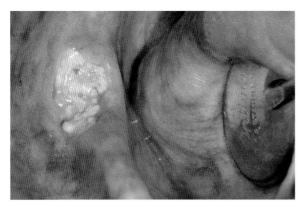
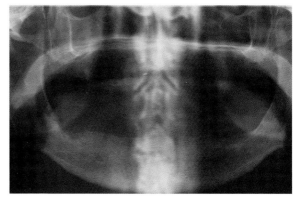

Figs 1-9 and 1-10   Osteoradionecrosis (ORN) in the posterior region of the right mandible up to the ascending ramus in an 84-year-old patient after radiotherapy for an oral cavity carcinoma.

cavity carcinomas (Figs 1-9 and 1-10). Around 30 years ago, a review article quoted an ORN incidence of 5% to 15% after doses of between 60 and 72 Gy. More recent studies with modern, slightly accelerated or hyperfractionated treatment regimens with doses of 69 to 81 Gy report a far lower ORN incidence of between < 1% and approximately 6%[59]. Intensity-modulated radiation therapy (IMRT) is likely to reduce the ORN rate further. In patients with oropharyngeal cancers receiving IMRT, ORN is relatively rare but does continue to occur over 5 years after treatment and the likelihood increases when there are additional risk factors such as smoking and BP medication[14].

Especially in the mandible, the risk of ORN after oral surgery is high if the applied radiation doses amounted to more than 40 Gy because the bone damage can persist for a lifetime. The risk of ORN is reduced if anti-infective prophylaxis (e.g. amoxicillin) is initiated not later than 24 hours prior to surgery and is continued for up to 2 weeks postoperatively. Tooth extraction in the formerly radiated field is performed atraumatically, all bone edges are smoothed, and a tight soft tissue coverage should ideally be performed without compromising on vascularization of the local bone, which may result in complications of wound healing. If the masticatory musculature and/or temporomandibular joints were located within the radiation field, trismus can develop even a long time after radiotherapy has been completed, which can additionally complicate the treatment[33].

Patients undergoing chemotherapy

Chemotherapy exerts a cytotoxic or cytostatic effect on cells with a high proliferation rate, malignant tumors, and metastases. Cytostatic agents inhibit tumor growth because they influence the replication cycle of the rapidly dividing cancer cells. As cytostatic agents usually do not differentiate between healthy cells in the body and cancer cells, the cells of the hematopoietic bone marrow, the hair follicles, and the epithelial cells of the oral mucosa are also inhibited. Reduced salivary flow, along with oral mucositis, candidiasis (Fig 1-11), a reduced sense of taste, nausea, and vomiting are among the most relevant side effects in patients undergoing or

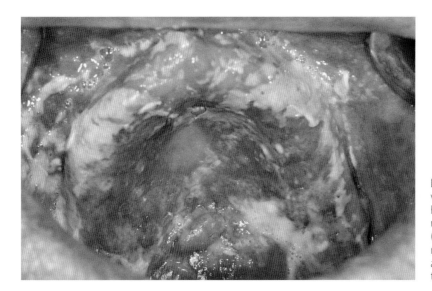

Fig 1-11   A 90-year-old patient with oral candidiasis. The patient has bronchial asthma and regularly uses a Symbicort inhaler (combination of sympathomimetic and glucocorticoid). In addition, she suffers from diabetes mellitus.

having had cytostatic therapy. Xerostomia and hyposalivation/oligosialia as well as intraoral ulcerations occur as early as the start of chemotherapy, which can have adverse effects on swallowing ability and hence food intake.

The bone marrow damage that occurs during ongoing chemotherapy commonly results in myelosuppression, causing a decrease in the number of white blood cells, which particularly affects neutrophilic granulocytes. This means that patients are more susceptible to infection during chemotherapy. Therefore, very good oral hygiene is all the more important. In addition, thrombocytopenia frequently occurs, which in turn can lead to an increased bleeding tendency. Leukemia or lymphoma patients with pancytopenia have a particularly high risk of bacterial dental infections. Patients with leukemia or a lymphoma undergo stem cell transplantation if radiotherapy or chemotherapy have not been successful enough or if they experience a relapse. In this immune situation, chronic periodontitis or apical periodontitis can lead to a systemic infection[3]. In this patient group, it is therefore advisable to eradicate dental foci of infection if at all possible before the appropriate oncologic treatment, after which close monitoring is important[30]. Oral surgery treatments should be avoided during ongoing chemotherapy, if at all possible. If there are acute symptoms and invasive oral surgery is unavoidable, the neutrophil granulocyte and platelet counts should be discussed with the attending oncologist. Antibiotic administration is indicated, depending on the findings. Once chemotherapy is completed, the majority of patients are again able to have normal dental treatment.

Infectious diseases

There is a potential risk of infection with every patient contact. The hygiene measures stipulated in practice are adequate to guarantee that staff are protected against the most common infectious diseases such as human immunodeficiency virus (HIV), hepatitis, herpes simplex virus (HSV-1 and HSV-2), and human papillomavirus (HPV). Appropriate vaccinations additionally protect staff against hepatitis A and B, and, ideally, influenza[9]. As a result of the severe acute respiratory syndrome (SARS)–coronavirus disease (COVID-19) pandemic, new additional hygiene measures were introduced in order to minimize contamination in the dental practice. Among these additional measures, the most important involve avoiding shaking hands, social distancing in the practice (waiting and break rooms), and wearing face masks at all times. Disinfectant is provided for patients at the entrance to dental practices, while reception staff are protected with a transparent acrylic screen. Furthermore, indoor ventilation is stepped up.

Since 2002, the number of **HIV** diagnoses in Switzerland has declined. Most HIV-infected patients in Switzerland are given antiretroviral treatment and hence no longer pose an acute risk of infection[10]. Nevertheless, with this group of patients, it is advisable to contact their general practitioner or infectiologist to check their immune status and infectiousness (viral load). It is mainly CD4+ lymphocytes that are relevant in HIV-infected patients because certain minimal quantities must be present for adequate immune defense. Neutropenia is also common among HIV-infected individuals. If leukopenia and/or neutropenia are present, prophylactic antibiotic use may be indicated before and at the time of a planned oral surgery procedure. During extraoral and intraoral examination, attention should be paid to any typical HIV-associated cutaneous or oral manifestations that may be present. Examples of such changes are lymphadenopathy, candidiasis, hairy leukoplakia, herpes infections, papillomas, aphthous ulcerations, Kaposi sarcoma or a necrotizing periodontal disease.

Infections with **HSV-1** and **HSV-2** are common: 70% of the Swiss population carry HSV-1, and 20% carry HSV-2. HSV-1 predominantly leads to infections in the oral and facial area (herpes labialis), and HSV-2 is primarily present in the genital area (herpes genitalis). HSV-1 and HSV-2 are transmitted by mucosal contact, by contact with infected skin or by smear infections. In principle, the prevailing hygiene measures taken in dental practices should provide adequate protection. However, it is advisable to postpone an appointment if a patient has acute labial herpes because contact with blisters and ulcers should be avoided[11].

HPVs are sexually transmitted and, although most types of HPV are harmless, they do cause a few cancerous conditions in the throat, pharyngeal, and genital area (cervical cancer). It is estimated that 70% to 80% of sexually active men and women are infected with HPV in the course of their lives, while two-thirds of the infections remain asymptomatic. There are many different types of HPV that infect the skin or mucosa. HPV is involved in the pathogenesis of various benign, exophytically growing tumors (e.g. verruca vulgaris, papillomas, focal epithelial hyperplasia) and is predominantly found on the tongue, soft palate, and lips[13].

Switzerland is a low-endemic country for **hepatitis** B virus (HBV) infection. According to the latest estimates, the viremic prevalence (hepatitis B surface antigen [HBsAg]) is given as 0.44% in the entire population with a low risk, and as 3.6% in those with a high risk. Seroprevalence for hepatitis C virus (HCV) infection (anti-HCV) is given as 0.7% in Switzerland for the entire population with a low risk, according to the latest estimates. HBV and HCV are mainly transmitted via blood but, depending on viral load, can also be detected in other bodily fluids (saliva, sperm, vaginal fluid, urine, tears, breast milk). Transmission of HBV and HCV is largely through sexual contact. However, iatrogenic transmission among health care staff is also possible. One of the sequelae of hepatitis infection is cirrhosis of the liver, which can lead to hemorrhagic diathesis because of the impaired hepatic function[9].

Immunosuppressed patients

A distinction is made between endogenous, exogenous, and iatrogenic immunosuppression in the case of immunosuppressed patients.

Endogenous immunosuppression may be the consequence of diseases such as leukemia or a variable immunodeficiency syndrome. Leukemia involves the uncontrolled proliferation of immature white blood cells, which displace the mature white blood cells (leukocytes), red blood cells (erythrocytes), and platelets (thrombocytes). In acute leukemia, due to the lack of mature functioning leukocytes, there is a greater susceptibility to infection and thrombocytopenia, which in turn increases the bleeding tendency. Variable immunodeficiency syndrome is the most common congenital immunodeficiency, in which the affected patients produce too few or no antibodies (IgA, IgM, IgG) because B lymphocytes are usually present but are not fully functioning.

HIV infection is an exogenous form of immunosuppression. Unlike leukemia, in which the body itself produces faulty white blood cells, in HIV infection the virus destroys functioning leukocytes (CD4+ lymphocytes).

The **iatrogenic** form of immunosuppression is caused by the administration of immunosuppressants, which reduce the body's immune defense in a variety of ways due to their mechanisms of action. There are various substances that influence the cellular and humoral immune response with a variety of mechanisms of action. Medications containing glucocorticoids or active substances such as cyclophosphamide, azathioprine, methotrexate or tumor necrosis factor (TNF) inhibitors are predominantly immunosuppressive. Immunosuppressants are principally indicated following allogeneic stem cell or organ transplantation, in autoimmune diseases (e.g. connective tissue diseases, chronic inflammatory bowel diseases or rheumatoid arthritis), and for cytostatic therapy. An increased susceptibility to infection is a typical side effect for patients undergoing immunosuppression.

Respiratory diseases

Dental practitioners frequently encounter patients with lung diseases in their practices.

Bronchial asthma and chronic obstructive pulmonary diseases (COPDs) are the most common respiratory conditions. Patients with bronchial asthma often have specific pharmacotherapy as on-demand treatment and usually basic anti-inflammatory therapy. Beta-2 sympathomimetics (e.g. Ventolin, Bricanyl, Symbicort, Seretide) or glucocorticosteroids (Pulmicort, Qvar) are commonly prescribed drugs for inhalation. Patients who regularly inhale glucocorticosteroids frequently develop oral candidiasis (Fig 1-11). Patients are asked to bring along the inhaler they use to any oral surgery treatment. In asthmatic diseases, certain analgesics such as Aspirin Cardio, Novalgin (metamizole), diclofenac or ibuprofen can decrease symptoms.

Smoking for several years (even after having quit) is a common cause of COPD. Depending on the severity of the disease, various pharmacologic therapeutic approaches are adopted, involving beta-2 sympathomimetics (Berodual, Bricanyl), anticholinergics (Atropair), glucocorticosteroids (Pulmicort, Qvar) or phosphodiesterase-4 inhibitors (Daxas). Long-term oxygen therapy is necessary in advanced-stage COPD. Essentially, patients with COPD must not be treated in the supine position in order to avoid dyspnea.

For patients with lung disease, it is important to check whether the oral surgery procedure would be better performed in a specialist clinic. Intravenous sedation may be indicated for asthmatics because it is not uncommon for bronchial asthma to be exacerbated by states of anxiety.

Allergies

It is important to pay attention to allergies in dental practice because they can affect not only patients but also members of staff. Allergies to latex, penicillin, chlorhexidine, and local anesthetics are being described with increasing frequency. **Latex** allergies are the most commonly reported. The prevalence is quoted as 3% to 17% for health care professionals and 1% to 6.5% for the general population. An allergy can manifest as a relatively harmless local reaction or be as serious as to cause anaphylaxis[7].

Penicillin allergy is the second most common allergy. Around 10% of the USA population state that they have an allergy to penicillin, with 90% to 95% not exhibiting clinically significant reactions. One reason for this contradictory finding might be that typical drug-specific side effects (e.g. nausea) resulting from taking penicillin are mistaken for an allergy. People can "grow out" of penicillin allergies over time: 80% of people lose their penicillin allergy after 10 years and 50% within 5 years[50,57]. It is estimated that potentially dangerous IgE-mediated reactions occur once to twice per 10,000 penicillin administrations[32]. If a penicillin allergy is suspected, however, the general practitioner should be consulted before any planned administration of penicillin[50,57].

The antiseptic **chlorhexidine** has a broad spectrum of antimicrobial activity against Gram-positive and Gram-negative pathogens, *Candida albicans*, and a few viruses. In the hospital setting, chlorhexidine is used for skin disinfection to prevent catheter-associated infections or to coat medical devices such as bladder or central venous catheters. In dentistry, chlorhexidine is found in products such as mouthwashes or gels. There are case reports of chlorhexidine allergies of varying degrees of severity; they can appear locally as harmless hypersensitivity but can also result in anaphylactic shock with a fatal outcome. The prevalence of chlorhexidine allergy is quoted as nearly 10% in the UK, Denmark, and Belgium[17].

True allergies to local anesthetics are very rare, with a prevalence of < 1%. Most side effects or incidents connected with local anesthetics are not of an allergic nature; they occur due to vasovagal complications (blood pressure decrease and sinus bradycardia), anxiety reactions, and hyperventilation or are caused by an adrenaline additive in the anesthetic (palpitations, tachycardia, hyperventilation)[24].

Neurodegenerative and mental disorders

Age brings with it many oral and systemic diseases as well as a decline in physiologic functions. The greater the cognitive impairment, the greater the frequency of impaired active mouth opening and swallowing difficulties. As a rule, however, the swallowing capacity of patients with cognitive impairment and those with dementia is good[19]. Patients with Parkinson's disease suffer from dysphagia in 18.5% to 100% of cases, depending on the test method used, and frequently suffer simultaneously from depression and anxiety disorders[56,60]. The pharmacokinetics and hence the mechanism of action of medications are altered in the elderly, for whom multimorbidity and polypharmacy are common. Particular attention should be paid to drug interactions. Limited mouth opening as well as cognitive and mental impairments might make it necessary to perform treatment under general anesthesia.

The most common mental disorder in children is ADHD (attention deficit hyperactivity disorder). Difficulties in concentrating and impulsive behavior are characteristic of children with ADHD. As recognizable hyperactivity does not always occur, a distinction is made between attention deficit disorder with hyperactivity (ADHD) and attention deficit disorder without hyperactivity (ADD). In Switzerland and across the world, an average of around 5% of schoolchildren meet the criteria for ADHD, with boys more frequently affected than girls. With the correct treatment, the symptoms of those affected with ADHD are mostly brought under control, and these individuals are able to lead a largely normal life[31]. ADHD can make oral surgery difficult and necessitate treatment under sedation or even general anesthesia.

People with autism spectrum disorder (ASD) see, hear, and feel the world differently and have difficulty empathizing with other people and communicating appropriately with them. They are often interested in a specific area; they focus on detail and find it difficult to adjust to new things or fully grasp a situation. Their movement patterns are often rather clumsy. Additional diagnoses such as speech disorder, intellectual disability, epilepsy, ADHD, Down syndrome or hyperlexia are sometimes found in those with ASD. There is still a lack of data regarding the prevalence of ASD. Around 1% of the population in Switzerland is diagnosed with the disorder. The rates range between 1% and 3% in other countries. Men and boys are more frequently diagnosed than women and girls. Oral surgery treatment can be carried out without any problems, depending on the severity of the ASD. However, the condition may also mean that surgery can only be performed under general anesthesia.

Pregnancy

The priority during pregnancy is the well-being of the mother and fetus. Around 15% of all pregnant women worldwide develop gestational diabetes (GD) during pregnancy due to various pregnancy hormones and a suboptimal diet. Whether or not periodontitis can significantly increase the risk of GD is a matter of some debate[1]. Pregnant women have a greater risk of caries and erosion as a result of altered saliva characteristics, higher concentrations of *mutans streptococci*, and frequently altered eating habits. Furthermore,

pregnant women suffer more commonly from gingivitis because of hormonal changes, and this can develop into periodontitis if the inflammation progresses[37]. One characteristic stomatologic phenomenon in pregnancy is pregnancy epulis (epulis gravidarum or pregnancy tumor), which usually recedes spontaneously after the baby is born and only rarely requires treatment (Figs 1-12 and 1-13).

Opinions differ on the extent to which the presence of periodontitis influences possible complications of pregnancy such as premature birth, pre-eclampsia, miscarriage or low birth weight. Routine dental measures such as diagnostic, preventive/prophylactic, restorative, and periodontal treatments should ideally be carried out in the second trimester[23]. In principle, elective oral surgery should be avoided during pregnancy. Urgent or emergency oral surgery treatments such as trauma, acute infections or bone/soft tissue pathologies are assessed and planned with due regard to optimal maternal health and minimal risk to the fetus[23,39]. Depending on the need for treatment, it is advisable to discuss the use of antibiotics with the attending gynecologist in view of the bacteremia likely to be associated with the procedure. During pregnancy, radiographs should only be taken after careful consideration of the risk–benefit ratio, and, if possible, should be avoided in the first trimester. It should be borne in mind that an untreated infection in the mother will have more impact on the fetus than a radiograph taken to detect that infection[43]. Morning appointments should be avoided for pregnant women, who often have frequent and excessive nausea in the mornings.

From the third trimester, treatments in the supine position should be avoided, if possible, so that the dorsally located blood vessels (inferior vena cava and aorta) are not compressed. The patient lying flat in the dental chair can cause dizziness, tachycardia, decreased blood pressure, and dyspnea (inferior vena cava syndrome).

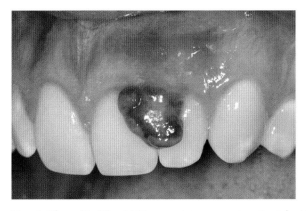 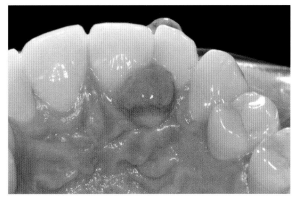

Figs 1-12 and 1-13 A 28-year-old pregnant patient (in the second trimester) with soft tissue proliferation that bleeds easily in the maxillary left central and lateral incisor region buccally (Fig 1-12) and palatally (Fig 1-13), which formed within a few days during pregnancy. This pregnancy epulis was not excised. The mucosal change regressed after the baby was born.

From an upright or semi-reclined position, the patient is placed in a slightly left lateral position in order to reduce the risk of this complication[23].

Any medication prescribed for pregnant women must be chosen so that the drug therapy does not harm the mother, embryo or fetus. Many medications can pass through the placental barrier unimpeded and hence enter the fetal circulation[44]. For this reason, drugs are only taken during pregnancy if they are absolutely essential. It is important to contact the attending gynecologist if a patient is taking longer-term medication. For analgesia, medications containing paracetamol should primarily be taken at a low dose and for a short time, if clearly indicated. However, these can pass through the placental barrier, and therefore liver damage to the fetus is possible. Analgesics containing the active ingredients acetylsalicylic acid, ibuprofen, and diclofenac should not be prescribed because they can cause an increased bleeding tendency in the mother and the fetus and can lead to closure of the *ductus arteriosus* in the fetus. Based on many years of experience, these authors suggest that antibiotics containing penicillin, cephalosporins, and beta lactamase inhibitors (clavulanic acid) are not problematic. Antibiotics from the tetracycline group are contraindicated. In terms of local anesthetics, the active substances articaine, bupivacaine or etidocaine can be used. Adrenaline is not able to pass through the placental barrier but can lead to underperfusion of the placenta, which in turn can result in reactive tachycardia in the fetus due to the lack of oxygen. Therefore, a low concentration (1:200,000) of the vasoconstrictor additive adrenaline should be selected[44]. Noradrenaline as well as felypressin and ornipressin are contraindicated[42].

Substance abuse

Substance abuse involving alcohol or tobacco, for instance, can promote intraoperative and postoperative complications. As mentioned above, alcohol abuse can result in acquired hemorrhagic diathesis because of cirrhosis of the liver. It can be difficult to get a clear and accurate history regarding alcohol consumption. It is sometimes advisable to measure preoperative blood levels for clotting factors in patients with known alcohol abuse, and intraoperative hemostatic measures should be planned for, in case they are needed.

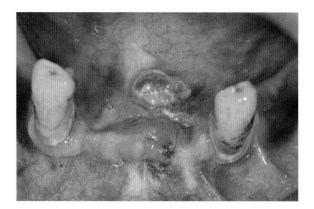

Fig 1-14 An 81-year-old patient with a white-red, partly verrucous, and exophytic change in the anterior part of the floor of the mouth and the adjacent crestal and buccal region. Initial histopathologic assessment revealed a moderately differentiated squamous cell carcinoma. The patient is a former smoker (approximately 40 pack-years).

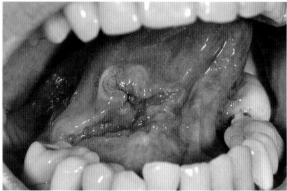

Fig 1-15 A 70-year-old smoker (approximately 40 pack-years) exhibits a hard, raised, and bulging tissue proliferation on the floor of the mouth and the right underside of the tongue, merging into an extensive, easily bleeding ulceration on the clearly hardened floor of the mouth. The patient had previously avoided dental check-ups due to her dental phobia and strong gag reflex. An initial histopathologic assessment revealed a well-differentiated, partly keratinized squamous cell carcinoma.

Cigarette smoking has multiple negative effects on oral health and also specifically increases the risk of oral cavity carcinomas (Figs 1-14 and 1-15), periodontal disease, and peri-implantitis. In recent years, tobacco has been consumed increasingly in the form of waterpipes (also known as hookahs, used to smoke shisha) and electronic cigarettes, known as e-cigarettes or vaping. Waterpipe smoking, in particular, is associated with periodontal diseases, alveolitis, and premalignant lesions as well as oral and esophageal carcinomas, just as much as tobacco smoking. Based on current knowledge, e-cigarettes do seem to be less harmful than conventional cigarettes, but their long-term health implications are still largely unknown[45,48].

Summary

Success and failure in oral surgery procedures are determined not only by surgical skills and individual experience but significantly by correct patient selection as well as precise preparatory measures and assessments. History taking is a key element in medical and dental activity, and it is particularly important to recognize at-risk patients and assess them properly. In particular, patients with polypharmacy and multimorbidity (primarily elderly individuals) present more complex general medical diagnoses and should receive holistic ("synoptic") care within the relevant medical disciplines. This approach helps to prevent complications and to achieve a successful treatment outcome for both the patient and dental practitioner.

References

1. Abariga SA, Whitcomb BW: Periodontitis and gestational diabetes mellitus: a systematic review and meta-analysis of observational studies. BMC Pregnancy Childbirth 2016;16:344.

2. Aframia DJ, Lalla RV, Peterson DE: Management of dental patients taking common hemostasis-altering medications. Oral Surg Oral Med Oral Pathol Oral Radiol Endod 2007;103(Suppl): S45.e1–e11.

3. Akintoye SO, Brennan MT, Graber CJ, McKinney BE, Rams TE, Barrett AJ, Atkinson JC: A retrospective investigation of advanced periodontal disease as a risk factor for septicemia in hematopoietic stem cell and bone marrow transplant recipients. Oral Surg Oral Med Oral Pathol Oral Radiol Endod 2002;94:581–588.

4. Ardekian L, Gaspar R, Peled M, Brener B, Laufer D: Does low-dose aspirin therapy complicate oral surgical procedures? J Am Dent Assoc 2000;131:331–335.

5. Bajkin BV, Popovic SL, Selakovic SD: Randomized, prospective trial comparing bridging therapy using low-molecular-weight heparin with maintenance of oral anticoagulation during extraction of teeth. J Oral Maxillofac Surg 2009;67:990–995.

6. Beirne OR: Evidence to continue oral anticoagulant therapy for ambulatory oral surgery. J Oral Maxillofac Surg 2005;63:540–545.

7. Binkley HM, Schroyer T, Catalfano J: Latex allergies: a review of recognition, evaluation, management, prevention, education, and alternative product use. J Athl Train 2003;38: 133–140.

8. Blinder D, Manor Y, Martinowitz U, Taicher S, Hashomer T: Dental extractions in patients maintained on continued oral anticoagulant: comparison of local hemostatic modalities. Oral Surg Oral Med Oral Pathol Oral Radiol Endod 1999;88:137–140.

9. Bundesamt für Gesundheit, Referenzzentren für blutübertragbare Inkfektionen im Gesundheitsbereich: Prävention blutübertragbarer Krankheiten auf Patienten: Empfehlungen für Personal im Gesundheitswesen mit Hepatitis B-, Hepatitis C- oder HIV-Inkfektion. Richtlinien und Empfehlungen. Bern: Bundesamt für Gesundheit, 2011.

10. Bundesamt für Gesundheit, Abteilung übertragbare Krankheiten: HIV, Syphilis, Gonorrhoe und Chlamydiose in der Schweiz im Jahr 2018: eine epidemiologische Übersicht. BAG-Bulletin 41 vom 7. Oktober 2019. www.bag.admin.ch (Accessed 15.11.2020).

11. Bundesamt für Gesundheit., Abteilung übertragbare Krankheiten: Herpes simplex (HSV-1, HSV-2). Letzte Änderung: 23.12.2019. www.bag.admin.ch (Accessed 15.11.2020).

12. Burwinkel M: Eingriffe an Blutungspatienten Teil 1: Systematik zur Risikoeinschätzung. Quintessenz 2013;64:339–350.

13. Candotto V, Lauritano D, Nardone M, Baggi L, Arcuri C, Gatto R, Gaudio RM, Spadari F, Carinci F: HPV infection in the oral cavity: epidemiology, clinical manifestations and relationship with oral cancer. Oral Implantol (Rome) 2017;10:209–220.

14. Caparrotti F, Huang SH, Lu L, Bratman SV, Ringash J, Bayley A, Cho J, Guiliani M, Kim J, Waldrin J, Hansen A, Tong L, Xu W, O'Sulivan B, Wood R, Goldstein D, Hope A: Osteoradionecrosis of the mandible in patients with oropharyngeal carcinoma treated with intensity-modulated radiotherapy. Cancer 2017;123:3691–3700.

15. Centers for medicare and medicaid services: Chronic conditions among medicare bene caries, Chartbook, 2012 Edition. Baltimore, 2012.

16. Charlesworth CJ, Smit E, Lee DSH, Alramadhan F, Odden MC: Polypharmacy among adults aged 65 years and older in the United States: 1988-2010. J Gerontol A Biol Sci Med Sci 2015;70:989–995.

17. Chiewchalermsri C, Sompornrattanaphan M, Wongsa C, Thongngarm T: Chlorhexidine allergy: Current challenges and future prospects. J Asthma Allergy 2020;13:127–133.

18. Cieślik-Bielewska A, Pelc R, Cieślik T: Oral surgery procedures in patients on anticoagulants. Preliminary report. Kardiol Pol 2005;63:137–140.

19. Delwel S, Scherder EJA, Perez RSGM, Hertogh CMPM, Maier AB, Lobbezoo F: Oral function of older people with mild cognitive impairment or dementia. J Oral Rehabil 2018;45:990–997.

20. Douketis JD, Hasselblad V, Ortel TL: Bridging anticoagulation in patients with atrial fibrillation. N Engl J Med 2016;374:93–94.

21. Eichhorn W, Burkert J, Vorwig O, Blessmann M, Cachovan G, Zeuch J, Eichhorn M, Heiland M: Bleeding incidence after oral surgery with continued oral anticoagulation. Clin Oral Investig 2012;16:1371–1376.

22. Evans IL, Sayers MS, Gibbons AJ, Price G, Snooks H, Sugar AW: Can warfarin be continued during dental extraction? Results of a randomized controlled trial. Br J Oral Maxillofac Surg 2002;40:248–252.

23. Flynn TR, Susarla SM: Oral and maxillofacial surgery for the pregnant patient. Oral Maxillofac Surg Clin North Am 2007;19:207–221.

24. Furci F, Martina S, Faccioni P, Faccioni F, Senna G, Caminati M: Adverse reaction to local anaesthetics: Is it always allergy? Oral Dis 2020. doi: 10.1111/odi.13310. Epub ahead of print.

25. Gaspar R, Brenner B, Ardekian L, Peled M, Laufer D: Use of tranexamic acid mouthwash to prevent postoperative bleeding in oral surgery patients on oral anticoagulant medication. Quintessence Int 1997;28:375–379.

26. Girotra C, Padhye M, Mandlik G, Dabir A, Gite M, Dhonnar R, Pandhi V, Vandekar M: Assessment of the risk of haemorrhage and its control following minor oral surgical procedures in patients on anti-platelet therapy: a prospective study. Int J Oral Maxillofac Surg 2014;43:99–106.

27. Grines CL, Bonow RO, Casey DE Jr, Gardner TJ, Lockhart PB, Moliterno DJ, O'Gara P, Whitlow P; American Heart Association; American College of Cardiology; Society for Cardiovascular Angiography and Interventions; American College of Surgeons; American Dental Association; American College of Physicians: Prevention of premature discontinuation of dual antiplatelet therapy in patients with coronary artery stents: a science advisory from the American Heart Association, American College of Cardiology, Society for Cardiovascular Angiography and Interventions, American College of Surgeons, and American Dental Association, with representation from the American College of Physicians. Circulation 2007;115:813–818.

28. Heidbuchel H, Verhamme P, Alings M, Antz M, Diener HC, Hacke W, Oldgren J, Sinnaeve P, Camm AJ, Kirchhof P: Updated European Heart Rhythm Association Practical Guide on the use of non-vitamin K antagonist anticoagulants in patients with non-valvular atrial fibrillation. Europace 2015;17:1467–1507.

29. Hoffmeister HM, Bode C, Darius H, Huber K, Rybak K, Silber S: Unterbrechung antithrombotischer Behandlung (Bridging) bei kardialen Erkrankungen. Kardiologe 2010;4:365–374.

30. Hong CHL, Hu S, Haverman T, Stokman M, Napeñas JJ, Braber JB, Gerber E, Geuke M, Vardas E, Waltimo T, Jensen SB, Saunders DP: A systematic review of dental disease management in cancer patients. Support Care Cancer 2018;26:155–174.

31. Hotz S: Kinder fördern. Handlungsempfehlungen zum Umgang mit AD(H)S im Entscheidungsprozess. Institut für Familienforschung und Beratung. Universität Fribourg, 2018.

32. International Rheumatic Fever Study Group: Allergic reactions to long-term benzathine penicillin prophylaxis for rheumatic fever. Lancet 1991;337:1308.

33. Jansma J, Vissink A, Spijkervet FK, Roodenburg JL, Panders AK, Vermey A, Szabó BG, Gravenmade EJ: Protocol for the prevention and treatment of oral sequelae resulting from head and neck radiation therapy. Cancer 1992;70:2171–2180.

34. Kämmerer PW, Frerich B, Liese J, Schiegnitz E, Al-Nawas B: Oral surgery during therapy with anticoagulants – a systematic review. Clin Oral Investig 2015;19:171–180.

35. Kämmerer PW und Al-Nawas B: S3-Leitlinie Zahnärztliche Chirurgie unter oraler Antikoagulation/Thrombozytenaggregationshemmung. AWMF-Registernummer: 083-018. Stand: August 2017.

36. Khan AA, Morrison A, Kendler DL, Rizzoli R, Hanley DA, Felsenberg D, McCauley LK, O'Ryan F, Reid IR, Ruggiero SL, Taguchi A, Tetradis S, Watts NB, Brandi ML, Peters E, Guise T, Eastell R, Cheung AM, Morin SN, Masri B, Cooper C, Morgan SL, Obermayer-Pietsch B, Langdahl BL, Dabagh RA, Davison KS, Sándor GK, Josse RG, Bhandari M, El Rabbany M, Pierroz DD, Sulimani R, Saunders DP, Brown JP, Compston J; International Task Force on Osteonecrosis of the Jaw: Case-Based Review of Osteonecrosis of the Jaw (ONJ) and Application of the International Recommendations for Management From the International Task Force on ONJ. J Clin Densitom 2017;20:8–24.

37. Laine MA: Effect of pregnancy on periodontal and dental health. Acta Odontol Scand 2002;60:257–264.

38. Masnoon N, Shakib S, Kalisch-Ellett L, Caughey GE: What is polypharmacy? A systematic review of definitions. BMC Geriatr 2017;17:230.

39. Muralidharan C, Merrill RM: Dental care during pregnancy based on the pregnancy risk assessment monitoring system in Utah. BMC Oral Health 2019;19:237.

40. Ockerman A, Bornstein MM, Leung YY, Li SKY, Politis C, Jacobs R: Incidence of bleeding after minor oral surgery in patients on dual antiplatelet therapy: a systematic review and meta-analysis. Int J Oral Maxillofac Surg 2020;49:90–98.

41. Ottesen C, Schiodt M, Gotfredsen K: Efficacy of a high-dose antiresorptive drug holiday to reduce the risk of medication-related osteonecrosis of the jaw (MRONJ): A systematic review. Heliyon 2020;6:e03795. doi:10.1016/j.heliyon.2020.e03795.

42. Pässler L, Pässler S: Die schwangere Patientin. Zahnmedizin up2date 2011;6:585–602.

43. Patcas R, Schätzle M, Lübbers HT: Nutzen-Risiko-Abwägung: Darf ich bei einer Schwangeren Röntgenbilder anfertigen? Zahnarzt Praxis 2011;5:19–21.

44. Pertl C, Heinemann A, Pertl B, Lorenzoni M, Pieber D, Eskici A, Amann R: Die schwangere Patientin in zahnärztlicher Behandlung. Umfrageergebnisse und therapeutische Richtlinien. Schweiz Monatsschr Zahnmed 2000;110:37–46.

45. Ramôa CP, Eissenberg T, Sahingur SE: Increasing popularity of waterpipe tobacco smoking and electronic cigarette use: Implications for oral healthcare. J Periodontal Res 2017;52:813–823.

46. Rankin A, Cadogan CA, Patterson SM, Kerse N, Cardwell CR, Bradley MC, Ryan C, Hughes C: Interventions to improve the appropriate use of polypharmacy for older people. Cochrane Database Syst Rev 2018: CD008165. Published online 2018 Sep 3. doi: 10.1002/14651858.CD008165.pub4.

47. Rechenmacher SJ, Fang JC: Bridging anticoagulation: Primum non nocere. J Am Coll Cardiol 2015;66:1392–1403.

48. Rehan HS, Maini J, Hungin APS: Vaping versus Smoking: A Quest for efficacy and safety of e-cigarette. Curr Drug Saf 2018;13:92–101.

49. Renton T, Woolcombe S, Taylor T, Hill CM: Oral surgery: part 1. Introduction and the management of the medically compromised patient. Br Dent J 2013;215:213–223.

50. Sacco KA, Bates A, Brigham TJ, Imam JS, Burton MC: Clinical outcomes following inpatient penicillin allergy testing: A systematic review and meta-analysis. Allergy 2017;72:1288–1296.

51. Safer DJ: Overprescribed medications for US adults: Four major examples. J Clin Med Res 2019;11:617–622.

52. Sánchez-Palomino P, Sánchez-Cobo P, Rodriguez-Archilla A, González-Jaranay M, Moreu G, Calvo-Guirado JL, Peñarrocha-Diago M, Gómez-Moreno G: Dental extraction in patients receiving dual antiplatelet therapy. Med Oral Patol Oral Cir Bucal 2015;20:616–620.

53. Scheller B, Levenson B, Joner M, Zahn R, Klauss V, Naber C, Schächinger V, Elsässer A, Arbeitsgruppe Interventionelle Kardiologie (AGIK) der Deutschen Gesellschaft für Kardiologie (DGK): Medikamente freisetzende Koronarstents und mit Medikamenten beschichtete Ballonkatheter – Positionspapier der DGK 2011. Der Kardiologe 2011;5:411–435.

54. Schellong SM, Haas S: Neue orale Antikoagulanzien und ihre Anwendung im perioperativen Umfeld. Anasthesiol Intensivmed Notfallmed Schmerzther 2012;47:266–272.

55. Schlitt A, Jámbor C, Spannagl M, Gogarten W, Schilling T, Zwißler B: Perioperativer Umgang mit Antikoagulanzien und Thrombozytenaggregationshemmern. Deutsches Ärzteblatt 2013;110:525–532.

56. Schrag A, Taddei RN: Depression and anxiety in parkinson's disease. Int Rev Neurobiol 2017;133:623–655.

57. Shenoy ES, Macy E, Rowe T, Blumenthal KG: Evaluation and management of penicillin allergy: a review. JAMA 2019;321:188–199.

58. Sindet-Pedersen S, Ramström G, Bernvil S, Blombäck M: Hemostatic effect of tranexamic acid mouthwash in anticoagulant-treated patients undergoing oral surgery. N Engl J Med 1989;320:840–843.

59. Studer G, Studer SP, Zwahlen RA, Huguenin P, Grätz KW, Lütolf UM, Glanzmann C: Osteoradionecrosis of the mandible: minimized risk profile following intensity-modulated radiation therapy (IMRT). Strahlenther Onkol 2006;182:283–288.

60. Umemoto G, Furuya H: Management of dysphagia in patients with parkinson's disease and related disorders. Intern Med 2020;59:7–14.

61. Václavík J, Táborský M: Antiplatelet therapy in the perioperative period. Eur J Intern Med 2011;22:26–31.

62. Wahl MJ: Myths of dental surgery in patients receiving anticoagulant therapy. J Am Dent Assoc 2000;131:77–81.

Optical magnifying aids

2

Fabio Saccardin, Thomas Connert

Optical magnifying aids such as loupes, operating microscopes, and endoscopes are indispensable in modern oral surgery. The magnified view of the working field allows the surgeon better detail detection and hence more precise working, especially on delicate structures. Furthermore, optical magnifying aids can also compensate for visual deficits, for instance, presbyopia (from about the age of 40), which leads to a decline in amplitude of accommodation. For this reason, it is advisable for practitioners to have their near vision tested every now and then during their careers and have the optics corrected accordingly (Figs 2-1 and 2-2). Another important aspect when using optical magnifying aids is improved ergonomics in relation to the patient. The individual systems of common magnification aids as well as their advantages and disadvantages are examined below.

Binocular loupes

In the case of dental loupes, two optics for the left and right eye are fixed onto the frame of a pair of spectacles. Compared with an operating microscope or endoscope, dental loupes have a far lower magnification factor, yet their key advantages are that they offer a larger overview of the working field, they are relatively inexpensive, and the viewing angle can be changed at any time without the user having to readjust or even remove the system. When utilizing the loupe system, it is not necessary to alter the working position or posture. However, dental loupes only contribute to better ergonomics if the directional angle of their optics is correct. To take the strain off the neck muscles, it is therefore important to ensure a forward and downward inclination of the optics (measured at the horizontal) when adjusting the loupe system. Loupes can be divided into Galilean and Keplerian (prismatic) systems, both with advantages and disadvantages.

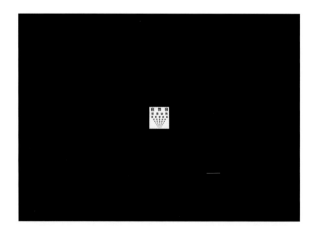

Fig 2-1 Near vision test (with tumbling E chart): The test should be viewed at 30 centimeters, the usual working distance for dental surgeons. However, despite the latest letterpress printing techniques, the quality of near vision tests is still limited by inadequate resolution.

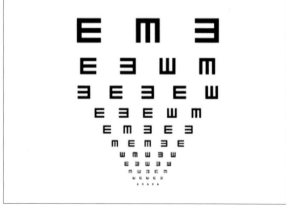

Fig 2-2 Enlarged version of the near vision test from Fig 2-1.

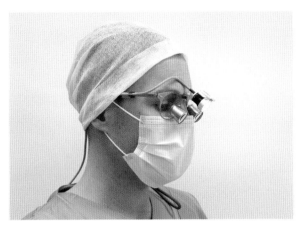

Fig 2-3 Example of a Galilean loupe system (loupes from ExamVision; light source from JADENT). The simple design and large field of vision are advantages but with the compromise of low magnification.

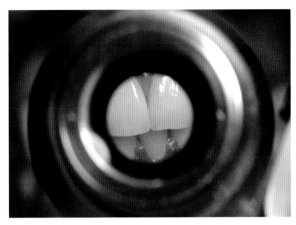

Fig 2-4 Field of vision of a Galilean loupe with ×2.5 magnification.

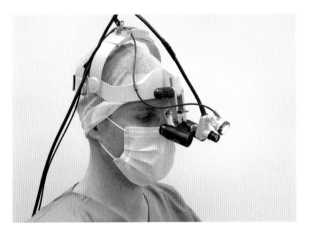

Fig 2-5 Example of a Keplerian loupe system (loupes from Carl Zeiss; light source with integrated full HD camera from StarMed). The optic system is much heavier and larger but can offer higher magnification than a Galilean loupe system.

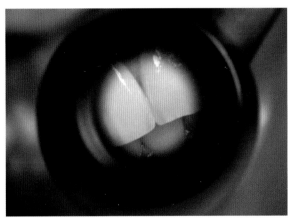

Fig 2-6 Field of vision of a Keplerian loupe with ×3.5 magnification.

The Galilean loupe system (Fig 2-3) has a cone-shaped optic system that consists of a convex and a concave lens, which for physical reasons only permits ×2.5 magnification (Fig 2-4). There are also Galilean loupes with ×1 to ×3.5 magnification but with the compromise of a limited field of vision and greater blurring around the edges. The advantages of Galilean loupe systems are that they are compact and lightweight while providing a relatively large field of vision. Furthermore, the working distance can be adjusted to individual ergonomic requirements. Their disadvantage is a comparatively low magnification factor.

Keplerian loupe systems typically have a cylindrical shape (Fig 2-5). The optic system consists of several convex lenses arranged one behind the other. As a result of the more complex design, up to ×8 magnification can be achieved. In oral surgery, however, ×3.5 to ×6

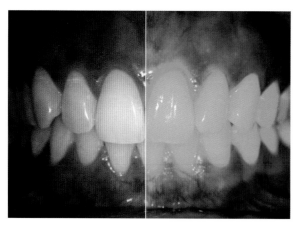

Fig 2-7 The white LED provides optimal illumination of the working field, while the green LED additionally intensifies the contrast with red. As a result, the fine blood vessels in the area of the mobile mucosa can be very clearly identified on the right of the image.

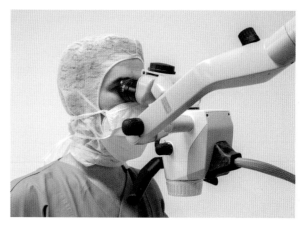

Fig 2-8 Example of an operating microscope (Extaro, Carl Zeiss).

magnification is recommended in order to minimize the influence of the limited depth of focus (Fig 2-6). The advantage of Keplerian loupe systems is stronger magnification but with the disadvantage of being much heavier to wear. For this reason, Keplerian loupes are usually fixed to the frame of the spectacles with an elastic band or with a head strap.

An external light source, which is generally fixed above the optic system or to the frame of the spectacles, ensures near-perfect illumination of the field of vision, thanks to the coaxial alignment. This eliminates the shadow that would usually be cast, depending on the adjustment angle of the chairside light source. Particularly when removing deeply fractured roots, direct illumination of the socket proves to be a decisive advantage. Modern light sources are mostly based on LED technology with rechargeable lithium ion batteries with a run time of several hours. Illumination levels of 60,000 lux or more can be achieved, depending on the manufacturer. However, glaring light can be tiring for the eyes. In addition, there are various optional modifications to the light source (Fig 2-7) such as attachable light filters or different-colored LEDs that can be switched on and off. Green light is especially important in oral surgery because it intensifies the contrast with red or with blood.

Operating microscope

The operating or surgical microscope (Fig 2-8) has become well established in dentistry, especially in the field of endodontics and periradicular surgery. With a magnification changer, objective, binocular tube, and eyepieces, its design is far more complex than that of dental loupes. One of its major advantages is a variably adjustable magnification up to factor 40. However, only × 4 to × 10 magnification is recommended in dentistry because otherwise the overall view would be small and the depth of focus would be reduced (Figs 2-9 and 2-10).

The field of vision can also be illuminated without casting a shadow, thanks to the coaxial alignment of the light source. Furthermore, some operating microscopes offer the option

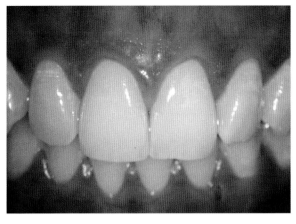

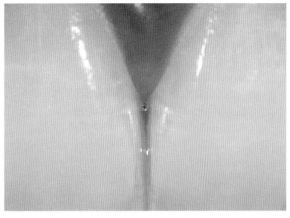

Fig 2-9   Field of vision of an operating microscope at ×4 magnification.

Fig 2-10   Field of vision of an operating microscope at maximal magnification.

Figs 2-11 and 2-12   Using a microscope allows the practitioner to adopt a beneficial ergonomic working posture with the spine upright. The armrests of the chair provide additional support to the forearms so that work can be carried out at elbow height. This relieves strain on neck and shoulder muscles. Ideally, practitioners should first position their own working chair, then the patient's chair, and finally the operating microscope.

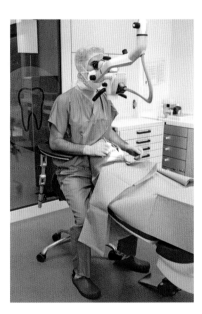

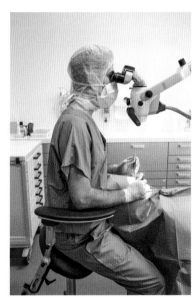

of mounting a camera in order to photograph or film the treatment. Working with an operating microscope also has ergonomic benefits. For instance, dental surgeons can alter their working distance by adjusting the objective lens to accommodate an upright sitting position (straight spine), thereby preventing musculoskeletal problems (Figs 2-11 and 2-12).

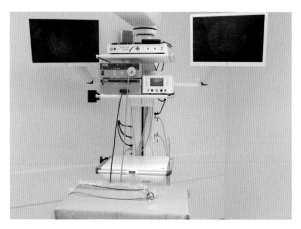

Fig 2-13   Endoscope unit with mobile stepped frame with camera system (Image1 S 4U, Karl Storz) and LED cold light source (POWER LED 175, Karl Storz). The teleotoscope lies on the operating table.

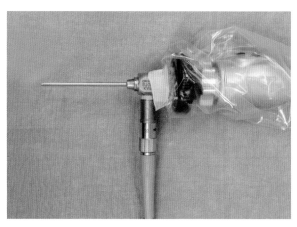

Fig 2-14   Teleotoscope (70-degree Hopkins, 3-mm diameter, 6-cm length, Karl Storz) with camera head and fiberoptic light transmission.

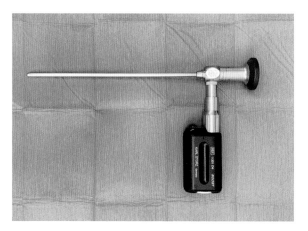

Fig 2-15   Teleotoscope (70-degree Hopkins II large-image lateral telescope, 4-mm diameter, 18-cm length, Karl Storz) with LED battery light source (Karl Storz).

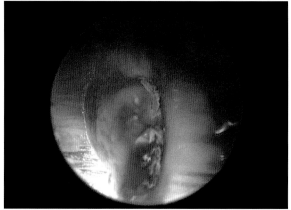

Fig 2-16   Monitor image during an apicoectomy (view of the resection area during retrograde cavity preparation): The microstructures can be seen extremely clearly.

Endoscope

The endoscope (Figs 2-13 and 2-14) was first used in dentistry in the 1970s. Initially, it was used for arthroscopy of the temporomandibular joint and for antroscopy of the maxillary sinus. Later, periradicular surgery particularly benefited from the introduction of the endoscope (but also the operating microscope) and could thus be developed from a microsurgical perspective. The success rates following apicectomies are higher under endoscopic control than when working with a loupe or entirely without magnification devices[1].

Rigid endoscopes (called teleotoscopes) are primarily used in dentistry. The complete endoscopy unit normally comprises four components: teleotoscope with image guide (including camera head), fiberoptic light transmission, light source (cold light source), and monitor. The components can be mounted on a mobile stepped frame and thus be positioned freely in the operating or treatment room. As well as the classic endoscopy unit, there are also smaller and more affordable all-in-one solutions. There are versions in which an LED battery light source is simply mounted on the teleotoscope, and the user looks directly through the eyepiece to view the image (Fig 2-15), and endoscopes in which all the components, including the monitor, are combined in a compact casing.

The magnification factor of the endoscope, unlike other magnifying devices, is not dependent on the optical system but on the distance between the endoscope and the object being viewed (Table 2-1). This means a magnification of more than ×100 can be achieved, and, when viewing the image on the monitor, even more than ×150 magnification (Fig 2-16). Since the endoscope is held in the hand and the viewer needs to look simultaneously at the monitor, handling requires a certain amount of practice. The advantages of the endoscope over the operating microscope are primarily much stronger magnification, direct viewing without (micro-)mirrors, minimally invasive access even in areas that are difficult to visualize (e.g. the molar region), and flexibility. For instance, the viewing angle of an endoscope can be quickly altered by slightly tipping or rotating the optic, and the magnification can be varied by changing the distance. Unlike the operating microscope, the endoscope allows the patient to move the head without any difficulty.

Table 2-1 The magnification factor of the endoscope is governed by the distance between the optic and the object being inspected.

Working distance [mm]	Magnification factor
40	×1
5	×8
2.5	×16
0.3	×132

Reference

1.   Setzer FC, Kohli MR, Shah SB, Karabucak B, Kim S: Outcome of endodontic surgery: a meta-analysis of the literature – Part 2: Comparison of endodontic microsurgical techniques with and without the use of higher magnification. J Endod 2012;38:1–10.

Recommended literature

Khayat B, Jouanny G: Optical aids and armamentarium. In Khayat B, Jouanny G (eds). Microsurgical Endodontics. Berlin: Quintesssence, 2019: 57–78.

Krastl G, Filippi A: Optische Vergrößerungshilfen im Rahmen periradikulärer Chirurgie. Endodontie 2008;17:123–131.

Perrin P, Eichenberger M, Neuhaus KW, Lussi A: Visual acuity and magnification devices in dentistry. Swiss Dent J 2016;126:222–235.

Perrin P, Neuhaus KW, Eichenberger M, Lussi A: Influence of different loupe systems and their light source on the vision in endodontics. Swiss Dent J 2019;129:922–928.

Zuhr O, Hürzeler M: Optische Hilfsmittel. In Zuhr O, Hürzeler M (Hrsg.): Plastisch-ästhetische Parodontal- und Implantatchirurgie: Ein mikrochirurgisches Konzept. Berlin: Quintessenz, 2016:43–47.

CO$_2$ laser

3

Fabio Saccardin

3 CO₂ laser

Laser (*Light Amplification by Stimulated Emission of Radiation*) is suitable for treatments not only on hard tissue (dental hard tissue, cartilage, and bone) but also on soft tissue (mucosa and submucosa). However, not all lasers are the same (Table 3-1). They are classified according to wavelength, absorption properties in tissue, penetration depth, length of laser exposure time, and their operating modes (continuous wave, chopped mode, pulsed mode, superpulse mode, ultrapulse mode, char-free mode, and free-running pulse mode). They have varying effects on tissue, depending on the type of laser and its setting parameters.

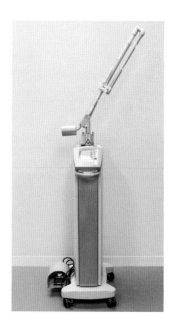

Fig 3-1 Mobile CO₂ laser unit with swiveling articulated arm (Spectra DENTA, Orcos Medical).

Table 3-1 Gas and solid-state lasers used in oral surgery.

	Hard tissue	**Soft tissue**
Gas laser	• CO₂ laser	• Gas laser • Argon laser • CO₂ laser • Helium-neon laser
Solid-state laser	• Er:YAG laser • Er,Cr:YSGG laser • Ho:YAG laser	• Diode laser • Er:YAG laser • Er,Cr:YSGG laser • Dye laser • Nd:YAG laser

Table 3-2 Indications and contraindications for CO₂ laser in oral surgery.

Indications	• Gingivectomy and gingivoplasty (gingival overgrowth) • Depigmentation of the gingiva • Frenulotomy/frenuloplasty (labial, buccal, lingual frenulum) • Pain relief for stomatitis, denture sores, herpes or aphthous lesions • Excision of precancerous lesions and benign neoplasias • Excision of (pseudo)cysts in soft tissue • Implant exposure • Decontamination of implant surfaces (peri-implantitis treatment) • Vestibuloplasty (preprosthetic surgery) • Coagulation (intraoperative and postoperative bleeding) • Scar correction • Abscess incision (only recommended as part of emergency treatment in patients with hemorrhagic diathesis)
Contra-indications	• Biopsy when malignancy is strongly suspected (in this case, direct referral is made to a specialist clinic for further diagnosis and treatment)

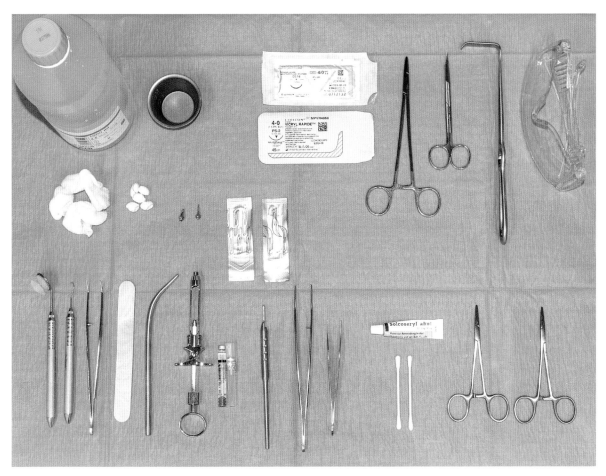

Fig 3-2 Equipment for soft tissue surgery with CO_2 laser: Ringer solution, various swabs, multipurpose bowl, laser attachments, scalpel, suture material, needle holders, dissecting scissors, retractor, safety glasses, dental mirror, cow horn forceps, tweezers, wooden spatula, surgical aspirator tip, local anesthetic, cotton buds, dental adhesive paste, and vessel clamps.

CO_2 laser (carbon dioxide laser) is both the oldest and the most important laser in oral surgery. At a wavelength of 10.6 µm, it reaches its maximal absorption in water. Since soft tissue contains more than 90% water, CO_2 laser is ideal for cutting oral soft tissue or removing it (ablation). It is therefore not surprising that CO_2 laser has a particularly broad spectrum of indications in stomatology (Table 3-2, Figs 3-1 and 3-2). At the same time, CO_2 laser can also be used to decontaminate surfaces such as implant surfaces during the course of peri-implantitis treatment.

Operating principles of CO_2 laser

With CO_2 laser, the laser beam is conducted in the hollow waveguide of the articulated arm by several mirrors and metallic surfaces without causing any damage in the process. As the laser beam encounters tissue, various effects on the surface and inside the tissue arise as a result of the interactions of individual photons of the laser beam with the molecular structures of the irradiated tissue (Fig 3-3). While a small proportion of the photons is initially reflected onto the tissue

3 CO₂ laser

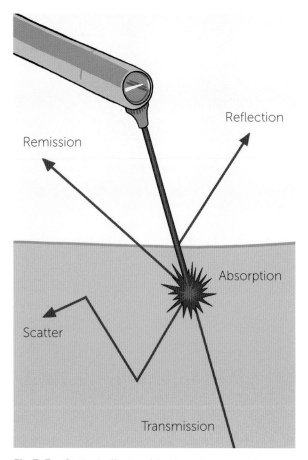

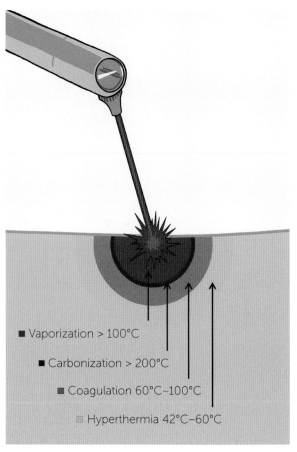

Fig 3-3 Optical effects of the laser beam on tissue.

Fig 3-4 (Photo)thermal effect of the laser beam on tissue.

surface, the rest of the photons penetrate inside the tissue. The photons are mainly absorbed there but are also scattered or reflected again. Theoretically, photons can escape again on the other side of the tissue (transmission radiation). Due to the optical effect of absorption, the molecules of the irradiated tissue enter a more energy-rich state, which gives rise to thermal energy. The resulting (photo)thermal effects ultimately allow tissue to be incised and removed with the CO₂ laser (Fig 3-4). Enzyme deactivation occurs in soft tissue above a temperature of 42°C, which can lead to irreversible cell damage within a few seconds to minutes. At temperatures between 60°C and 100°C, protein denaturation results in coagulation, with the resulting cell necrosis. If the soft tissue is heated above 100°C, the water it contains starts to boil, and vaporization of the liquid cell components and intercellular substance ensues. If the temperature continues to increase, carbonization occurs from 200°C, all tissue components vaporize above 300°C, and smoke is given off. The maximal achievable temperature is dependent on the local accumulation of heat and on dissipation of the heat of a certain tissue to its surroundings, and is described in physics by the term *thermal relaxation time*. So that the heat generated

36

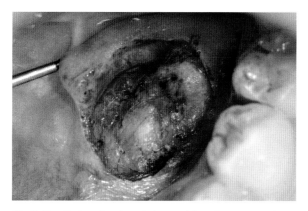

Fig 3-5 Carbonized and almost bloodless wound surface after excision of an extravasation mucocele on the floor of the mouth by CO_2 laser.

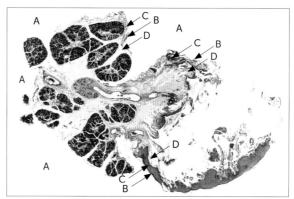

Fig 3-6 Histopathologic image of the extravasation mucocele: ablation zone (A), carbonization zone (B), necrosis/coagulation zone (C), and edema zone (D).

in the tissue can be better dissipated, and consequently the degree of thermal heat damage can be reduced, the laser should be used in pulsed mode, which means high energy density and short pulse duration (superpulse mode or ultrapulse mode/char-free mode). This aspect is relevant because when a biopsy is taken by CO_2 laser, histopathologic usability of the biopsied or excised specimen must be guaranteed since the thermal tissue damage at the resection margin is 0.5 mm on average (Figs 3-5 and 3-6). Furthermore, there is evidence in the literature that heat generation can also give rise to cytologic atypias as well as artefacts, which ultimately lead to incorrect diagnoses. Consequently, it is advisable to maintain a safety margin of 1 mm around the future biopsy or excised material, especially with laser biopsy, to identify the benign or malignant nature of a specimen. It is also important to inform the pathologist that the tissue specimen was obtained using CO_2 laser.

CO_2 laser is normally used without making contact with the tissue. The tissue penetration depth for optimum absorption (= minimum absorption depth) is 0.1 mm. The laser beam has a coagulating effect and thereby seals blood vessels with a diameter of up to 0.5 mm. This guarantees a virtually blood-free view of the surgical site and additionally reduces the risk of postoperative bleeding and hematoma formation. Especially in patients with hemorrhagic diathesis (see Section 1), the risk of intraoperative and postoperative bleeding is thus reduced, although merely using CO_2 laser is no substitute for the necessary preoperative risk assessment or consultation with the patient's attending physician. Furthermore, the coagulating effect also seals lymph vessels, which reduces the degree of postoperative swelling. During the cutting process, the zoom on the laser attachment should, generally, be closed so that the laser beam remains focused and hence a precise incision path is guaranteed (Figs 3-7 to 3-13, Video 3-1). The tissue is kept taut by tension and needs to be kept moist in the process. For ablation, the zoom is opened, and the laser beam is hence defocused. The tissue dehydrated by the laser beam is repeatedly wiped with moist stick swabs. After CO_2 laser treatment has been performed, the open wound surfaces are usually left to secondary wound healing. In the process, the surface of the wound area might be carbonized

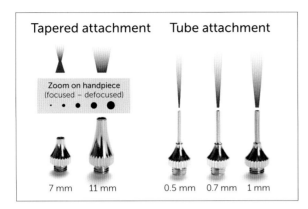

Fig 3-7   Various attachments/tips for a CO₂ laser handpiece (Spectra DENTA 2, Orcos Medical).

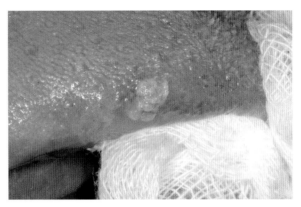

Fig 3-8   Clinical situation: Sharply defined and raised papillomatous tissue overgrowth on the right margin of the tongue of a 29-year-old patient.

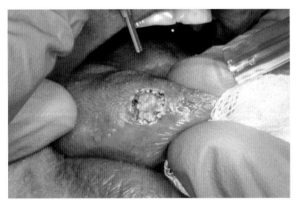

Fig 3-9   Following local anesthesia, the CO₂ laser is used to section the epithelial layer in a circle around the lesion.

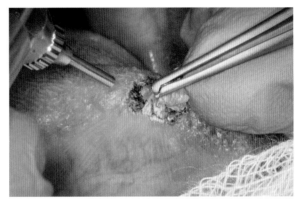

Fig 3-10   The lesion is then carefully raised with surgical tweezers so that the CO₂ laser can reach the deeper tissue layers.

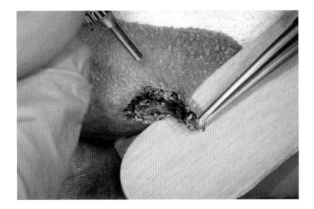

Fig 3-11   The lesion can now be detached from the underlying musculature. The wooden spatula serves to protect the surrounding soft tissue.

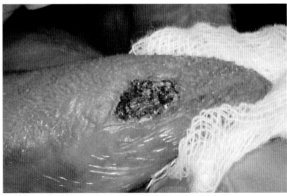

Fig 3-12   Finally, the surface of the excised site can be carbonized with the defocused laser beam (wound dressing).

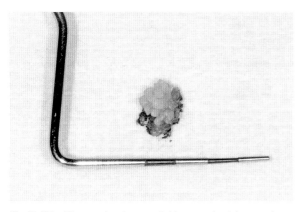

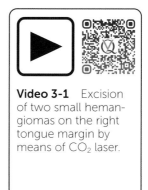

Video 3-1 Excision of two small hemangiomas on the right tongue margin by means of CO_2 laser.

Fig 3-13 The excised material is sent for histopathologic evaluation (to ascertain whether it is malignant or benign). The diagnosis in this case was squamous papilloma (human papillomavirus 6, low risk).

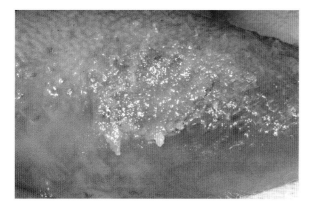

Fig 3-14 The wound area can additionally be covered with dental adhesive paste (here: Solcoseryl, MEDA Pharmaceuticals).

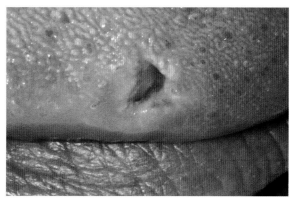

Fig 3-15 Wound situation 2 weeks after excision. Wound healing was delayed in this case due to the mechanical irritation caused by the teeth (when eating, drinking, swallowing, and speaking).

by the defocused laser beam, which does delay wound healing but can be utilized as a type of wound dressing. The wound area can additionally be covered with dental adhesive paste (e.g. Solcoseryl, MEDA Pharmaceuticals) (Fig 3-14).

To decontaminate implant surfaces during peri-implantitis treatment, the CO_2 laser is swept over the implant surface intermittently for a few seconds in continuous mode with low energy density. The zoom usually remains open.

To achieve optimal results with CO_2 laser, a specific treatment protocol with the appropriate setting parameters can be found in the

literature for nearly every indication. The treatment protocol for the Spectra DENTA 2 CO_2 laser from Orcos Medical is presented here by way of example (Table 3-3).

Wound healing

During postoperative checks it is important to bear in mind that the healing process for a laser wound differs from that of a scalpel wound (Fig 3-15). A laser wound generally has a delayed inflammatory reaction, the intensity

Table 3-3 Treatment protocol with the recommended setting parameters for a CO$_2$ laser (Spectra DENTA 2, Orcos Medical).

Indication	Attachment	Mode [CW = continuous wave, CF = char-free mode]	Frequency [Hz]	Pulse duration [µs]	Power [W]	Zoom	Comments
Abscess incision	Taper	CW			4	1	
Aphthae	Taper	CF	20	180–250		1	Sweep over surface several times
De-epithelialization	Taper	CF	120	150		1–2	
Epulis	Taper	CF	100–180	500		2	Then coagulation with CW (2–3 W) as far as the periosteum
Fibroma	Taper	CF	140–180	450		1	Lift with grasping instrument or suture
Frenectomy (labial and buccal frenulum)	Taper	CF	140–180	450–500		1–3	Then coagulation with CW (2–3 W)
Frenectomy (lingual frenulum)	Taper	CF	140–180	450–700		2	Local anesthetic with vaso-constrictor due to possible bleeding
Gingival overgrowth	Tube (1 mm)	CF	120–180	350–450		1	Keep laser tip parallel to the tooth axis
Hemangioma	Tube (1 mm)	CF	180	500–700		2	Safety margin of approximately 1 mm
Herpes	Taper	CF	20	180–250		1	Irradiate each site at least 3× (finally 250 µs)

Table 3-3 (continued)   Treatment protocol with the recommended setting parameters for a CO_2 laser (Spectra DENTA 2, Orcos Medical).

Indication	Attachment	Mode [CW = continuous wave, CF = char-free mode]	Frequency [Hz]	Pulse duration [µs]	Power [W]	Zoom	Comments
Implant exposure	Taper	CF	140–180	450		3	On implant surface only with CW (maximum 3 W)
Crown lengthen-ing (gingiva)	Tube (1 mm)	CF	100–180	350–500		1	Keep laser tip parallel to the tooth axis (option to use a metal spatula for protection)
Coagulation	Taper	CW			4–8	5	Sweep in a circle around vessel, then coagulate in the center
Mucocele	Taper or tube (0.7 mm)	CF	160–180	450		1–2	In vertical direction at maximal point of mucocele
Peri-implantitis (decontami-nating implant surface)	Taper	CW			3	1	Sweep over implant surface until dry
Denture sore	Taper	CF	20	150–300		1	Sweep over surface several times
Flabby ridge	Taper	CW			5	1	Then coagulation with CW (2–3 W)
Vestibuloplasty (in edentulous patients)	Taper	CF	160–180	500		3	Spare periosteum and bone
Vestibuloplasty (in dentate patients)	Tube (0.7 mm)	CF	140–180	250–450		1	Suture split flap apical to the periosteum

of which is variably described in the literature. Whereas some studies reported a rather mild inflammatory reaction from a laser wound, others observed from day 2 or 3 postoperatively a much more extensive inflammatory reaction with pronounced infiltrate compared with a scalpel wound. However, after the first postoperative week, the degree of inflammation is identical for both types of wounds, and the inflammatory reaction subsides after 2 weeks at the latest. Complete re-epithelialization can be expected after only 2 weeks with a scalpel wound, whereas this tends to occur later with a laser wound, after about 2 to 4 weeks. In terms of neovascularization, a laser wound will show a smaller number of newly formed blood vessels than a scalpel wound in the first 2 to 4 days, but the numbers converge for both types as the healing process continues. Furthermore, less wound contraction and scar formation is likely with a laser wound. One possible explanation might be the lower number of myofibroblasts within the laser wound during the healing process. Irrespective of whether CO$_2$ laser or a scalpel is used, the tissue elasticity of the oral mucosa is postoperatively more reduced than before the surgical procedure, although this is less marked with a laser wound than a scalpel wound (1.75-fold versus 3-fold).

Table 3-4 Direct comparison of CO$_2$ laser with conventional scalpel (advantages and disadvantages).

	CO$_2$ laser	Scalpel
Advantages	• Sterility maintained during the surgical procedure • Almost bloodless view of the surgical site • Lower risk of bleeding in patients with hemorrhagic diathesis (Caution: Using CO$_2$ laser, however, is no substitute for preoperative risk assessment) • Time saving (surgical wound closure is rarely necessary) • Less postoperative bleeding • Less postoperative swelling • Less postoperative pain • Less scarring • Hardly any wound infections	• Faster healing process based on primary wound healing
Disadvantages	• Longer healing process based on secondary wound healing • High purchase costs of CO$_2$ laser equipment • Special infrastructure necessary (laser/operating room, laser marking, safety glasses, etc) • Additional training and education	• Loss of substance • Suture removal necessary if nonresorbable suture material is used • More frequent scarring

CO_2 laser compared with a scalpel

CO_2 laser definitely has certain advantages over the conventional scalpel (Table 3-4). An almost bloodless view of the surgical site is a key benefit of CO_2 laser. Furthermore, there is greater patient acceptance of CO_2 lasers because postoperatively fewer incidents of bleeding or less bleeding as well as less hematoma, pain, and swelling are likely. However, depending on size and localization, the clinical appearance of a laser wound may be very striking for patients because of the carbonization layer, and it also may be worrying and alarming for some patients. For this reason, the postoperative wound situation should be addressed in the preoperative discussion. It is a matter of debate in the literature whether CO_2 laser compared with a conventional scalpel can reduce the risk of hematogenic and/or lymphogenic spread of cancer cells when malignant tumors are excised[1].

Safety aspects

Working with lasers requires intensive study and regular attendance at training events. Furthermore, there are innumerable regulations and safety guidelines that must be taken into account (e.g. UVV German Accident Prevention Regulations – Laser Radiation; Swiss Accident Insurer, SUVA, Information on Safe Handling of Lasers, Swissmedic Laser; USA: ANSI Z136.1 Standard for the Safe Use of Lasers, IEC 825-1, Safety of Laser Products).

One important aspect that is often not rigorously implemented is the wearing of safety glasses or eye protectors (in accordance with EN 207). Optical glasses provide no eye protection; on the contrary, if the laser beam strikes the glasses, sudden heating can shatter them, and splinters of glass can hence get into the eyes. For this reason, those performing the treatment as well as auxiliary staff who are in the same room and obviously patients themselves must wear eye protection.

Reference

1. Wiegand S, Wiemers C, Murthum T, Zimmermann AP, Bette M, Mandic R, Werner JA: Risk of lymph node metastases after en bloc cold steel, en bloc laser-, and piecemeal laser surgical resection of auricular VX2 carcinoma. Lasers Med Sci 2013;28:1137–1141.

Recommended literature

Bornstein MM, Suter VG, Stauffer E, Buser D: The CO_2 laser in stomatology. Part 1. Schweiz Monatsschr Zahnmed 2003;113:559–570.

Bornstein MM, Suter VG, Stauffer E, Buser D: The CO_2 laser in stomatology. Part 2. Schweiz Monatsschr Zahnmed 2003;113:766–785.

Moritz A: Orale Lasertherapie. Berlin: Quintessenz, 2006.

Westermann U, Podmelle F. Kapitel 10: Laseranwendung in der ZMK-Heilkunde. In: Schwenzer N, Ehrenfeld M (eds). Zahnärztliche Chirurgie (5. unveränderte Auflage). New York: Thieme, 2019:274–286.

Piezoelectric surgery

4

Fabio Saccardin, Sebastian Kühl

4 Piezoelectric surgery

Piezoelectric surgery (in Ancient Greek, *piezen* means to press) was developed in the 1980s thanks to advances in conventional ultrasound technology in order to make oral surgery procedures on bone more tissue-preserving than the popular methods at the time such as rotary instruments, hammer and chisel, and bone saws (Fig 4-1). The operating technique is based on the piezoelectric effect, also known as the piezo effect. This effect arises from the elastic deformation of piezo crystals as electric voltage is applied. The resulting piezoelectric vibration in the ultrasonic range (25,000 to 35,000 Hz) enables precise cutting or removal of hard tissue because the frequency is attuned to hard tissue structures such as bone and dental hard tissue but not to soft tissue structures. This makes it possible to separate bone and dental hard tissue

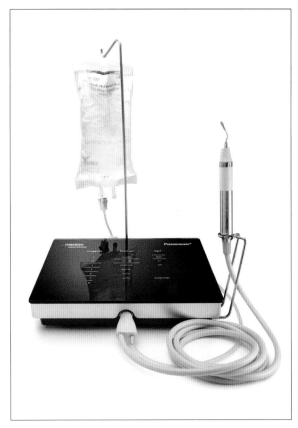

Fig 4-1 Example of a piezoelectric surgery unit (Piezosurgery touch, Mectron Medical Technology).

without having any appreciable influence on soft tissue. The indications for piezoelectric surgery therefore are basically confined to use on bone and dental hard tissue (Table 4-1).

When using a piezoelectric surgical instrument, it is important to ensure that the tip of the instrument remains in constant motion due to forward and backward movements, and to exert only a small amount of pressure on the bone (approximately 150 g) in order to avoid overheating. Furthermore, excessive pressure is counterproductive because the vibration decreases, and hence cutting efficiency is reduced. Various stainless steel piezoelectric surgical inserts for the handpiece, depending on the indication, are available on the dental market (Fig 4-2). These essentially differ in their shape (straight/angled, serrated, conical, round, spatula-shaped, cylindrical, etc) and their surface finish (uncoated, diamond-coated, titanium-coated). The piezoelectric surgical device must include the intended setting parameters for the particular piezoelectric surgical inserts.

The piezoelectric surgical instrument has a broad spectrum of indications, especially in dentoalveolar surgery. The tissue-preserving surgical technique can be useful when performing osteotomies close to nerves, such as surgical extractions of wisdom teeth in the mandible. To date, it has not been scientifically proven that the risk of injury to the inferior alveolar nerve and lingual nerve can be reduced by the use of a piezoelectric surgical instrument compared with rotary instruments[1]. However, one study reveals that inadvertent contact between a piezoelectric surgical instrument and a nerve does not sever the nerve but merely compresses it, and this hardly ever happens, in contrast to rotary instruments[5]. If the epineurium and perineurium remain intact, the nerve tissue is usually able to regenerate well. It is additionally reported that there is less postoperative pain and swelling as well as reduced jaw opening during surgical

Table 4-1 Indications and contraindications for piezoelectric surgery.

Indications	<ul><li>Osteotomy or osteoplasty (e.g. in the case of tooth extractions, exostoses, cysts, tumors) in the immediate vicinity of an anatomical structure to be preserved and/or in a surgical site that is difficult for rotary instruments to access</li><li>Corticotomy (surgically supported tooth movement in orthodontics)</li><li>Implant bed preparation</li><li>Bone augmentation (autogenous bone block, autogenous bone chips, ridge-splitting technique, sinus floor elevation)</li><li>Explantation</li><li>Apicoectomy (retrograde root canal preparation)</li><li>Resective and regenerative periodontal surgery</li><li>Surgical crown lengthening</li></ul>
Contraindications	<ul><li>Patients with a cardiac pacemaker (following manufacturer's instructions)</li></ul>

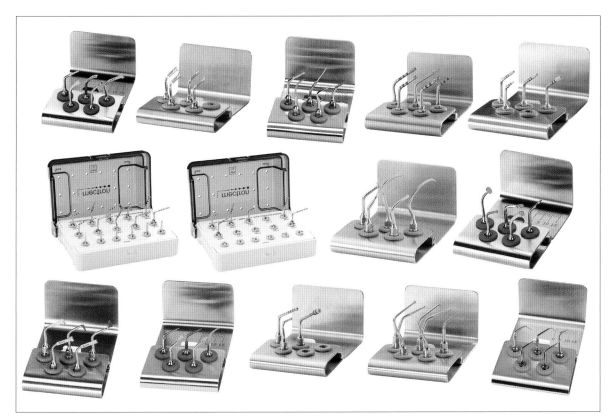

Fig 4-2 Depending on the indication, different piezoelectric surgical inserts are required for the handpiece, which are available on the dental market mostly as a kit (Mectron Medical Technology).

third molar extraction with piezoelectric surgical instruments than with rotary instruments[1].

Piezoelectric surgery is particularly valuable in periradicular surgery (Figs 4-3 to 4-5, Video 4-1). Thanks to the introduction of microsurgical operating principles in the 1990s, the success rates for apicoectomies have significantly improved (59% vs 94%)[4] (see Section 10).

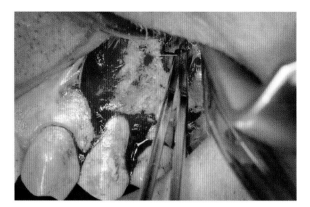

Fig 4-3   After incision (in this case, an intrasulcular vertcial releasing incision) and mobilization of the mucoperiosteal flap, an access osteotomy is performed with subsequent resection of the root apex and its removal.

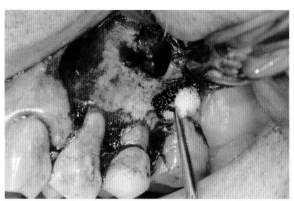

Fig 4-4   To exclude a longitudinal fracture at the root, the resection surface is stained with methylene blue (2%) and inspected by endoscope. A longitudinal fracture was excluded in this case.

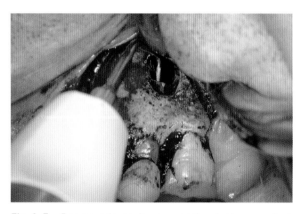

Fig 4-5   Retrograde cavity preparation is then carried out with the aid of the piezoelectric surgical instrument. Finally, the smear layer is removed with a gel containing EDTA (PrefGel®, Straumann), and the cavity is dried with absorbent points and filled with mineral trioxide aggregate (TotalFill BC RRM, FKG Dentaire).

Video 4-1   Piezoelectric surgery-assisted apicoectomy with retrograde filling in a maxillary left second premolar.

Axially correct and sufficiently deep (approximately 3 mm) retrograde preparation of root canals can now be performed with the aid of angled and diamond-coated micro inserts. Furthermore, a smaller access osteotomy can be created, and an acute bevel of the resection surface (> 20 degrees) is not required. It has not yet been fully ascertained whether ultrasonic-operated micro inserts cause clinically relevant (micro)cracks in the root[3].

Piezoelectric surgical devices are also now used in implantology for implant bed preparation. Previous in vitro studies showed comparable results to conventional preparation with pilot and spiral drills in terms of primary stability and heat generation. A disadvantage is that piezoelectric surgical preparation of the implant bed takes significantly longer, and therefore piezoelectric surgery provides no real added value in this indication. However, the use of piezoelectric

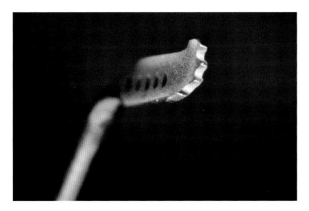

Fig 4-6 Specifically shaped piezoelectric surgical insert for selective osteotomizing around the implant. The black dots act as a depth check.

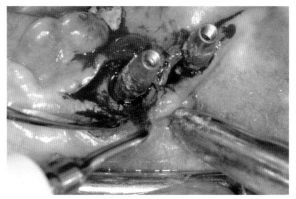

Fig 4-7 A minimal, circular osteotomy around the implant being removed is performed using special piezoelectric surgical inserts. The piezoelectric surgical instrument is kept in constant motion, and little pressure is applied to the bone.

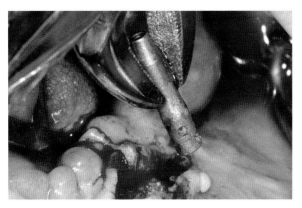

Fig 4-8 In this case, after osteotomy by piezoelectric surgery, the implant could be mobilized with a lever, then removed with diamond-coated forceps.

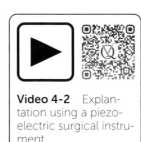

Video 4-2 Explantation using a piezoelectric surgical instrument.

surgery in implantology is greatly beneficial in explantation. Implants often cannot be explanted simply by using a special explantation kit (e.g. BTI implant explantation set, Biotechnology), which involves screwing a small self-cutting screw in a counterclockwise direction into the implant being removed, wedging it, and removing it with a ratchet. An extensive osteotomy with rotary instruments, especially a trephine drill, should be avoided because it can cause sizeable bone

defects. Especially if another implant placement is planned, the explantation should be as tissue-preserving as possible. In these cases, it is advisable to use specially designed piezoelectric surgical inserts to perform a minimally invasive osteotomy circumferentially around the implant to be removed (Figs 4-6 to 4-8, Video 4-2).

Piezoelectric surgery is also appropriate for use in bone augmentation (e.g. ridge-splitting techniques, autogenous bone blocks, sinus

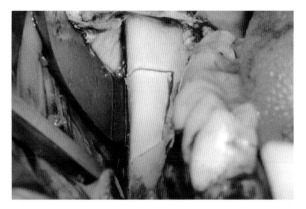

Fig 4-9 After incision and visualization of the external oblique line, the piezoelectric surgical instrument is used to cut through the cortical bone, and a defined breaking point for bone block harvesting is thereby created.

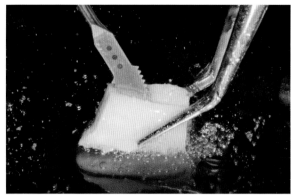

Fig 4-10 In view of the thick and very compact cortical bone, the bone block had to be additionally thinned in this case.

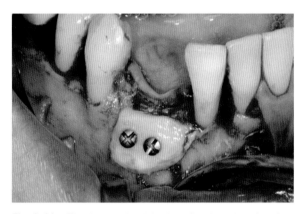

Fig 4-11 The bone block is then fixed to the alveolar bone with two osteosynthesis screws.

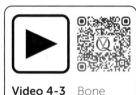

Video 4-3 Bone block harvesting at the oblique line with specially designed piezoelectric surgical inserts.

floor elevation). Especially in the ridge-splitting technique and for bone block harvesting, piezoelectric surgical instruments have helped to significantly reduce the risk of injury to adjacent anatomical structures compared with classic methods involving rotary instruments, hammer and chisel or bone saws. There are piezoelectric surgical saws specially designed for the purpose that have differently angled inserts, allowing for ease of access and a precise osteotomy (Figs 4-9 to 4-11, Video 4-3).

Piezoelectric surgical instruments are also very advantageous when performing sinus floor elevations (Figs 4-12 to 4-14, Video 4-4). A meta-analysis showed that the creation of a lateral window with the aid of a piezoelectric surgical instrument markedly reduced the risk of perforating the sinus membrane compared with an osteotomy performed solely with a rotary instrument (8% vs 24%)[2]. The basic recommendation is to create a window, first with rose burs, then with diamond burs, until the sinus membrane is

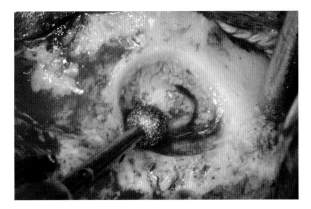

Fig 4-12 A window is first prepared with a rotary instrument (a rose bur and then a diamond bur) until only a wafer-thin bone lamella of the laterofacial maxillary sinus wall exists.

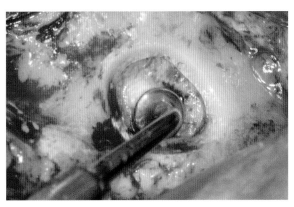

Fig 4-13 Then, the piezoelectric surgical instrument is used to break through the remaining bone lamella and the sinus membrane is carefully lifted in a circular manner.

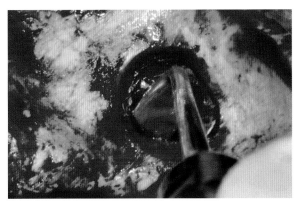

Fig 4-14 The sinus membrane is then carefully detached from the inner wall of the maxillary sinus with hand instruments. During preparation, it should be ensured that the instrument tip is in continuous contact with the bone in order to minimize the risk of perforation.

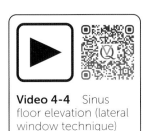

Video 4-4 Sinus floor elevation (lateral window technique) with the aid of piezoelectric surgery.

clearly visible (Fig 4-12). Only then should the membrane be gently separated from the inner wall with a piezoelectric surgical insert (e.g. "elephant foot" or diamond-coated ball). In this situation, the piezoelectric effect and the frequency matched to hard tissue are a major advantage. While the insert cuts through individual bony bridges, there is a very low risk of damaging the sinus membrane because of the specific vibration frequency (Fig 4-13). Another advantage is that the view onto the surgical site is greatly improved because of the cavitation effect and the continuous irrigation with sterile isotonic saline. As soon as the membrane has been detached in a complete circle with the piezoelectric surgical insert, preparation can continue with hand instruments (Fig 4-14).

To summarize, the key advantages of piezoelectric surgery lie in precise and minimally invasive cutting or removal of hard tissue, the low risk of injury from inadvertent contact with the surrounding soft tissue or with other anatomically

Table 4-2 Advantages and disadvantages of piezoelectric surgical instruments compared with conventional methods such as rotary instruments, hammer and chisel or bone saws.

Advantages	<ul><li>Precise and minimally invasive osteotomy</li><li>Lower risk of injury from inadvertent contact with surrounding soft tissue or with other anatomically significant neighboring structures (neurovascular bundles, sinus membrane, etc)</li><li>Less thermal necrosis affecting the bone</li><li>Almost bloodless view due to the cavitation effect</li><li>Greater safety (even difficult-to-access surgical sites can be better reached with angled and exchangeable piezoelectric surgical inserts)</li><li>Fewer postoperative complaints (pain, swelling, reduced jaw opening)</li></ul>
Disadvantages	<ul><li>Cannot be used in patients with a cardiac pacemaker</li><li>Longer operating time</li></ul>

significant neighboring structures (neurovascular bundles, sinus membrane, etc) as well as an almost bloodless view of the surgical site due to the cavitation effect of the piezoelectric surgical instrument and the additional irrigation with sterile isotonic saline (Table 4-2). However, use of a piezoelectric surgical instrument requires a substantially longer operating time.

References

1. Bailey E, Kashbour W, Shah N, Worthington HV, Renton TF, Coulthard P: Surgical techniques for the removal of mandibular wisdom teeth. Cochrane Database Syst Rev 2020;7:1–162.

2. Jordi C, Mukaddam K, Lambrecht JT, Kühl S: Membrane perforation rate in lateral maxillary sinus floor augmentation using conventional rotating instruments and piezoelectric device – a meta-analysis. Int J Implant Dent 2018;4:3.

3. Palma PJ, Marques JA, Casau M, Santos A, Caramelo F, Falacho RI, Santos JM: Evaluation of root-end preparation with two different endodontic microsurgery ultrasonic tips. Biomedicines 2020;8:383.

4. Setzer FC, Shah SB, Kohli MR, Karabucak B, Kim S: Outcome of endodontic surgery: a meta-analysis of the literature – part 1: Comparison of traditional root-end surgery and endodontic microsurgery. J Endod 2010; 36:1757–1765.

5. Schaeren S, Jaquiéry C, Heberer M, Tolnay M, Vercellotti T, Martin I: Assessment of nerve damage using a novel ultrasonic device for bone cutting. J Oral Maxillofac Surg 2008;66:593–596.

Recommended literature

Vercellotti T (ed): Essentials in Piezosurgery: Clinical Advantages in Dentistry. Mailand: Quintessence Publishing, 2009.

Vercellotti T (ed): Piezoelectric Bone Surgery: A New Paradigme. Batavia: Quintessence Publishing, 2020.

Cone beam computed tomography

Dorothea Dagassan-Berndt

5

Cone beam computed tomography (CBCT) has revolutionized dental radiology due to the fascination with three-dimensionality. The technology is capable of visualizing the whole head or parts thereof in all three planes with a single coordinated rotation of the x-ray tube and the sensor[1,11]. In the process, the volume recorded can be oriented in any chosen plane. The curved shape of the jawbones and the number of complex, widely varied anatomical structures that occur close together in the head make this feature essential for an appropriate diagnosis[10]. For this reason, CBCT is being increasingly used in dentistry. Surprisingly, the number of manufacturers is also still increasing, whereas there are only a small number of major manufacturers of CT devices[6].

CBCT technology was introduced into dentistry around 25 years ago, with three different devices. These three devices differed in terms of the size of the field of view (FoV)[1,11].

Nowadays, most devices offer different FoV sizes, which makes the use of CBCT very versatile. The indication for a CBCT scan is critical to the choice of FoV and other important parameters. Several professional bodies at the national and international level have drawn up scientific guidelines on indications for CBCT use[3-5,14,15]. Within dentistry, oral surgery generates the most frequent applications of CBCT[2]. It is very important to precisely establish the indication for the use of CBCT in oral surgery, and to guarantee that the technology is implemented with due regard to radiation safety aspects.

The imaging techniques of dental radiology operate within a low-dose range. Among all the imaging methods used in dentistry, CBCT is associated with the highest dose. The range of possible doses applied is very wide, and its maximal levels may extend to the medium-dose range[9,16]. It is hence all the more important to follow the ALARA principle (*As Low As Reasonably Achievable*), established in 1977[13]. Thus, national legislation in the area of radiation protection stipulates that ionizing rays must be used in accordance with the latest technologic standards and regulations.

This section outlines and explains the most important setting options and parameters of CBCT devices. Other aspects covered are the way the dose is delivered to the patient and how the dose can be reduced.

Region of interest

When three-dimensional (3D) imaging is indicated, the area requiring 3D visualization needs to be identified on the basis of the case history and clinical findings. It is therefore important to formulate a suspected diagnosis together with associated differential diagnoses in order to define the area that needs to be scanned. This is known as the region of interest (RoI). The necessary quality and hence the selected parameters of a CBCT scan will depend on the suspected and differential diagnoses.

Field of view

The above-mentioned RoI is then translated into the scan volume provided by CBCT devices, known as the FoV. This is the area that will be scanned. Scan volume is categorized as small, medium, and large (Figs 5-1 to 5-3). Small volumes depict individual teeth with their neighboring structures and are between approximately 4 × 4 cm and 6 × 6 cm in size (Fig 5-1). Medium volumes can visualize the entire maxilla or mandible with adjacent anatomical structures (e.g. the maxillary sinus) or segments with their surrounding tissue, with or without the temporomandibular joint (Fig 5-2). Large volumes scan both the maxilla and mandible with a large proportion of relevant neighboring anatomical structures (Fig 5-3).

CBCT technology makes it possible to use various shutter systems to limit small volumes in all three planes and hence reduce the dose applied to the patient. Choosing the smallest possible FoV is hence an important measure in terms of individual radiation protection. Since most CBCT scan volumes are cylindrical, the FoV is given in terms of the equivalent diameter and height of the cylinder.

Voxel

Voxel is a word coined from *volumetric* and *pixel* and describes the smallest possible 3D cube of a scan volume. It is hence the 3D equivalent of a pixel. In CBCT, the voxels are isotropic. This means that a "sharp" image can be obtained in all three planes. In addition, the volume can be individually oriented, depending on what is being scanned, while achieving the same image quality. The size of voxels is given as the edge length in mm or μm.

Milliampere

Milliampere (mA) is the strength of current and correlates with the number of electrons at the cathode. This number correlates directly with the effective dose delivered to the patient.

Kilovolt

Kilovolt (kV) is the voltage that is applied between cathode and anode when the x-rays are generated and determines the penetration capacity of the x-rays and hence the level of contrast.

Scan mode

Most CBCT units offer different scan modes that dictate the number of images, the scanning time or the voxel size selected (e.g. low-dose, standard, high-resolution, high-definition, high-fidelity). This setting also has a direct influence on the effective dose delivered to the patient and should be selected according to the indication for a CBCT scan. The higher the resolution, the more images per roatation. The longer the scanning time, the higher the effective dose delivered to the patient.

The above points have an effect on the image quality of a CBCT scan. Other parameters influencing scan quality are the sensor used, reconstruction algorithms, filters, orbits, and patient compliance. These different parameters give rise to a wide variety of CBCT devices, and it is often too complex for the technology to be understood in its entirety. Ultimately, it is important to utilize the available features of a CBCT device to suit the situation of the individual patient.

Patients

Oral surgery patients vary in age from infants to the elderly and present with a wide range of issues (see Section 1). Once again, it is essential to observe the principles of radiation protection. Particularly when using CBCT on children, specific principles of radiation protection and scanning protocols must be followed[8].

Applications

General rules about the settings for the most common indications for CBCT scans covered in this book are discussed below. Generally, a distinction is made between two distinct indications for CBCT investigations in oral surgery.

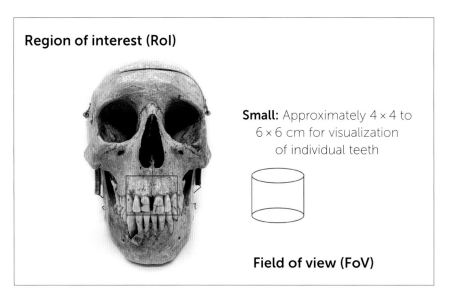

Region of interest (RoI)

Small: Approximately 4 × 4 to 6 × 6 cm for visualization of individual teeth

Field of view (FoV)

Fig 5-1   Small field of view (FoV) in dentistry/oral surgery for visualization of individual teeth and their surrounding tissue.

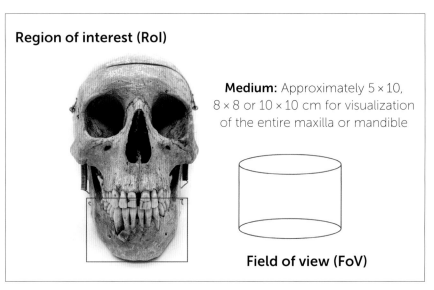

Region of interest (RoI)

Medium: Approximately 5 × 10, 8 × 8 or 10 × 10 cm for visualization of the entire maxilla or mandible

Field of view (FoV)

Fig 5-2   Medium FoV in dentistry/oral surgery for visualization of the entire maxilla or mandible or segments and their surrounding tissue.

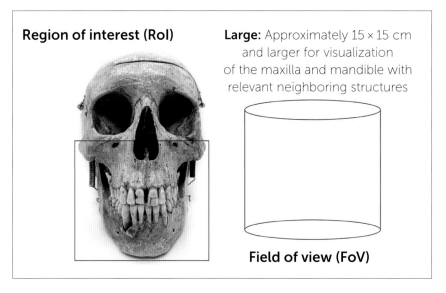

Region of interest (RoI)

Large: Approximately 15 × 15 cm and larger for visualization of the maxilla and mandible with relevant neighboring structures

Field of view (FoV)

Fig 5-3   Large FoV in dentistry/oral surgery for visualization of the maxilla and mandible with relevant neighboring structures.

Anatomical visualization for orientation at the surgical site

This classically includes visualization of impacted and displaced teeth, especially third molars, and their location in relation to neighboring anatomical structures. These cases involve the visualization of relatively large anatomical structures such as teeth, alveolar bone, the mandibular canal or the bordering bony structures of the maxillary sinus or paranasal sinuses. This category also covers the visualization of bone for planning implants or osseous anchorage. These structures are several millimeters or even centimeters in size and hence do not require scanning at maximal resolution. Standard or low-dose settings are entirely adequate for this purpose, as is the use of larger voxels and the reduction of the scan rotation (e.g. 180 instead of 360 degrees). As previously mentioned, especially in cases involving children, all the necessary measures must be taken to reduce radiation exposure.

Visualization of pathologic structures for diagnosis and assessment of treatment extent

The visualization of pathologic structures and their investigation involves establishing their localization and obtaining a detailed picture of the structure. The smallest changes in radiopacity, the internal structure and composition, and the precise visualization of neighboring structures will provide information about pathologic processes. This will make it possible to match a pathologic structure to a diagnosis.

Furthermore, the extent and involvement of neighboring structures (resorptions, infiltrations, etc) will dictate the appropriate treatment. For this reason, good to very good image quality is absolutely essential, which in all cases correlates with a higher dose. Therefore, it is very important to choose the smallest FoV possible in order to justify the increased dose in terms of optimal image quality.

CBCT scans are not usually indicated for soft tissue surgery because the technology only depicts hard tissue. In addition, CBCT does not include Houndsfield units, which would allow differentiation of the different types of tissue. One of the few indications for the use of CBCT in soft tissue is for localizing foreign bodies.

Identification of infections due to hard tissue changes can sometimes be challenging. For instance, inflammatory reactions are visible after 3 weeks at the earliest. In a few cases, if a diagnosis could not be made in the acute phase of the inflammation, and the required treatment could not be implemented, CBCT can be used at a later stage in the treatment[7].

To summarize, a detailed general medical history, a specific history, and a precise record of clinical dental findings are required to decide whether CBCT is indicated and to justify its use. The volume and parameters chosen should ensure that CBCT is performed according to the ALADAIP principle (As Low as Diagnostically Acceptable, being Indication-oriented and Patient-specific)[12]. For the broad range of oral surgery procedures, CBCT thus offers excellent support in selected cases.

5   Cone beam computed tomography

References

1.   Arai Y, Tammisalo E, Iwai K, Hashimoto K, Shinoda K: Development of a compact computed tomographic apparatus for dental use. Dentomaxillofac Radiol 1999;28:245–248.

2.   Carter JB, Stone JD, Clark RS, Mercer JE: Applications of cone-beam computed tomography in oral and maxillofacial surgery: an overview of published indications and clinical usage in United States academic centers and oral and maxillofacial surgery practices. J Oral Maxillofac Surg 2016;74:668–679.

3.   Carter L, Farman AG, Geist J, Scare WC, Angelopoulos C, Nair M, Hildebolt CF, Tyndall D, Shrout M: American Academy of Oral and Maxillofacial Radiology executive opinion statement on performing and interpreting diagnostic cone beam computed tomography. Oral Surg Oral Med Oral Pathol Oral Radiol 2008;106:561–562.

4.   Dula K, Bornstein MM, Buser D, Dagassan-Berndt D, Ettlin DA, Filippi A, Gabioud F, Katsaros C, Krastl G, Lambrecht JT, Lauber R, Lübbers HAT, Pazera P, Türp JC: SADMFR Guidelines for the use of cone-beam computed tomography / digital volume tomography. Swiss Dent J 2014;124:1170–1183.

5.   Dula K, Benic GI, Bornstein MM, Dagassan-Berndt D, Filippi A, Hicklin S, Kissling-Jeger F, Lübbers HT, Sculean A, Sequeira-Byron P, Walter C, Zehnder M: SADMFR Guidelines for the use of cone-beam computed tomography / digital volume tomography – Endodontics, Periodontology, Reconstructive Dentistry, Pediatric Dentistry. Swiss Dent J 2015;125: 945–953.

6.   Gaeta-Araujo H, Alzoubi T, Vasconcelos KF, Orhan K, Pauwels R, Casselman JW, Jacobs R: Cone beam computed tomography in dento-maxillofacial radiology: a two-decade overview. Dentomaxillofac Radiol 2020;29:20200145.

7.   Gander T, Dagassan-Berndt D, Mascolo L, Kruse AL, Grätz KW, Lübbers HAT: Gesichtsschmerzen – eine seltene Ursache. Retinierte untere Weisheitszähne als Ursache für zunächst «unklare» Gesichtsschmerzen. Ein Fallbericht. Schweiz Monatsschr Zahnmed 2013;123: 767–777.

8.   Kühnisch J, Anttonen V, Duggal MS, Loizides Sypridonos M, Rajasekharan S, Sobczak M, Stratigaki E, VanAcker JWG, Aps JKM, Horner K, Tsiklakis K: Best clinical practice guidance for prescribing dental radiography in children and adolescents: an EAPD policy document. Eur Arch Paediatr Dent 2020;21:375–386.

9.   Ludlow JE, Timothy R, Walker C, Hunter R, Benavides E, Samuelson DB, Scheske MJ: Effective dose of dental CBCT – a meta-analysis of published data and additional data for nine CBCT units. Dentomaxillofac Radiol 2015;44:20140197.

10.   Lübbers HT, Matthews F, Damerau G, Kruse AL, Obwegeser JA, Grätz KW, Eyrich GK: No plane is the best one – the volume is! Oral Surg Oral Med Oral Pathol Oral Radiol 2012;113:421.

11.   Mozzo P, Procacci C, Tacconi A, Martini PT, Andreis IA: A new volumetric CT machine for dental imaging based on the cone-beam technique: preliminary results. Eur Radiol 1998;8:1558–1564.

12.   Oenning AC, Jacobs R, Pauwels R, Stratis A, Hedesiu M, Salmon B, Dimitra Research Group Cone-beam CT in paediatric dentistry: DIMITRA project position statement. Pediatr Radiol 2018;48:308–316.

13.   Recommendation of the International Commission on Radiological Protection ICRP Publication 26. Oxford: Pergamon Press, 1977.

14.   Sedentexct Radiation Protection 172: Cone Beam CT for Dental and Maxillofacial Radiology – evidence-based guidelines. Publ Eur Communities 2012:156.

15.   Schulze R et al.: S2K-Leitlinie Dentale digitale Volumentomographie. https://www.awmf.org/uploads/tx_szleitlinien/083-005l_S2k_Dentale_Volumentomographie_2013-10-abgelaufen.pdf

16.   Schulze R: Strahlendosis bei der röntgenologischen Bildgebung für implantologische Fragestellungen im Vergleich: Intraoral-, Panorama-schichtaufnahme, DVT und CT. Implantologie 2009;17:377–386.

Alveolar stabilization

6

Michael Payer, Ronald E. Jung

Atrophy of the surrounding alveolar bone will occur after tooth extraction as well as after structural and morphologic soft tissue changes[27]. The resulting three-dimensional loss of volume can cause esthetic limitations during implant-prosthetic rehabilitation and therefore necessitates regeneration of the hard and soft tissue.

As part of the periodontium, the alveolar process surrounds the erupted tooth and contains lamellar bone, known as bundle bone, in the inner portion of the socket[4]. Bundle bone usually has a layer thickness of approximately 0.2 to 0.4 mm, and, just like cementum, its existence is strongly tooth-bound[26].

In the anterior maxilla, the average thickness of the buccal bone lamella is likely to be < 1 mm. A study by Januario et al found a maximum layer thickness of 0.5 mm in 50% of the sites in the anterior maxilla measured by CBCT[14]. This means the buccal bone lamella and the bundle bone in the esthetic zone have roughly the same dimension, and after tooth extraction, significant remodeling and resorption processes are to be expected[16]. Generally, but especially in the esthetic zone with a view to tissue preservation, it is imperative for tooth extraction to be as tissue preserving and atraumatic as possible (Figs 6-1 to 6-4)[17,23].

Hence, before tooth extraction, the clinician should already have a clear idea of further therapeutic measures, including alveolar treatment. A distinction is usually made between three different therapeutic approaches:

- Spontaneous healing of the extraction socket,
- Immediate implant placement,
- Techniques for preservation of hard and soft tissue:
  - Socket preservation for fully preserved extraction sockets or four-walled sockets,
  - Ridge preservation for sockets with deficient bone walls or defects affecting three or four walls.

This section examines decision making about which measures seem expedient for which patients based on the available evidence-based data.

Spontaneous healing

A systematic literature analysis of 20 human studies showed that hard and soft tissue resorption processes of approximately 11% to 22% (-1.24 ± 0.11 mm) in the vertical direction and 29% to 63% (-3.79 ± 0.23 mm) in the horizontal direction are to be expected within the first 6 to 7 months after tooth extraction[28]. Thereafter, additional dimensional loss of around 0.5% to 1% per year occurs. To summarize, based on the clinical trials evaluated, it was found that dimensional loss of the alveolar ridge of up to 50% can be expected after spontaneous healing of single-tooth extraction sockets, with bone resorption mainly taking place in the buccal direction[15] (Fig 6-5). Furthermore, quantitative analyses showed that > 1-mm residual bone thickness of a socket leads to less horizontal resorption than thinner bone thicknesses[6].

Immediate implant placement

Immediate implant placement can be performed using a flap or flapless technique, with or without additional tissue regeneration measures. The tissue changes following immediate implant placement have been examined in clinical trials. For example, after immediate implant placement with a flap and without augmentation measures in 18 patients/21 teeth, Botticelli et al observed resorption processes of 56% in the buccal and 30% in the lingual direction after 4 months[8]. These remodeling processes after immediate implant placement were confirmed in several other studies[1-3,11,20,24].

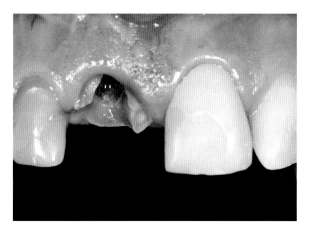
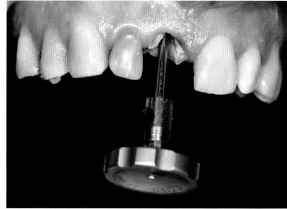
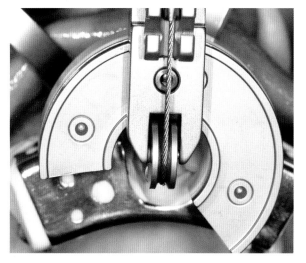
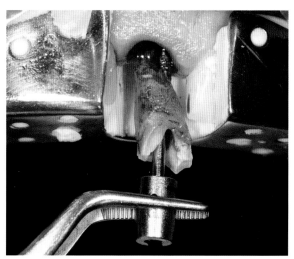

Figs 6-1 to 6-4 Tissue-preserving tooth extraction using the Benex Extraction System (Helmut Zepf Medizintechnik and Hager & Meisinger).

The results with immediate implant placement combined with simultaneous augmentation measures have also been examined in clinical trials. In a randomized, controlled clinical trial by Chen et al, patients were subdivided into three groups: 10 patients received immediate implant placement without further bone build-up, 10 patients underwent simultaneous guided bone regeneration (GBR) with bovine hydroxyapatite, and 10 patients received GBR with bovine hydroxyapatite and a collagen membrane[10]. At the 4-year follow-up, horizontal resorption of 48.3% was observed in the group without GBR, whereas there was significantly less resorption in

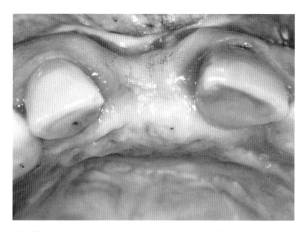

Fig 6-5 Extensive loss of dimension of the alveolar ridge, mainly in the buccal direction (6 months after extraction of the maxillary right central incisor and spontaneous healing).

the other two groups with GBR: 15.8% horizontal resorption in the group with bovine hydroxyapatite, and 20% resorption in the group that received bovine hydroxyapatite and a collagen membrane.

The following can therefore be said about immediate implant placement: Implants placed immediately after tooth extraction cannot prevent resorption processes in the area of the extraction socket. These seem to take place to a similar extent as in untreated postextraction sockets. Simultaneously performed GBR measures with and without a collagen membrane very probably result in a significant reduction of resorption processes in the horizontal direction after tooth extraction[16].

Alveolar stabilization options

Various techniques and materials aimed at preserving hard and/or soft tissue or the alveolar contour after tooth extraction is the subject of many scientific studies.

Generally, the following options for alveolar stabilization are described in the literature: autogenous soft and hard tissue augmentation materials, the use of a combination of biomaterials for hard and soft tissue augmentation, and lastly, the use of autologous blood products (e.g. platelet-rich fibrin [PRF]) or cellular therapeutic approaches[22]. The purpose of these techniques is to limit the resorption processes and to stimulate hard and soft tissue healing so that dental implants can subsequently be inserted in prosthetically correct positions without further augmentation measures[19]. From the clinical perspective, the decision to carry out socket-preserving measures is dependent on the following factors:

■ Planned implant placement timing,
■ Quantity and quality of the soft tissue available in the area of the extraction socket,

■ Anticipated implant survival and success rate.

From the patient's point of view, immediate implant placement is obviously the ideal approach; in practice, however, this technique is frequently limited by hard or soft tissue deficits.

The following healing times after ridge preservation measures are described in the literature[9]:
■ Optimization of soft tissue (6- to 8-week healing phase after tooth extraction),
■ Optimization of hard and soft tissue (4- to 6-month healing phase),
■ Optimization of hard tissue (healing phase of > 6 months).

Preservation of soft tissue

In terms of materials, subepithelial connective tissue grafts harvested from the palatal area, free mucosal grafts or substitute materials, and resorbable membranes are available to support wound healing and wound closure[25]. These techniques are generally performed with minimal coronal flap advancement or without flap formation in the so-called flapless technique in order to preserve or harvest keratinized mucosa[7]. The scientific evidence regarding these techniques is heterogenous and includes preclinical as well as clinical studies[16].

Preservation of hard and soft tissue

Deficits of hard and soft tissue can be observed in many patients following tooth extraction. In these cases, clinical procedures known as socket seal combination techniques seem expedient for preserving hard and soft tissue, with healing times of 4 to 6 months (Videos 6-1 and 6-2). This involves filling the socket with biomaterials to replace the bone, and sealing with an autogenous soft tissue graft or a soft tissue substitute[21]. Clinical trials showed that this technique, using xenogeneic bone substitute materials in combination with free mucosal grafts from the palate, known as mucosal patches, as well as with collagen matrices as a soft tissue substitute, demonstrated less resorption after a healing period of 4 to 6 months than control groups with spontaneous healing or bone substitute material without sealing. Both horizontal and vertical resorption processes were minimal and enabled dental implants to be inserted with high implant survival rates after 12 months[16]. It was shown histologically that bone substitute materials do slow down healing but clearly contribute significantly to minimal postextraction loss of volume[18]. It was additionally demonstrated that soft tissue substitutes in the form of collagen matrices can be used successfully for socket sealing and thus help to simplify the technique and reduce morbidity[21].

As previously mentioned, the healing phase for soft tissue-preserving measures is roughly 6 to 8 weeks. Only minimal new bone formation, but complete soft tissue sealing of the extraction socket, is likely during this period[13,18]. Biomaterials to fill the socket are primarily intended to maintain the position of autogenous grafts or biomaterials that are placed at the soft tissue level. It is difficult to compare the different techniques because of the above-mentioned heterogeneity of the studies. Soft tissue substitute materials do appear to reduce postoperative morbidity; however, due to the lack of evidence to date, the use of autogenous soft tissue grafts continues to be regarded as the gold standard in alveolar stabilization at the soft tissue level after tooth extraction[29,30].

The results of another systematic literature analysis also confirm that socket preservation measures reduce horizontal bone resorption by 1.99 mm on average (95% confidence interval [CI]: 1.54 to 2.44; $P < 0.001$), vertical buccal resorption by 1.72 mm (95% CI: 0.96 to 2.48; $P < 0.001$), and vertical lingual resorption by 1.16 mm (95% CI: 0.81 to 1.52; $P < 0.001$)

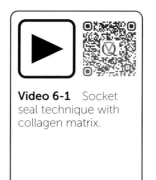

Video 6-1 Socket seal technique with collagen matrix.

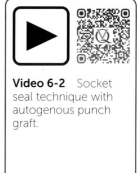

Video 6-2 Socket seal technique with autogenous punch graft.

compared with tooth extraction alone. The following techniques were compared:

- Bovine bone particles + socket seal,
- Constructs, consisting of 90% bovine bone particles and 10% porcine collagen,
- Porcine corticocancellous bone particles + socket seal,
- Allograft particles + socket seal,
- Alloplastic materials with or without socket seal,
- Autologous blood products,
- Cell therapies,
- Recombinant human bone morphogenetic protein-2 (rhBMP-2),
- Socket seal alone.

This literature analysis did not resolve whether any of the ridge preservation techniques employed was superior. Nevertheless, particulate xenogeneic or allogeneic hydroxyapatite substitute materials, covered with a resorbable collagen membrane or a collagen sponge, showed the most promising results with regard to horizontal volume preservation[6]. Furthermore, another literature review and meta-analysis revealed an additional horizontal bone loss of 2.37 mm ($P > 0.001$) in the horizontal direction and 1.10 mm in the vertical direction in spontaneously healing sockets with a buccal bone defect compared with extraction sockets in which ridge preservation measures were performed[12].

As regards cellular therapeutic approaches, their complexity, invasiveness, and not least their cost should be borne in mind, given that their clinical advantage over other techniques is still uncertain[22].

Chairside methods for producing autologous blood products such as PRF for single use or in combination with substitute materials seem more feasible. However, the literature still does not demonstrate the advantage of these methods over other techniques[5].

Preservation of hard tissue

In cases of significant bone loss of more than 50% of the buccal bone lamella, surgical techniques to preserve hard tissue with longer healing times have been described in the literature. These mainly use bone substitute materials and collagen membranes and involve flap formation with partial or complete wound closure. There are also reports in the literature of the application of bone substitutes followed by complete wound closure by means of coronal flap advancement or rotation flap or the use of bone substitutes without wound closure. However, a systematic literature analysis found the least evidence for the latter technique[31].

Meta-analyses did in fact show significantly lower vertical and horizontal resorption rates for ridge preservation techniques versus control groups[16]. Furthermore, Mardas et al showed in a systematic literature analysis that, as a result of alveolar preservation techniques employed, the need for further augmentation measures at the time of implant placement was significantly lower (0% to 15%) than for spontaneously healing sockets (0% to 100%)[19].

Despite the many clear advantages of socket preservation techniques in terms of lower vertical and horizontal soft and hard tissue resorption rates and hence a reduced need for augmentation at the time of implant placement, the advantages of these techniques with regard to implant survival and implant success rates cannot be clearly concluded from the literature[19]. In addition, none of the quoted clinical trials and meta-analyses revealed any advantages of ridge preservation techniques over control groups with respect to the feasibility of implant placement. It should nevertheless be remembered that feasibility alone should not be the decisive factor in the evaluation, but instead it should be the possibility of placing the implant in the prosthetically correct position[16].

To summarize, with respect to preservation of hard tissue volume, it can therefore be stated that the available data from the literature support alveolar preservation measures at the time of tooth extraction in daily practice. In addition, at the level of implant-related parameters, no other clinical advantages can be deduced for the above-mentioned measures, which are usually associated with flap formation and healing phases of more than 6 months.

Clinical decision making

Especially in the esthetic zone, whether alveolar preservation should be carried out and which measures to utilize should be considered prior to tooth extraction. Jung et al presented the following decision-making concept[16]:

- If implant placement is possible within 0 to 2 months postextraction, measures for socket preservation are not indicated,
- If soft tissue optimization is not required, the socket should be left to heal spontaneously, and the implant should be placed 6 to 8 weeks after extraction (type 2 or

delayed immediate implant placement) or at the time of tooth extraction (type 1 or immediate implant placement)[9] (Figs 6-6 to 6-13),

- In the case of a soft tissue deficit, a soft tissue preservation measure should be taken, usually involving the use of autogenous soft tissue grafts and bone substitute materials (Figs 6-14 to 6-33),
- If implant placement is not possible within 2 months after extraction, alveolar preservation techniques should be carried out,

- If less than 50% of buccal bone is missing, a flapless technique using slowly resorbable bone substitute and autogenous soft tissue graft materials or collagen matrices should be used (Figs 6-34 to 6-43),
- If more than 50% of buccal bone is missing, ample data are available on the use of techniques of GBR involving flap formation[16] (Figs 6-44 to 6-56).

6 Alveolar stabilization

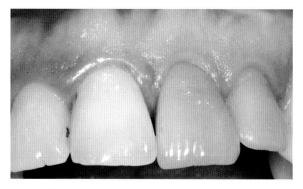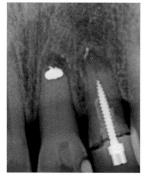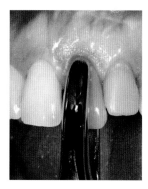

Figs 6-6 to 6-8 Extraction of the maxillary left central and lateral incisors due to root fracture following trauma.

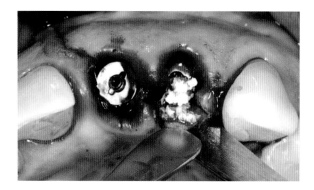

Fig 6-9 Immediate implant placement with simultaneous augmentation with hydroxyapatite.

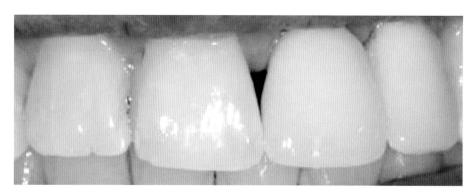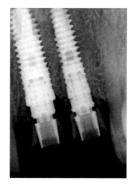

Figs 6-10 and 6-11 Provisional immediate restoration.

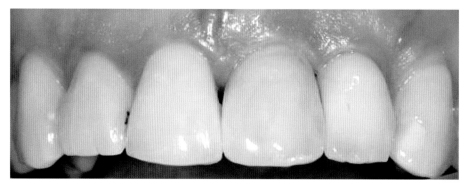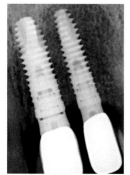

Figs 6-12 and 6-13 Clinical and radiographic situation 8 years after implant placement.

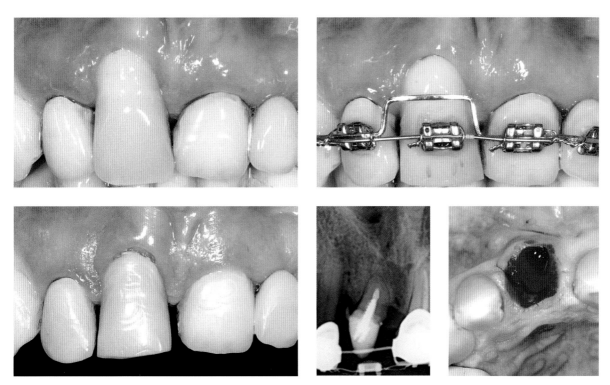

Figs 6-14 to 6-18 Orthodontic extrusion and extraction of the maxillary right central incisor with buccal recession (Miller Class I).

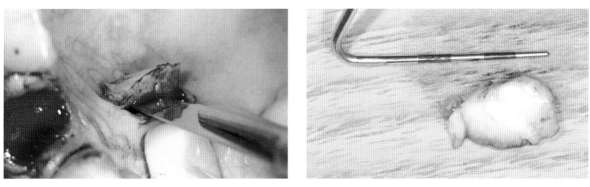

Figs 6-19 and 6-20 Harvesting of an autogenous mucosal graft from the palate.

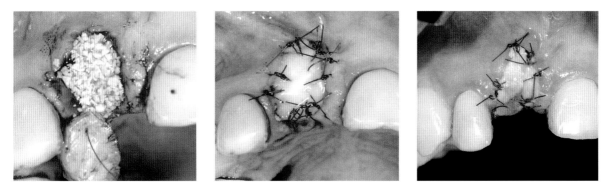

Figs 6-21 to 6-23 Flapless ridge preservation technique using a slowly resorbable bone substitute and socket seal with an autogenous mucosal graft.

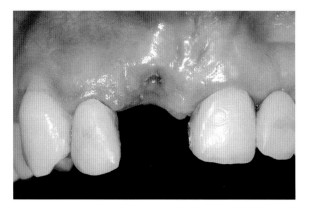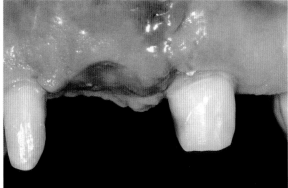

Figs 6-24 and 6-25 Clinical situation 3 and 6 months after tooth extraction.

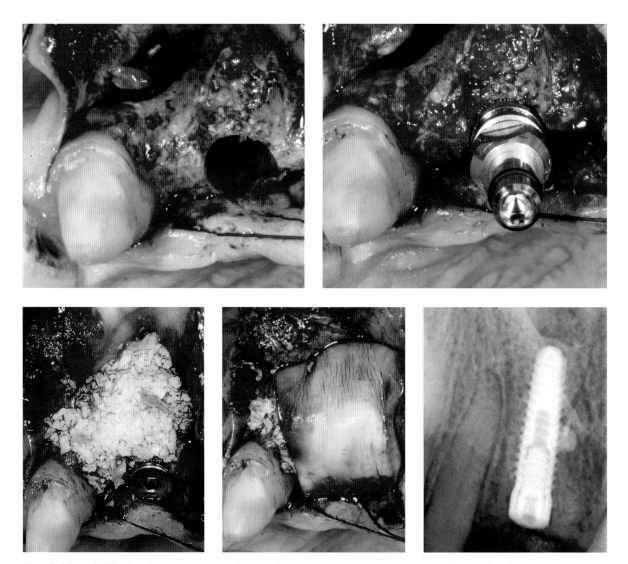

Figs 6-26 to 6-30 Implant placement with simultaneous contour augmentation 6 months after tooth extraction.

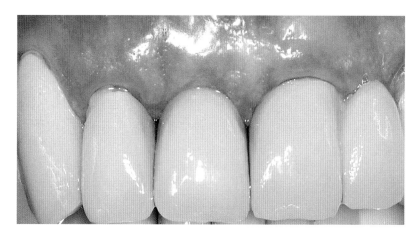

Fig 6-31 Provisional crown restoration 3 months after implant placement.

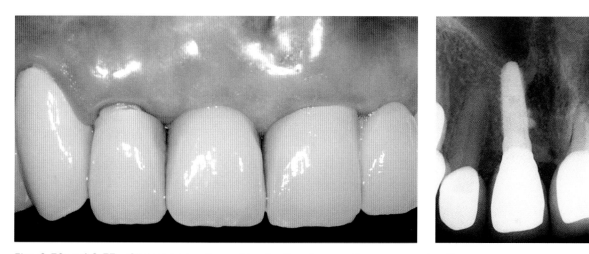

Figs 6-32 and 6-33 Clinical and radiographic situation 5 years after crown restoration.

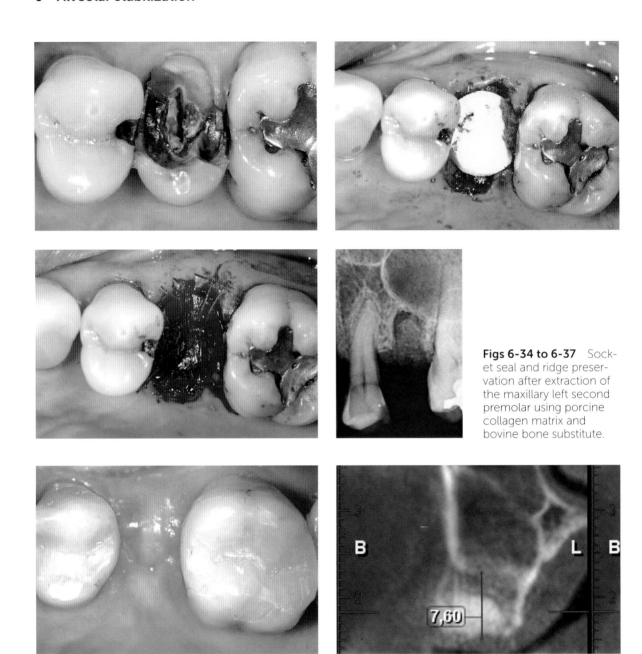

Figs 6-34 to 6-37 Socket seal and ridge preservation after extraction of the maxillary left second premolar using porcine collagen matrix and bovine bone substitute.

Figs 6-38 and 6-39 Clinical situation and radiographic measurement 6 months after tooth extraction.

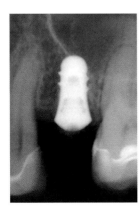

Fig 6-40 Radiographic situation after implant placement.

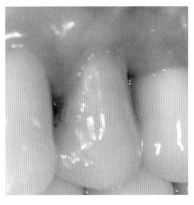 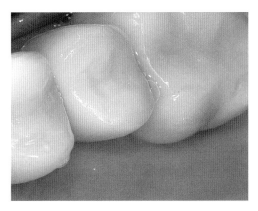 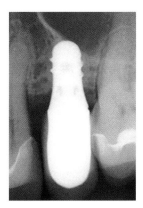

Figs 6-41 to 6-43 Prosthetic restoration 3 years after implant placement.

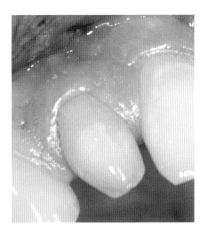 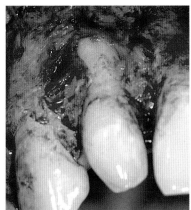 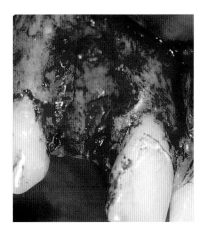

Figs 6-44 to 6-46 Extraction of the maxillary right lateral incisor due to root fracture following trauma.

Figs 6-47 and 6-48 Guided bone regeneration (GBR) with a flap due to loss of > 50% of buccal bone in the course of tooth extraction.

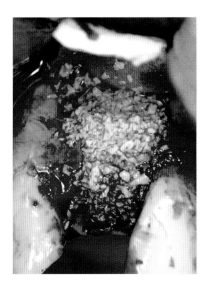 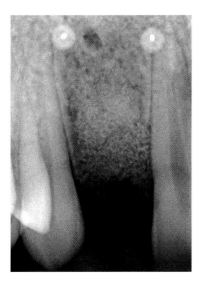

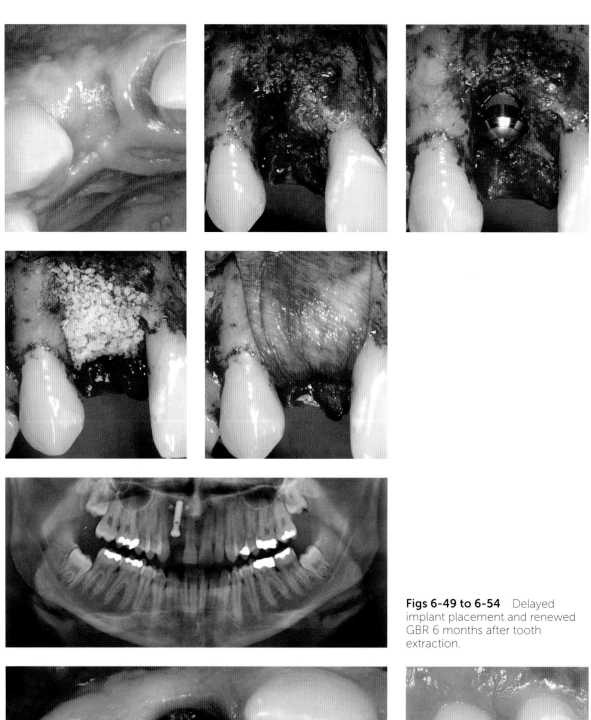

Figs 6-49 to 6-54 Delayed implant placement and renewed GBR 6 months after tooth extraction.

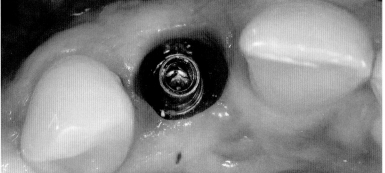

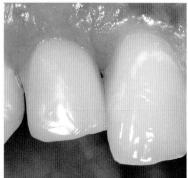

Figs 6-55 and 6-56 Prosthetic restoration 3 months after implant placement.

References

1. Araujo MG, Sukekava F, Wennstrom JL, Lindhe J: Ridge alterations following implant placement in fresh extraction sockets: an experimental study in the dog. J Clin Periodontol 2005;32:645–652.

2. Araujo MG, Sukekava F, Wennstrom JL, Lindhe J: Tissue modeling following implant placement in fresh extraction sockets. Clin Oral Implants Res 2006;17:615–624.

3. Araujo MG, Wennstrom JL, Lindhe J: Modeling of the buccal and lingual bone walls of fresh extraction sites following implant installation. Clin Oral Implants Res 2006;17:606–614.

4. Araujo MG, Silva CO, Misawa M, Sukekava F: Alveolar socket healing: what can we learn? Periodontol 2000 2015;68:122–134.

5. Areewong K, Chantaramungkorn M, Khongkhunthian P: Platelet-rich fibrin to preserve alveolar bone sockets following tooth extraction: A randomized controlled trial. Clin Implant Dent Relat Res 2019;21:1156–1163.

6. Avila-Ortiz G, Chambrone L, Vignoletti F: Effect of alveolar ridge preservation interventions following tooth extraction: A systematic review and meta-analysis. J Clin Periodontol 2019;46(Suppl 21):195–223.

7. Barone A, Borgia V, Covani U, Ricci M, Piattelli A, Iezzi G: Flap versus flapless procedure for ridge preservation in alveolar extraction sockets: a histological evaluation in a randomized clinical trial. Clin Oral Implants Res 2015;26:806–813.

8. Botticelli D, Berglundh T, Lindhe J: Hard-tissue alterations following immediate implant placement in extraction sites. J Clin Periodontol 2004;31:820–828.

9. Chen ST, Wilson TG Jr, Hammerle CH: Immediate or early placement of implants following tooth extraction: review of biologic basis, clinical procedures, and outcomes. Int J Oral Maxillofac Implants 2004;19(Suppl):12–25.

10. Chen ST, Darby IB, Reynolds EC: A prospective clinical study of non-submerged immediate implants: clinical outcomes and esthetic results. Clin Oral Implants Res 2007;18:552–562.

11. Ferrus J, Cecchinato D, Pjetursson EB, Lang NP, Sanz M, Lindhe J: Factors influencing ridge alterations following immediate implant placement into extraction sockets. Clin Oral Implants Res 2010;21:22–29.

12. García-González S, Galve-Huertas A, Aboul-Hosn Centenero S, Mareque-Bueno S, Satorres-Nieto M, Hernández-Alfaro F: Volumetric changes in alveolar ridge preservation with a compromised buccal wall: a systematic review and meta-analysis. Med Oral Patol Oral Cir Bucal 2020;25:e565–e575.

13. Jambhekar S, Kernen F, Bidra AS: Clinical and histologic outcomes of socket grafting after flapless tooth extraction: a systematic review of randomized controlled clinical trials. J Prosthet Dent 2015;113:371–382.

14. Januario AL, Duarte WR, Barriviera M, Mesti JC, Araujo MG, Lindhe J: Dimension of the facial bone wall in the anterior maxilla: a cone-beam computed tomography study. Clin Oral Implants Res 2011;22:1168–1171.

15. Jung RE, Philipp A, Annen BM, Signorelli L, Thoma DS, Hammerle CH, Attin T, Schmidlin P: Radiographic evaluation of different techniques for ridge preservation after tooth extraction: a randomized controlled clinical trial. J Clin Periodontol 2013;40:90–98.

16. Jung RE, Ioannidis A, Hämmerle CHF, Thoma DS: Alveolar ridge preservation in the esthetic zone. Periodontology 2000 2018;77:165–175.

17. Leblebicioglu B, Hegde R, Yildiz VO, Tatakis DN: Immediate effects of tooth extraction on ridge integrity and dimensions. Clin Oral Investig 2015;19:1777–1784.

18. Lindhe J, Cecchinato D, Donati M, Tomasi C, Liljenberg B: Ridge preservation with the use of deproteinized bovine bone mineral. Clin Oral Implants Res 2014;25:786–790.

19. Mardas N, Trullenque-Eriksson A, MacBeth N, Petrie A, Donos N: Does ridge preservation following tooth extraction improve implant treatment outcomes: a systematic review: Group 4: Therapeutic concepts & methods. Clin Oral Implants Res 2015;26(Suppl 11):180–201.

20. Matarasso S, Salvi GE, Iorio Siciliano V, Cafiero C, Blasi A, Lang NP: Dimensional ridge alterations following immediate implant placement in molar extraction sites: a six month prospective cohort study with surgical re-entry. Clin Oral Implants Res 2009;20:1092–1098.

21. Meloni SM, Tallarico M, Lolli FM, Deledda A, Pisano M, Jovanovic SA: Postextraction socket preservation using epithelial connective tissue graft vs porcine collagen matrix. 1-year results of a randomised controlled trial. Eur J Oral Implantol 2015;8:39–48.

22.   Moreno Sancho F, Leira Y, Orlandi M, Buti J, Giannobile WV, D'Aiuto F: Cell-based therapies for alveolar bone and periodontal regeneration: concise review. Stem Cells Transl Med 2019;8:1286–1295.

23.   Oghli AA, Steveling H: Ridge preservation following tooth extraction: a comparison between atraumatic extraction and socket seal surgery. Quintessence Int 2010;41:605–609.

24.   Sanz M, Cecchinato D, Ferrus J, Pjetursson EB, Lang NP, Lindhe J: A prospective, randomized-controlled clinical trial to evaluate bone preservation using implants with different geometry placed into extraction sockets in the maxilla. Clin Oral Implants Res 2010;21:13–21.

25.   Sisti A, Canullo L, Mottola MP, Covani U, Barone A, Botticelli D: Clinical evaluation of a ridge augmentation procedure for the severely resorbed alveolar socket: multicenter randomized controlled trial, preliminary results. Clin Oral Implants Res 2012;23:526–535.

26.   Schroeder HE. The Periodontium. Berlin, Heidelberg: Springer, 1986.

27.   Schropp L, Wenzel A, Kostopoulos L, Karring T: Bone healing and soft tissue contour changes following single-tooth extraction: a clinical and radiographic 12-month prospective study. Int J Periodontics Restorative Dent 2003;23: 313–323.

28.   Tan WL, Wong TL, Wong MC, Lang NP: A systematic review of post-extractional alveolar hard and soft tissue dimensional changes in humans. Clin Oral Implants Res 2012;23(Suppl 5):1–21.

29.   Thoma DS, Sancho-Puchades M, Ettlin DA, Hammerle CH, Jung RE: Impact of a collagen matrix on early healing, aesthetics and patient morbidity in oral mucosal wounds – a randomized study in humans. J Clin Periodontol 2012;39:157–165.

30.   Thoma DS, Buranawat B, Hammerle CH, Held U, Jung RE: Efficacy of soft tissue augmentation around dental implants and in partially edentulous areas: a systematic review. J Clin Periodontol 2014;41(Suppl 15):77–91.

31.   Vignoletti F, Matesanz P, Rodrigo D, Figuero E, Martin C, Sanz M: Surgical protocols for ridge preservation after tooth extraction. A systematic review. Clin Oral Implants Res 2012;23(Suppl 5):22–38.

Autologous dental hard tissue

7

Puria Parvini, Frank Schwarz

Preclinical and clinical trials have shown that tooth root augmentation is a possible option for alveolar ridge augmentation as an alternative to an autogenous bone block[12-14,16]. The transplantation of teeth to replace lost teeth has been an established concept for many years[10,11]. Various experimental studies demonstrated that extracted teeth have a structural biologic potential[2] to assist the regeneration of bone defects[1,3,4,7]. Like the composition of bone, dentin consists of an inorganic portion (dentin 69.3% versus bone 62%) and an organic portion (dentin 17.5% versus bone 25%), which in turn consists of 90% type I collagen[5,9]. It was shown that, even in the presence of root fragments, successful implant integration can be achieved, which involves deposition of newly formed cementum and the formation of periodontal fibers in the area in contact with the implant surface[6,8,17], and that histologically osseointegration of titanium implants ensues[15].

Specific risks

The risks of (surgical) extraction of teeth used for augmentation coincide with the usual general risks, which should be explained to the patient at least 24 hours before the surgical procedure.

The patient should also be informed about the possibility of the loss of the augmentation material.

Preoperative diagnostics

The patient should have one or more caries-free, partly or fully impacted third molar or other teeth that fulfill the indication criteria for tooth extraction.

For imaging diagnostics, a panoramic radiograph or CBCT scan is recommended for visualizing the bone defects and the tooth to be extracted (Figs 7-1 to 7-3).

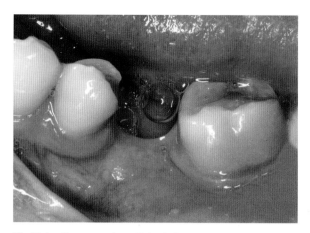

Fig 7-1   Preoperative clinical situation.

Step-by-step clinical procedure

After the patient has rinsed with a local antiseptic (e.g. chlorhexidine), local anesthesia is carried out depending on the region of the tooth being extracted and the region being augmented. After a mucoperiosteal flap has been raised, the recipient bed is exposed (Fig 7-4). The dimensions of the bone defect can then be measured. The tooth serving as the augmentation material is extracted as atraumatically as possible (Fig 7-5) and is then prepared. The crown is first separated horizontally from the root portion in the region of the cementoenamel junction with a Lindemann bur or a cutting disc (Figs 7-6 and 7-7).

For multirooted teeth, vertical separation of these roots takes place. The pulp is left in the case of healthy or periodontally damaged teeth. The surface of the augmentation material facing the soft tissue remains unchanged; it has been found that an intact cementum is less prone to replacement resorption, and hence the volume of the augmented contour can be guaranteed[15]. If teeth are periodontally damaged, however, complete preservation of the cementum cannot be achieved because intensive scaling and

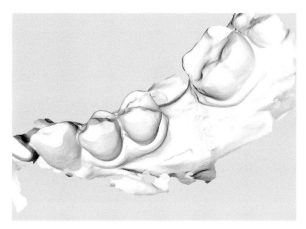

Fig 7-2 Preoperative intraoral scan.

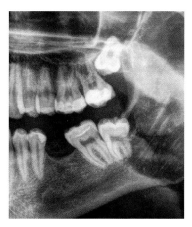

Fig 7-3 Panoramic radiograph of the preoperative situation.

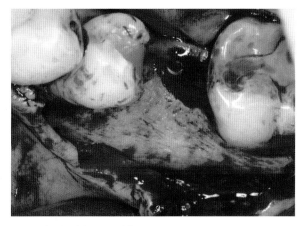

Fig 7-4 Incision and formation of the mucoperiosteal flap, then exposure of the bone defect.

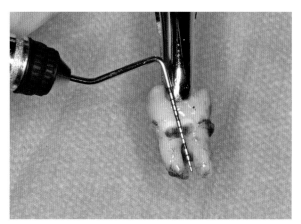

Fig 7-5 Tooth after extraction.

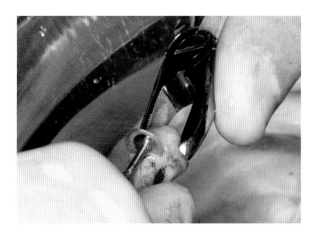

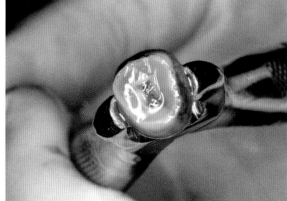

Figs 7-6 and 7-7 Separation of the crown from the root at the cementoenamel junction.

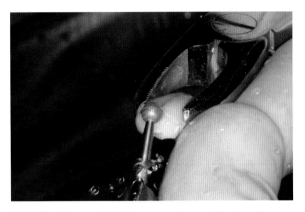

Fig 7-8   Removal of the cementum at the basal contact zone until dentin exposure is achieved.

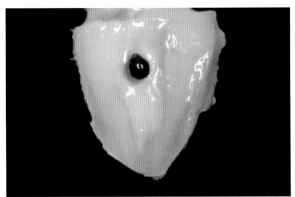

Fig 7-9   Preparation of the augmentation material for the osteosynthesis screw and visualization of the basal contact zone, which has been completely freed of cementum.

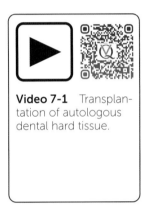

Video 7-1   Transplantation of autologous dental hard tissue.

piezoelectric surgical instruments. The primary objective of the surgical protocol is to promote ankylosis and remodeling of the tooth root at the residual recipient bed (Fig 7-8). The vestibular cortical bone at the recipient site can be perforated using a Lindemann bur. After adaptation of the augmentation material, a drill hole is prepared with a round bur for the screw head of the osteosynthesis set (Fig 7-9). Then, a gliding hole in the tooth root augmentation material and an air hole in the recipient site are prepared in order to stabilize the block with the aid of an osteosynthesis screw (Figs 7-10 and 7-11, Video 7-1).

root planing is required before and after tooth extraction to ensure complete removal of all bacterial deposits. The areas of the root augmentation material that will be in contact with the residual bone in the recipient bed are completely freed of cementum at the basal contact zones until dentin exposure is achieved. For preparation, all the instruments available for hard tissue preparation can be used, for example, fissure drills, Lindemann burs, round burs of different diameters, diamond-tipped round burs or

Wound care and closure

After successful fixation of the augmentation material, wound closure takes place with anchoring and adaptation sutures. It is advisable to use a multilayer suturing technique for closure such as a combination of interrupted sutures with mattress sutures or a double-loop suture (Fig 7-12). In the same way as for surgical tooth extraction, 5-0 or 6-0 diameter monofilament suture material can be used with an atraumatic needle.

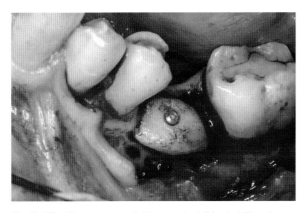

Fig 7-10 The augmentation material is stabilized with an osteosynthesis screw. The perforation of the cortical bone at the recipient site can be identified.

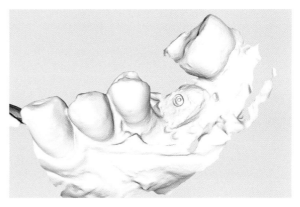

Fig 7-11 Intraoral scan after fixation of the augmentation material.

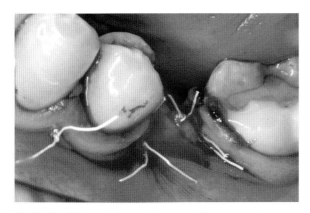

Fig 7-12 Wound closure by a multilayer suturing technique.

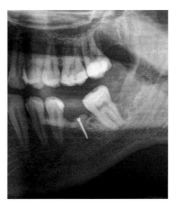

Fig 7-13 Postoperative control radiograph.

Postoperative controls and course

A postoperative radiograph can be taken in order to document the patient's progress (Fig 7-13). Sutures are usually removed after 8 to 10 days (Fig 7-14). Accompanying antibiotic administration is not absolutely necessary and is dependent on the patient's particular history. Analgesics are prescribed as required, depending on the history and based on the patient's body weight.

Implant placement

After a healing time of 6 months, a radiograph is taken prior to implant placement. In the case of a dental panoramic radiograph, it is advisable to take the image with a measuring aid (e.g. calibration ball). A three-dimensional (3D) image (e.g. CBCT scan) is also useful for the purpose of precise 3D planning prior to implant placement (Figs 7-15 to 7-17). A mucoperiosteal flap is raised to expose the implant site (Figs 7-18 and 7-19).

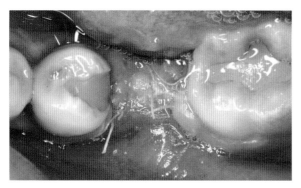

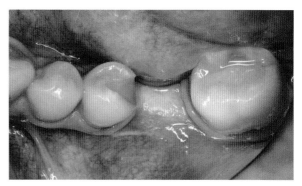

Fig 7-14 Wound check and suture removal 8 to 10 days postoperatively.

Fig 7-15 Clinical situation after 6 months of healing time.

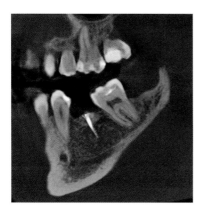

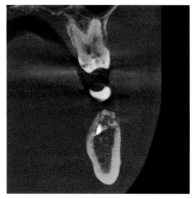

Figs 7-16 and 7-17 Three-dimensional images after 6 months of healing time.

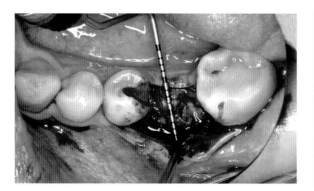

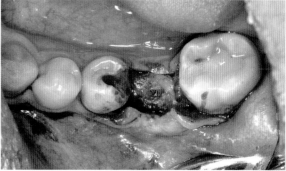

Figs 7-18 and 7-19 Reopening after 6 months. Exposure of the tooth root augmentation material after the raising of a mucoperiosteal flap.

The osteosynthesis screw can then be removed. If a bleeding site is identifiable after the removal of the screw, this is indicative of the remodeling process of the augmentation material (Fig 7-20).

Implant placement follows the standard protocol for that particular implant system (Figs 7-21 and 7-22); whether subgingival or transgingival healing is to take place is dependent

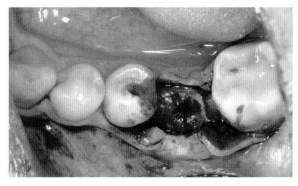

Fig 7-20 After removal of the osteosynthesis screw, a bleeding site can be detected in the root augmentation material.

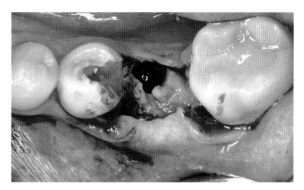

Fig 7-21 Implant site preparation.

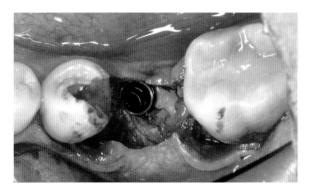

Fig 7-22 Implant in situ.

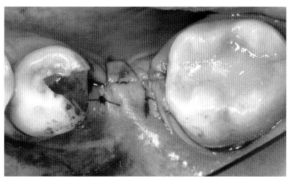

Fig 7-23 Wound closure.

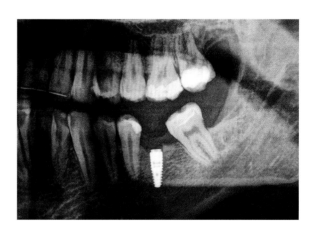

Fig 7-24 Control radiograph after implant placement.

on the primary stability at implant placement and/or patient compliance (Fig 7-23). A control radiograph is taken after implant placement (Fig 7-24). After osseointegration of the implant

has occurred, subsequent prosthetic treatment can be carried out as with standard implant placement.

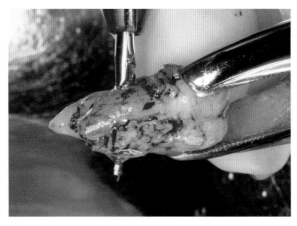

Fig 7-25 Holding the tooth with diamond-tipped extraction forceps and separating the unused tooth root with a Lindemann bur.

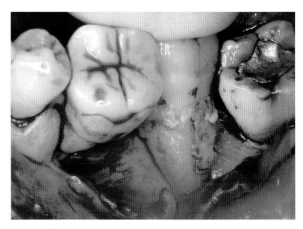

Fig 7-26 Try-in of the root augmentation material (still attached to the tooth crown) at the recipient site.

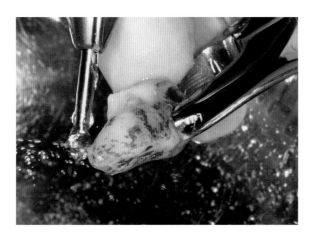

Fig 7-27 Preparation of the tooth root congruent with the defect at the recipient site.

Modification of root augmentation material preparation

The smaller the root augmentation material, the more challenging the fixation during preparation. If there are very tight spaces and significant bone resorption, preparation of the root augmentation material can be modified for easier handling in order to ensure a short and efficient operating time.

Step-by-step clinical procedure

It is advantageous to use extraction or fixation forceps with diamond-coated tips in order to prevent the tooth from slipping out of the tips of the forceps during preparation with a Lindemann bur or round bur. After tooth extraction, in the case of multirooted teeth, the most suitable root for augmentation is first selected, and the root not being used is separated using a Lindemann bur or cutting disc (Fig 7-25). The root being used for augmentation remains attached to the

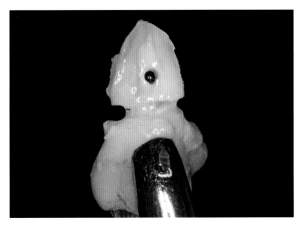

Fig 7-28 Prepared root augmentation material with intended separation site and sliding hole (still attached to the tooth crown).

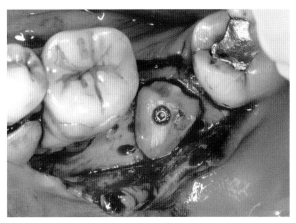

Fig 7-29 Fixed root augmentation material after separation of the tooth crown.

tooth crown for the time being, making it easier to carry out the subsequent try-in at the recipient site (Fig 7-26). The aim is to achieve maximal congruence between the root augmentation material and the recipient site. The tooth root is prepared as described above (Fig 7-27). For orientation and easier subsequent separation, an intended separation point can be prepared that is appropriate for the defect (Fig 7-28). Intraoral preparation of the air and sliding holes at the recipient site is faster and easier to perform with the modified procedure. The graft is fixed with an osteosynthesis screw, and then the tooth crown can be separated from the augmentation material (Fig 7-29). Tension-free flap closure then takes place.

References

1. Andersson L: Dentin xenografts to experimental bone defects in rabbit tibia are ankylosed and undergo osseous replacement. Dent Traumatol 2010;26:398–402.

2. Andersson L, Ramzi A, Joseph B: Studies on dentin grafts to bone defects in rabbit tibia and mandible; development of an experimental model. Dent Traumatol 2009;25:78–83.

3. Atiya BK, Shanmuhasuntharam P, Huat S, Abdulrazzak S, Oon H: Liquid nitrogen-treated autogenous dentin as bone substitute: an experimental study in a rabbit model. Int J Oral Maxillofac Implants 2014;29: e165–e170.

4. Bormann KH, Suarez-Cunqueiro MM, Sinikovic B, Kampmann A, von See C, Tavassol F, Binger T, Winkler M, Gellrich NC, Rucker M: Dentin as a suitable bone substitute comparable to ss-TCP- an experimental study in mice. Microvasc Res 2012;84:116–122.

5. Brudevold F, Steadman LT, Smith FA: Inorganic and organic components of tooth structure. Ann N Y Acad Sci 1960;85:110–132.

6. Buser D, Warrer K, Karring T: Formation of a periodontal ligament around titanium implants. J Periodontol 1990;61:597–601.

7. Catanzaro-Guimaraes SA, Catanzaro Guimaraes BP, Garcia RB, Alle N: Osteogenic potential of autogenic demineralized dentin implanted in bony defects in dogs. Int J Oral Maxillofac Surg 1986;15:160–169.

8. Hurzeler MB, Zuhr O, Schupbach P, Rebele SF, Emmanouilidis N, Fickl S: The socket-shield technique: a proof-of-principle report. J Clin Periodontol 2010;37:855–862.

9. Linde A: Dentin matrix proteins: composition and possible functions in calcification. Anat Rec 1989;224:154–166.

10. Nordenram A: Autotransplantation of teeth. A clinical and experimental investigation. Acta Odontol Scand 1963;21(Suppl 33): 7–76.

11. Pape HD, Heiss R: History of tooth transplantation [in German]. Fortschr Kiefer Gesichtschir 1976;20:121–125.

12. Parvini P, Sader R, Sahin D, Becker J, Schwarz F: Radiographic outcomes following lateral alveolar ridge augmentation using autogenous tooth roots. Int J Implant Dent 2018;4:31.

13. Ramanauskaite A, Sahin D, Sader R, Becker J, Schwarz F: Efficacy of autogenous teeth for the reconstruction of alveolar ridge deficiencies: a systematic review. Clin Oral Investig 2019;23:4263–4287.

14. Schwarz F, Hazar D, Becker K, Sader R, Becker J: Efficacy of autogenous tooth roots for lateral alveolar ridge augmentation and staged implant placement. A prospective controlled clinical study. J Clin Periodontol 2018;45:996–1004.

15. Schwarz F, Mihatovic I, Golubovic V, Becker J: Dentointegration of a titanium implant: a case report. Oral Maxillofac Surg 2013;17:235–241.

16. Schwarz F, Schmucker A, Becker J: Initial case report of an extracted tooth root used for lateral alveolar ridge augmentation. J Clin Periodontol 2016;43:985–989.

17. Warrer K, Karring T, Gotfredsen K: Periodontal ligament formation around different types of dental titanium implants. I. The self-tapping screw type implant system. J Periodontol 1993;64:29–34.

Decoronation

8

Andreas Filippi

Ankylosed teeth with advanced replacement resorption cannot be extracted conventionally but only by osteotomy. This results in relatively large bone defects with subsequent sagittal and possibly vertical bone loss because there is no clear boundary between root and bone. In these cases, decoronation guarantees that the entire width of the alveolar process is preserved for the purpose of preparing for implant or prosthetic treatment. If decoronation is performed while the jaw is still growing, bone apposition onto the resection surface will additionally improve the vertical bone supply (Figs 8-1 to 8-3).

Indications

Decoronation is only indicated for advanced, usually trauma-related, replacement resorption (osseous replacement) (Figs 8-4 to 8-7) prior to planned removable or fixed restorations (bonded or conventional partial dentures) and implant placement. Decoronation is not to be confused with a coronectomy, in which the teeth have a vital periodontium[1].

Contraindications

Absolute or temporary contraindications mostly arise from a patient's general history. Bearing in mind planned further care, decoronation is not indicated if the clinical gap that is formed will be closed by orthodontic space closure or by tooth transplantation (see Section 11). In these cases, the root must be surgically removed in its entirety. Decoronation is also not indicated if a tooth is not ankylosed or not extensively ankylosed. The latter is typically indicated by a nonphysiologically high percussion sound (tap note) from the tooth, negative vertical Periotest values (Fig 8-8) or progressive infraposition in the growing jaw, where the tooth root is still almost entirely visible on a current single-tooth radiograph. Such teeth generally can be extracted completely and without difficulty using forceps (Figs 8-9 to 8-14).

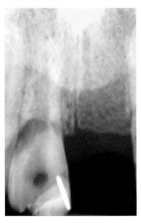

Fig 8-1   Trauma-related advanced replacement resorption at the maxillary right central incisor in the growing jawbone.

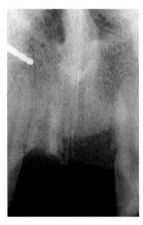

Fig 8-2   Radiographic situation immediately after decoronation.

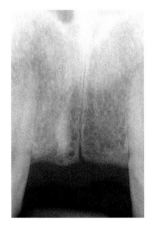

Fig 8-3   Radiographic situation 1 year after decoronation showing typical vertical bone apposition on the resection surface.

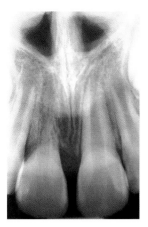
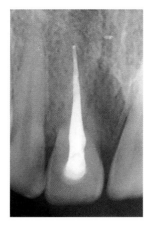
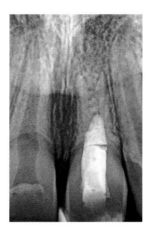
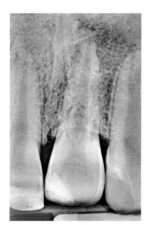

Figs 8-4 to 8-7   Examples of trauma-related advanced replacement resorption in the growing jawbone.

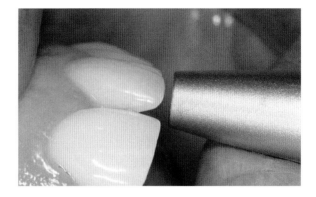

Fig 8-8   The vertical Periotest measurement is more sensitive than the horizontal one.

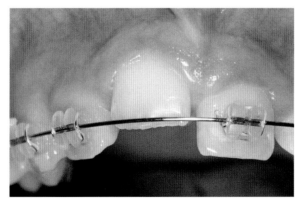
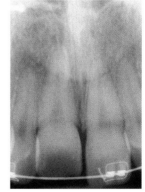

Figs 8-9 and 8-10
Typical trauma-related infraposition due to ankylosis in the growing jaw; however, the contours of the tooth root can be fully identified two-dimensionally.

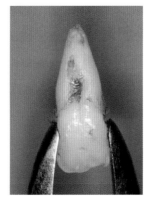
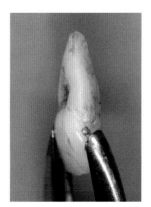

Figs 8-11 and 8-12   Problem-free tooth extraction despite ankylosis because of mostly limited resorption lacunae.

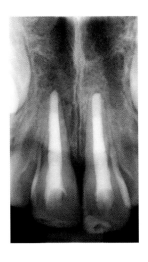
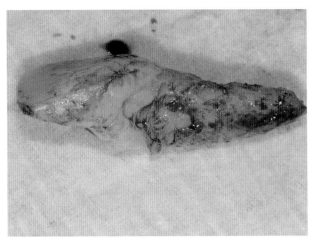

Figs 8-13 and 8-14 A non-preservable maxillary right central incisor due to trauma-related ankylosis, in infraposition. Due to limited resorption lacunae, the tooth is extracted intact without difficulty.

Step-by-step clinical procedure

After appropriate local anesthesia, a sharp surgical bur (e.g. Lindemann bur) is used to separate the crown from the root along the gingival contour (scalloped), which gives the decoronation technique its name (Figs 8-15 to 8-20). Any enamel remnants that might be left in the area of the cementoenamel junction (Fig 8-21) are then fully removed with a round bur (Fig 8-22) because enamel is not remodeled into bone. The resection surface then slightly resembles the crater of a volcano. If a root canal filling is present, incrementally smaller round burs from coronal to apical are used to remove it completely under direct vision (Fig 8-23). An intraoperative control radiograph is not usually required. Remaining parts of the root (root dentin, cementum) are not removed. If possible, primary soft tissue closure completes the procedure (Figs 8-24 to 8-42). This can be performed with soft tissue harvested from the palate (punch) or by soft tissue coverage; in the case of the latter, only if there is enough buccal keratinized gingiva available.

Secondary wound healing should be avoided, especially if the cervical parts of the root are still more or less intact. In that case, it is not uncommon for a nonepithelializing crestal indentation to persist.

Postoperative controls and course

Postoperative controls are the same as those following surgical tooth extraction. Suture removal takes place after about a week. A few weeks later, prosthetic restoration of the space can be started, provided that the emergence profile has been created, for example, with a removable provisional restoration (Figs 8-43 to 8-47). Implant-based treatment might be initiated if the progression of replacement resorption is observed on radiographs (Figs 8-48 to 8-58).

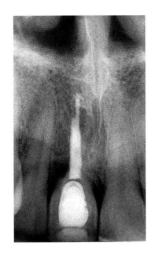

Fig 8-15 Trauma-related advanced replacement resorption at the maxillary right central incisor in a 19-year-old patient.

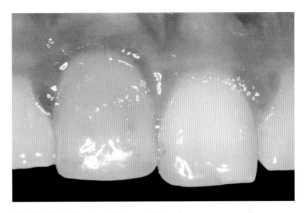

Fig 8-16 The tooth has clinically corresponding infraposition due to vertical anterior jaw growth.

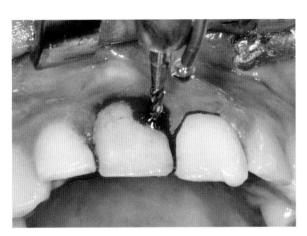

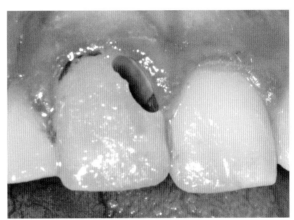

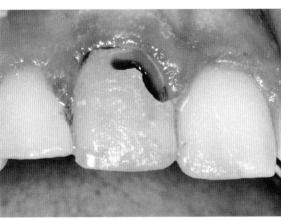

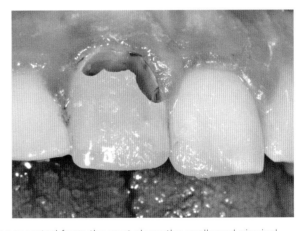

Figs 8-17 to 8-20 Under local anesthesia, the crown is separated from the root along the scalloped gingival contour using a sharp surgical bur.

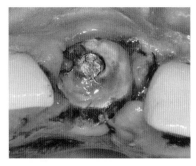

Fig 8-21 View of the resection surface with enamel remnants in the area of the cementoenamel junction.

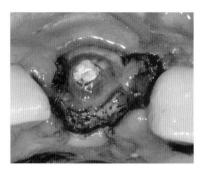

Fig 8-22 Situation after removal of the enamel remnants with a round bur.

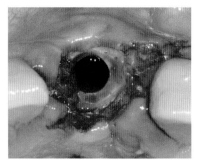

Fig 8-23 Situation after complete removal of the root canal filling with incrementally smaller rose burs down to the apex.

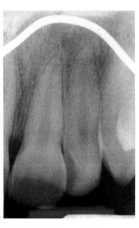

Fig 8-24 In a different case, radiographic situation of the maxillary left central incisor in a 13-year-old patient, before a severe dislocation injury leading to replacement resorption.

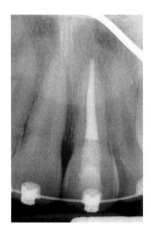

Fig 8-25 Radiographic situation after the severe dislocation injury, repositioning, and root canal treatment in the patient, now aged 14 years.

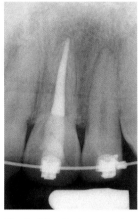

Fig 8-26 Radiographic situation 3 years after the dental trauma showing distinct replacement resorption at the maxillary left central incisor.

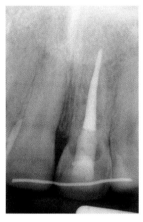

Fig 8-27 Radiographic situation nearly 4 years after dental trauma showing progression of replacement resorption at the maxillary left central incisor.

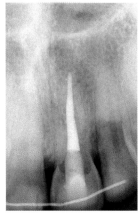

Fig 8-28 Radiographic situation 6 years after dental trauma in the patient, now aged 20 years, shortly before decoronation.

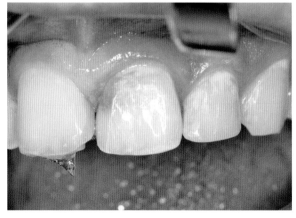

Fig 8-29 Preoperative clinical situation: Reddish discoloration in the gingival area due to underlying resorption at the crown of the maxillary left central incisor.

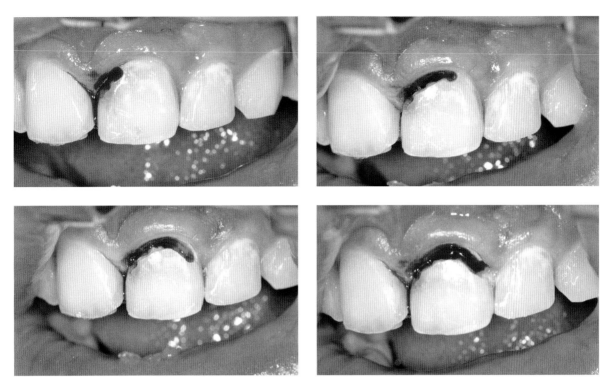

Figs 8-30 to 8-33 Separating the crown from the root along the gingival contour using a sharp surgical bur.

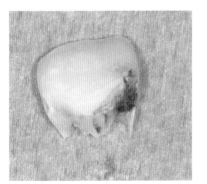

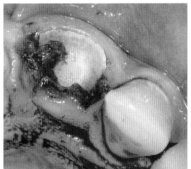

Fig 8-34 Crown after decorona-tion.

Figs 8-35 and 8-36 Removing persistent enamel portions with a large round bur.

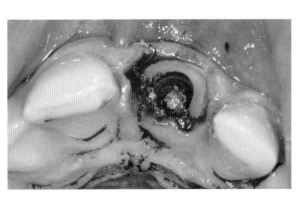

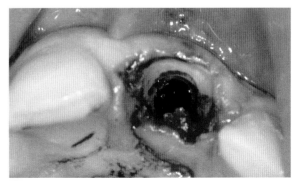

Figs 8-37 and 8-38 Completely removing the root canal filling with incrementally smaller rose burs from coronal to apical.

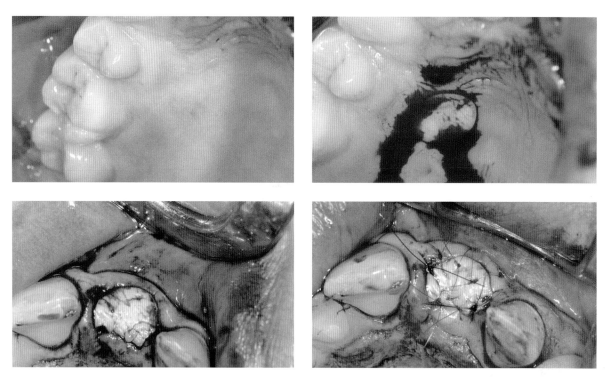

Figs 8-39 to 8-42   Harvesting a palatal punch for primary wound closure and fixation with thin, monofilament suture material.

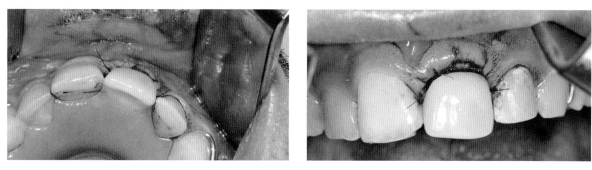

Figs 8-43 and 8-44   Postoperative placement of an interim prosthesis for the wound healing phase.

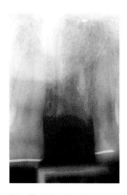 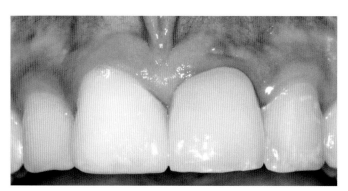 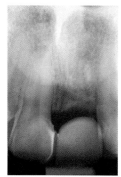

Fig 8-45   Radiographic situation after decoronation.

Fig 8-46   Bonded partial denture in place after completion of wound healing (image courtesy of Prof Dr N. U. Zitzmann).

Fig 8-47   Radiographic check of bone remodeling after placement of the bonded partial denture.

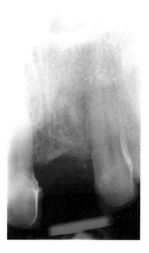
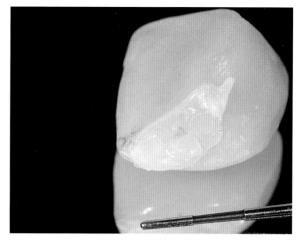

Figs 8-48 and 8-49 Fracture of the bonded partial denture 3.5 years after decoronation, caused by another dental trauma at the age of 24 years (images courtesy of Prof Dr N. U. Zitzmann).

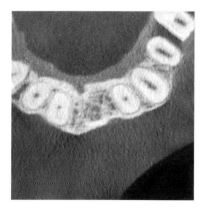
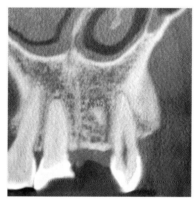
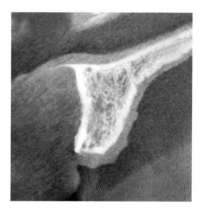

Figs 8-50 to 8-52 CBCT planning prior to implant placement with hypodivergent growth of about 95 degrees in the area of the angle of the jaw associated with a low risk of later infraposition of the implant: Good bone supply exists in all three planes.

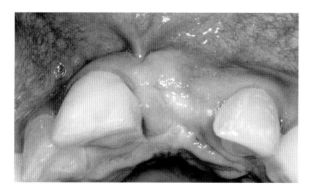
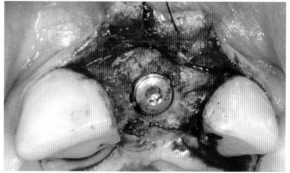

Figs 8-53 and 8-54 Implant placement in the maxillary left central incisor region 4 years after decoronation, given ample sagittal bone supply.

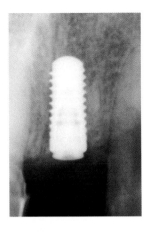

Fig 8-55   Radiographic check-up after implant placement and subgingival healing.

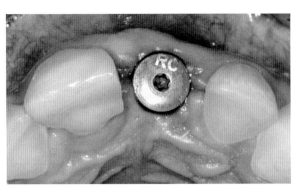

Fig 8-56   Situation 10 days after implant exposure and insertion of a gingiva former.

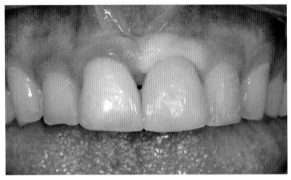

Fig 8-57   Situation after placement of the provisional implant crown for soft tissue shaping (image courtesy of Prof Dr N. U. Zitzmann).

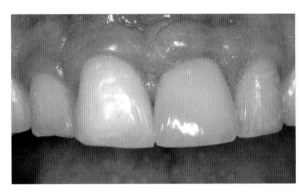

Fig 8-58   Situation approximately 6 years after decoronation and approximately 1.5 years after placement of the implant crown (image courtesy of Prof Dr N. U. Zitzmann).

Reference

1   Filippi, A, Saccardin F, Kühl S: Das kleine 1x1 der Oralchirurgie. Berlin: Quintessenz, 2020.

Recommended literature

Filippi A, Pohl Y, von Arx T: Decoronation of an anky-losed tooth for preservation of alveolar bone prior to implant placement. Dent Traumatol 2001;17:93–95.

Malmgren B. Decoronation: how, why, and when? J Calif Dent Assoc 2000;28:846–854.

Sapir S, Kalter A, Sapir MR: Decoronation of an anky-losed permanent incisor: alveolar ridge preserva-tion and rehabilitation by an implant supported porcelain crown. Dent Traumatol 2009;25: 346–349.

Zürcher A, Zitzmann N, Filippi A: Dekoronation als präimplantologische Maßnahme. Quintessenz 2019;70:432–439.

Surgical exposure and orthodontic alignment

Sebastian Kühl

Indications

Surgical exposure and orthodontic alignment of teeth is always indicated 1) if a tooth is no longer expected to erupt normally because it is impacted or ectopic after physiologic exfoliation has taken place and/or root growth is completed, and 2) if tooth alignment is appropriate and desirable for functional and esthetic reasons (Figs 9-1 to 9-3). This indication primarily relates to the maxillary canines, followed by the mandibular second premolars, maxillary incisors, and mandibular canines[2]. The cause can be genetic, systemic, and/or of anatomical origin.

In most cases, the location of an impacted and ectopic tooth can be identified clinically by palpation (bulge on the mucosa) and radiologically from orthoradial and eccentric single-tooth radiographs. However, it is advisable to perform CBCT, particularly in close proximity to relevant anatomical structures and especially when they are to be preserved, but also when resorption affecting the impacted and ectopic tooth or the adjacent tooth root is suspected. The aim of surgical exposure is to aid the eruption of an impacted and ectopic tooth and to shorten the orthodontic treatment time. Furthermore, in many cases, exposure and alignment can be used in addition to treatment of a follicular cyst (Fig 9-4).

Contraindications

Absolute contraindications mainly arise from the general medical history when patients cannot undergo surgery due to their general state of health (e.g. undergoing chemotherapy or diagnosed with terminal-stage cancer). Provisional triple anticoagulation that will be switched to bi- or monotherapy in the foreseeable future is an example of a temporary contraindication. Acute local infections may also be regarded as a temporary contraindication because sufficient depth of anesthesia during the surgical procedure might not be achievable, and the risk of a postoperative wound infection might be increased. Since the patient's cooperation is essential for exposure and alignment, young age also has to be considered a temporary contraindication. Finally, ankylosis or primary failure of eruption of a tooth being aligned may also be classified as a contraindication[4]. However, this is not always diagnostically predictable, which means it is more of a complication than a contraindication.

Specific risks

The specific risks arise from the nature of the procedure and specific anatomy. In this respect, most exposures involve surgical uncovering of the tooth crown by osteotomy, so the specific risks can take the form of injuries to vital neighboring structures such as nerves, blood vessels or adjacent roots caused by rotary instruments. Generally, however, these are very rare and avoidable with precise knowledge of the patient's anatomy. In case of doubt, preoperative CBCT can provide clarity with regard to the precise localization of neighboring anatomical structures (e.g. adjacent roots, nasal floor, mental foramen). As with any surgical procedure, the general risks in the form of pain, swelling, wound infections, and bleeding have to be accepted. One particular risk is associated with premature loosening or detachment of the bonded attachment (bracket with fixed chain for orthodontic alignment). As this is attached with an adhesive bond, and it is impossible to create an absolutely dry field with rubber dam when placing the attachment, the bond to the tooth might be lost, especially during intensive application of force, and this might make repeat surgery necessary. To prevent soft tissue complications during

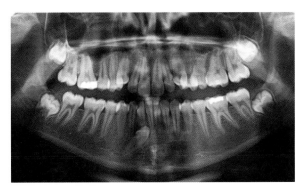

Fig 9-1 Impacted and ectopic canine in the right mandible.

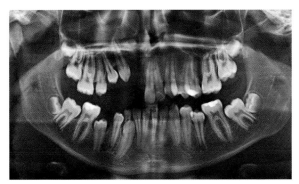

Fig 9-2 Several impacted and ectopic teeth in the maxilla and mandible; canines and premolars are typically affected.

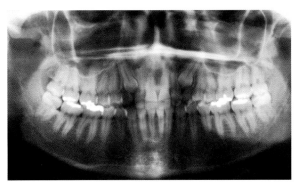

Fig 9-3 Typical impaction and displacement of maxillary canines.

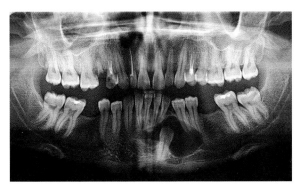

Fig 9-4 Sizeable follicular cyst pericoronal to the impacted and ectopic mandibular left canine. The cyst can be treated at the same time via exposure and alignment of the canine.

tooth alignment, after the surgery the other end of the orthodontic chain should already lie at the target area of the tooth being aligned. Another risk during exposure and alignment is associated with the fact that, in rare cases, teeth cannot be moved because of ankylosis or primary failure to erupt. Surgical loosening of these teeth with a lever has not proved successful because such teeth will usually ankylose (again) in a very short time. In this situation, surgical extraction of the impacted and ectopic tooth is usually the only possible option.

Step-by-step clinical procedure

In the maxilla, vestibular and palatal infiltration anesthesia is chosen, in the same way as for tooth extractions. If the tooth is palatally displaced and access is from the palatal direction, anesthesia should take place on both sides at the greater palatine foramen and in the area of the incisive foramen. Placing a small amount of local anesthetic in the area of the anticipated tooth crown has also proved effective because the presence of a vasoconstrictor can reduce

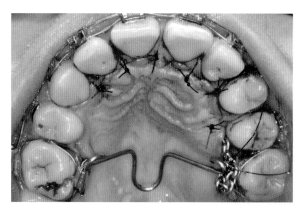

Fig 9-5   The chain has not been placed directly in the maxillary left canine region, into which the canine will be moved. The maxillary left first premolar first has to be moved away from the adjacent lateral incisor.

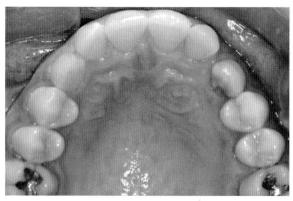

Fig 9-6   Both maxillary canines are palatally displaced (see panoramic radiograph in Fig 9-3). The incision should be intrasulcular for palatal access, taking into account the neurovascular bundle in the area of the incisive foramen.

Video 9-1   Surgical exposure and bonding of an orthodontic attachment in the mandible.

bleeding and hence improve the relative isolation during adhesive bonding of the attachment. In the case of palatal access, the only purpose of vestibular infiltration anesthesia is to ensure that papillary adaptation can be shaped painlessly with an intrasulcular incision. Consequently, the anesthetic dose can be reduced to a minimum.

When access is vestibular, the area to be exposed is numbed by infiltration anesthesia in the same way as for tooth extraction. Once again, it is advisable to use a local anesthetic with a vasoconstrictor, which reduces the blood flow

and hence optimizes the relative isolation when bonding the attachment. Palatally, usually in the quadrant where surgery is being performed, local anesthetic is placed in the region of the greater palatine foramen and the incisive foramen. Here, too, anesthesia aids pain-free adaptation of the papillae after intrasulcular incision from the vestibular direction.

In the mandible, infiltration anesthesia in the area of the mental foramen is generally sufficient. Lingual infiltration anesthesia in the area is imperative, just as for tooth extractions. Alternatively, if the depth of anesthesia is inadequate, a nerve block in combination with vestibular infiltration anesthesia can be chosen.

The incision is made after local anesthesia has taken place. The incision path and access are determined by the localization of the impacted tooth. In principle, palatally displaced teeth should be exposed from the palatal direction, and vestibularly displaced teeth from the vestibular direction. Regardless of which of the two directions of access is chosen, two aspects are particularly important: 1) Whenever possible, the incision should be intrasulcular so that the chain is always surrounded by keratinized gingiva,

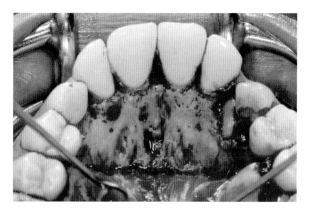

Fig 9-7 Raising the mucoperiosteal flap, taking into account the neurovascular bundle at the incisive foramen.

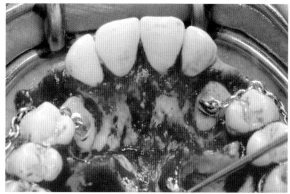

Fig 9-8 After extraction of the retained primary teeth, the tooth crowns are exposed with round burs. After fixing the attachment, the orthodontic chains are aligned with the location determined by the orthodontist.

and 2) Upon exposure, the chain should already be placed in the future location of the tooth being aligned or where the orthodontic direction of traction will be applied (Figs 9-5 and 9-6, Video 9-1). This requires good interdisciplinary consultation. A paramarginal incision should only be considered if the impacted and ectopic tooth lies very close to the adjacent tooth root so that later there will be insufficient bone support when the mucoperiosteal flap is being repositioned. As a result, the risk of wound dehiscence and later recession affecting the neighboring tooth can be reduced.

In the case of palatal access, the incision usually extends over one to two teeth in the mesial and distal direction, for the purpose of horizontal releasing in order to ensure adequate mobilization of the mucoperiosteal flap. The neurovascular bundle in the area of the incisive foramen can be sharply severed with a scalpel blade when the mucoperiosteal flap is being dissected (Fig 9-7).

No permanent sensory disorders are to be expected here[3]. The impacted teeth are then exposed with round burs (e.g. rose burs) or a piezoelectric surgical device so that the largest circumference of the tooth crown is no longer covered by bone (Fig 9-8). Exposure of the tooth crown must never extend beyond the cementoenamel junction because this can eventually lead to bone loss and gingival recession. Luxating the impacted and ectopic tooth with a lever should also be avoided because it carries the risk of ankylosis and root resorption[1].

Adhesive bonding of the attachment follows. The dental follicle is only removed to the extent that relative isolation will be guaranteed because there is evidence in the literature that remaining parts of the dental follicle can encourage imminent eruption of a tooth[5]. The attachment should ideally be placed incisally or occlusally (depending on the direction of traction). There are two reasons for this: Firstly, this location is readily accessible to the oral surgeon in most cases, and secondly, no unwanted rotation of the tooth will occur later during orthodontic alignment. To fit the attachment, the enamel is first etched with phosphoric acid under relative isolation, then fixed with a bonding agent. A bonding agent is also required for the attachment. Care must be taken to ensure that the attachment is coated with enough composite

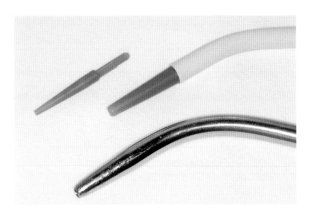

Fig 9-9 Microsurgical aspirators, with relative isolation, can keep blood away from the bonding zones during adhesive fixation of the attachment.

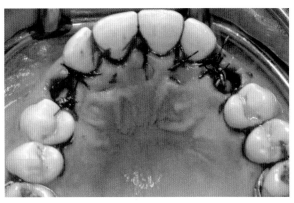

Fig 9-10 Wound closure with interrupted sutures in the area of the papillae. The chain is also fixed at the end with an interrupted suture.

and the enamel is not contaminated with blood during the bonding process. For this purpose, microsurgical aspirators such as those used for apicoectomies (see Section 10) have proved very effective (Fig 9-9). Any excess composite should be removed well before it sets because, once it sets, access can frequently be limited due to lack of space. Additionally, the edges of the attachment can be coated with low-viscosity composite so that there is mechanical retention as well as adhesive bonding. Before wound closure, traction should be applied to the chain to check whether the bond strength is adequate. Wound closure with sutures then takes place (Fig 9-10).

Like palatal access, vestibular access is via an intrasulcular incision, or in edentulous areas on the middle of the alveolar ridge, hence crestally, so that there is sufficient keratinized gingiva on the vestibular aspect. CBCT, by identifying the correct location of the impacted teeth, can make a significant contribution to incision and surgical exposure (Figs 9-11 to 9-14). Vertical releasing incisions are made at a minimum distance of 3 mm from the tooth crowns being exposed. After dissection of the mucoperiosteal flap, the tooth crowns are exposed by osteotomy using round burs. Once again, the osteotomy should ideally extend to the largest circumference of the tooth crown. Exposure is followed by etching and fixation of the attachment with relative isolation (Figs 9-15 to 9-17).

Wound closure is adaptive, with interrupted sutures for both vestibular and palatal access. Either interrupted sutures or vertical mattress sutures can be used for the papillae (see Figs 9-10 and 9-18). A tight seal is not absolutely essential. To prevent soft tissue complications during tooth alignment, by this stage the other end of the chain should already lie at the target area of the tooth being aligned. The orthodontist normally stipulates whether the chain should pass below the mucoperiosteal flap or above it (due to an iatrogenic perforation on the mucoperiosteal flap). In the first 12 to 24 hours after palatal access, use of a palatal protector may be appropriate depending on the size of the mucoperiosteal flap in order to counteract any postoperative swelling and bleeding (i.e. for patient comfort).

Postoperative controls and course

Check-ups following surgical procedures generally take place on the second day postoperatively because intervention-related problems are most significant at this stage (Fig 9-19). During

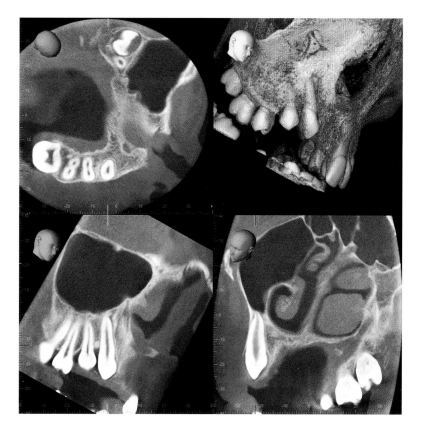

Fig 9-11 CBCT to localize the impacted maxillary right canine and first premolar (see panoramic radiograph in Fig 9-2). The incision must be made in the middle of the alveolar ridge (crestally), and the relieving incisions must be made at a distance of at least 3 mm from the impacted tooth crowns.

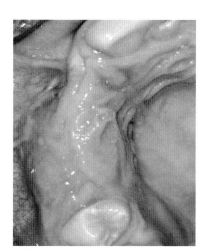 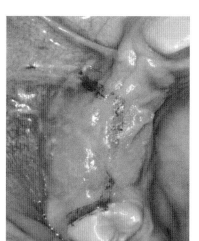 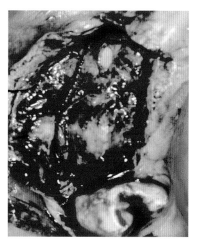

Figs 9-12 to 9-14 Vestibular access via a crestal incision and mesial and distal vertical releasing incisions at a sufficient distance from the impacted teeth.

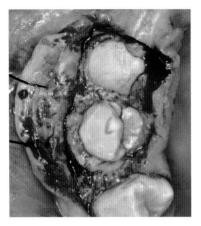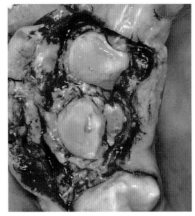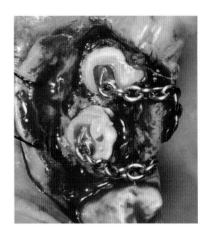

Figs 9-15 to 9-17   Exposing the tooth crowns down to the largest circumference with round burs, followed by etching and fixation of the attachment.

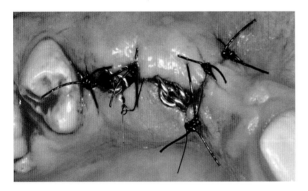

Fig 9-18   Adaptive wound closure with interrupted sutures. The chains are also fixed with interrupted sutures.

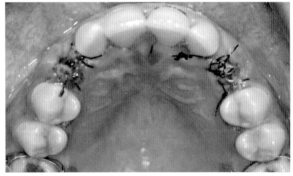

Fig 9-19   Plaque is visible on the sutures 2 days after exposure. Despite instructions, the patient was afraid to clean the area.

the check-up, wound disinfection can be carried out with 1% hydrogen peroxide or with povidone iodine. It is important to encourage patients to resume their habitual hygiene measures and clean the wounds with a relatively soft toothbrush.

References

1.   Becker A, Abramovitz I, Chaushu S: Failure of treatment of impacted canines associated with invasive cervical root resorption. Angle Orthod 2013;83:870–876.

2.   Bishara SE: Impacted maxillary canines: A review. Am J Orthod Dentofac Orthop 1992;101:159–171.

3.   Filippi A, Pohl Y, Tekin U: Sensory disorders after separation of the nasopalatine nerve during removal of palatal displaced canines: prospective investigation. Br J Oral Maxillofac Surg 1999;37:134–136.

4.   Fleury JE, Deboets D, Assaad-Auclair C, Maffre N, Sultan P: La canine incluse. Mise au point à propos de 212 observations. Principes gènèraux de traitement. Revue de Stomatologie et de Chirurgie Maxillo-Faciale 1985;86:122–131.

5.   Koutzoglou SI, Kostaki A: Effect of surgical exposure technique, age, and grade of impaction on ankylosis of an impacted canine, and the effect of rapid palatal expansion on eruption: A prospective clinical study. Am J Orthod Dentofacial Orthop 2013;143:342–352.

Apicoectomy

10

Sebastian Kühl, Andreas Filippi

Indications

An apicoectomy is indicated if an apical event in the form of apical periodontitis or a radicular cyst cannot be explored and hence treated via coronal root canal access (Fig 10-1). This is generally the case when, for example, a tooth root is fitted with a pin that cannot be removed for endodontic retreatment (orthograde access) (Fig 10-1). An apicoectomy may also be indicated, however, if success is not achieved despite endodontic retreatment (Fig 10-2) or there is a recurrence after the apicoectomy has been carried out (Fig 10-3). In this situation, the cause might lie in the apical delta, which the clinician is trying to eliminate by performing the apicoectomy[4], or in recurrences which might have originated from an insufficient orthograde or retrograde filling or an inadequate restoration (see Fig 10-3). In the case of multirooted teeth, it is justifiable to resect the affected root alone. A study showed that only 8.1% of nontreated roots displayed radiographic signs of apical periodontitis after 5 years[2].

Contraindications

Absolute contraindications mainly arise from the general medical history when patients cannot undergo surgery due to their general state of health (e.g. undergoing chemotherapy or diagnosed with terminal-stage cancer). Provisional triple anticoagulation that will be switched to bi- or monotherapy in the foreseeable future is an example of a temporary contraindication. Local infections may also be regarded as a temporary contraindication because an adequate depth of anesthesia during the surgical procedure might not be achievable. An apicoectomy is contraindicated if the tooth root exhibits a longitudinal fracture in the case of advanced marginal periodontitis or a complex periodontal-endodontic lesion. In this situation, the tooth must be extracted.

Specific risks

The specific risks arise from the nature of the procedure and the patient's specific anatomy. In this regard, it is important to preserve vital neighboring structures such as the mental nerve in the mandibular premolar region or the inferior alveolar nerve in the molar region. Making a mistake regarding which root requires treatment due to a lack of orientation is another risk, which must be absolutely avoided. In the maxillary posterior region, there is a risk of perforation of the maxillary sinus and consequently displacement of the resected root apex into the sinus (Fig 10-4). Most inflammatory processes are associated with increased blood flow. Hence, slightly increased local bleeding is not uncommon, especially at the start of an apicoectomy, but this bleeding can usually be stopped effectively. Furthermore, as with any surgical procedure, the general risks in the form of pain, swelling, wound infections, and bleeding have to be accepted.

Step-by-step clinical procedure

In the maxilla, it is advisable to inject local anesthetic into the vestibule mesial and distal to the root apex being resected[1]. Intraoperative bleeding can be reduced with the use of a vasoconstrictor (adrenaline/epinephrine 1:100,000), which optimizes the overall view and the working of materials used for retrograde sealing of the neo-apex. In addition, palatal infiltration anesthesia should be carried out because the infection will frequently have extended so far palatally that painless removal of granulation tissue by curettage or enucleation of the cyst

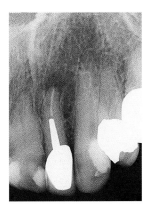

Fig 10-1 Apical periodontitis in the form of an apical radiolucency. Orthograde access to the apex is not possible due to a post and core.

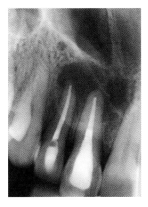

Fig 10-2 Despite endodontic retreatment of the maxillary right central and lateral incisors, the apical radiolucency is unchanged after 6 months.

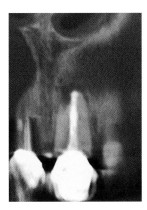

Fig 10-3 Despite a root canal filling and a previously performed apicoectomy, the apical radiolucency has not diminished and there are clinical symptoms (pain and fistula).

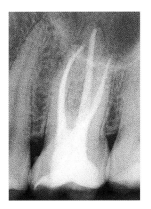

Fig 10-4 As a result of the anatomical proximity to the maxillary sinus, there is a risk in the maxillary posterior region of displacing the resected root apex into the maxillary sinus.

in this area is not possible without palatal local anesthesia.

In the mandible, a distinction must be made between the anterior and posterior regions. In the mandibular anterior region, it is usually enough to inject local anesthetic into the vestibule mesial and distal to the apex being resected, and additionally carry out lingual infiltration anesthesia[1]. In the mandibular posterior region, especially the molar region, a nerve block of the inferior alveolar nerve is additionally indicated in order to achieve adequate freedom from pain. Despite the nerve block, mesial and distal infiltration into the vestibule is also required in order to adequately anesthetize the mucosa and create bloodless conditions at the surgical site. Once again, it is advisable to use a local anesthetic with a vasoconstrictor (adrenaline/epinephrine 1:100,000).

The incision is made after local anesthesia has taken place. The incision path and access are dictated by the localization of the apex being resected. In principle, the incision should be intrasulcular in the region of the root being

resected, and a vertical releasing incision should be placed at the line angle of the neighboring tooth (Figs 10-5 and 10-6). For esthetic reasons, this vertical releasing incision should be made as distally as possible in the anterior region, whereas in the posterior region it should be made to the mesial neighboring tooth for reasons of visibility (Fig 10-7). After a mucoperiosteal flap has been raised, the root apex is located and exposed with round burs (Figs 10-8 and 10-9, Video 10-1).

This is followed by a resection of the root of about 3 mm using diamond or tungsten carbide burs (Fig 10-10). A bevel toward the vestibular aspect should be avoided or reduced to a minimum (< 20 degrees)[8]. Any apical soft tissue (cyst or granulation tissue) should be curetted at the latest after the resection of the root tip. The part of the root now visible is stained with methylene blue (Fig 10-11) in order to exclude a longitudinal fracture. In principle, magnifying aids (ideally an operating microscope or endoscope, see Section 2) should be used for every apicoectomy because they have a great influence on treatment outcome[5,6].

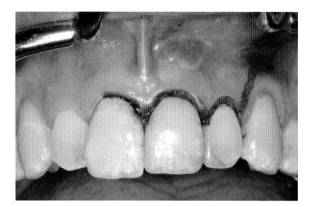

Fig 10-5   An intrasulcular incision is made in the anterior region and a vertical releasing incision is made in the distal third of the neighboring tooth for esthetic reasons.

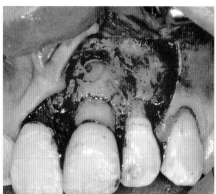

Fig 10-6   After raising the mucoperiosteal flap.

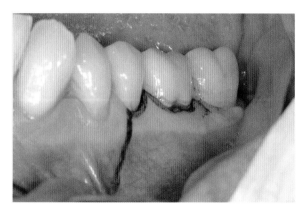

Fig 10-7   In the posterior region, the releasing incision is made to the mesial neighboring tooth because it aids visibility and the esthetic demands are lower.

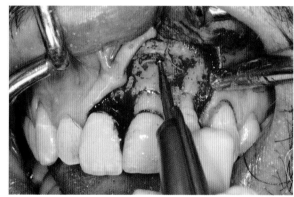

Fig 10-8   The root apex is exposed with a rose bur.

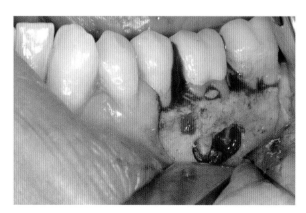

Fig 10-9   Exposed root apices.

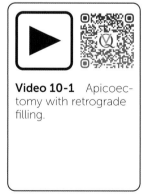

Video 10-1   Apicoectomy with retrograde filling.

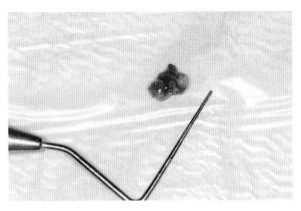

Fig 10-10 The root tip is resected at least 3 mm from the apex (the same patient as in Fig 10-7).

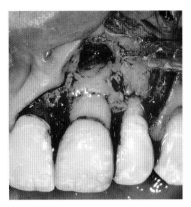

Fig 10-11 A loose retrograde filling is revealed as the cause of recurrence. The lack of tightness is very clearly highlighted by the methylene blue.

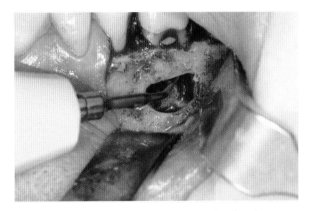

Fig 10-12 Retrograde cavity preparation by piezo-electric surgery.

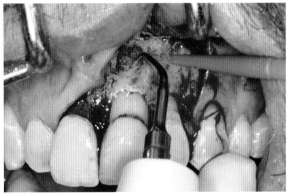

Fig 10-13 Diamond-coated piezoelectric surgery insert for retrograde preparation of the cavity.

With the aid of special diamond-coated piezoelectric surgery inserts (see Section 4), retrograde preparation of a cavity along the root canal can be carried out (Figs 10-12 and 10-13). For guidance, it is helpful to orient the tip of the piezoelectric surgery insert in the direction of the incisal edge or occlusal surface of the tooth. The retrograde cavity should then be 3-mm deep, if possible. Where there are orthograde-positioned posts extending into the apical third of the root, the cavity is prepared as far as the post.

The smear layer, an abrasion film of hydroxy-apatite-collagen detritus that arises with any kind of preparation, is removed with chelate-forming substances such as pH-neutral 25% ethylene-diaminetetraacetic acid (EDTA; PrefGel®, Straumann). For this purpose, sterile absorbent points are cut into 4- to 5-mm–long pieces, which are then coated to carry the EDTA and inserted into the retrograde cavity (Figs 10-14 to 10-16). This is allowed to take effect for 1 minute, and then the gel is rinsed off with sterile isotonic saline.

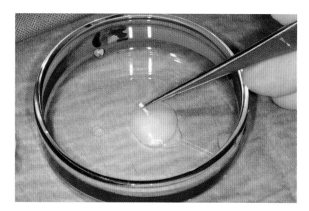

Fig 10-14   Coating the cut-to-size sterile absorbent point with ethylenediaminetetraacetic acid (EDTA; PrefGel®).

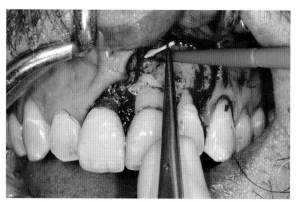

Fig 10-15   The prepared sterile absorbent points used to apply the EDTA can be tailored to any shape.

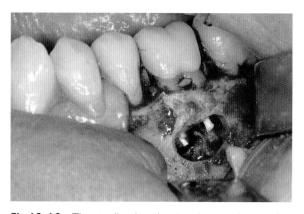

Fig 10-16   The sterile absorbent points are inserted into the retrograde cavity to apply the EDTA.

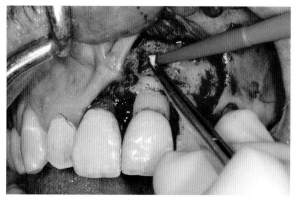

Fig 10-17   A paper point is used to dry the retrograde cavity.

The same short absorbent points are used to dry the retrograde cavity before and after conditioning (Fig 10-17).

What are known as hydraulic silicate cements (HSCs) are employed nowadays as retrograde filling material. This group of products is biocompatible and offers excellent tightness and setting properties in the humid environment. However, they are difficult to handle because they must be neither too fluid nor too solid when mixed. Special syringe systems (e.g. the MAP System, PD Dental) have proved useful for

application into the retrograde cavity (Figs 10-18 and 10-19). During the surgical procedure, all the working steps should be checked with a magnifying aid (ideally an operating microscope or endoscope, see Section 2) (Figs 10-20 to 10-26).

Before wound closure, the resection cavity is cleaned and thoroughly flushed with sterile isotonic saline (Fig 10-27). Wound closure in the area of the releasing incision involves the use of interrupted sutures (Figs 10-28 and 10-29). Suture material with a 4-0 or 5-0 diameter should be used here, if possible. The papillae are

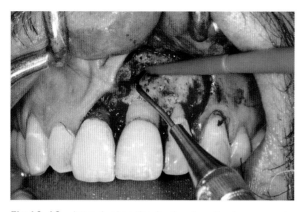

Fig 10-18 Introducing the hydraulic silicate cement (HSC) in a retrograde fashion with a special syringe system.

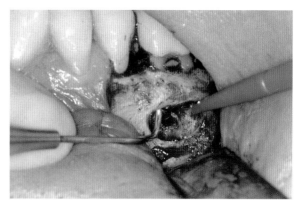

Fig 10-19 Applying the HSC using a special syringe system.

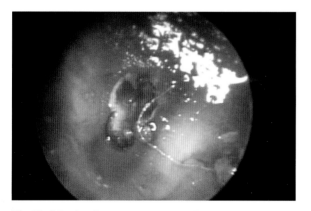

Fig 10-20 Inadequate root canal filling visible with an endoscope.

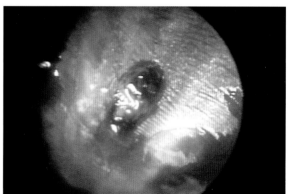

Fig 10-21 After staining with methylene blue, the insufficiency of the root canal filling is visible with an endoscope.

fixed using vertical mattress sutures and a 3-0 diameter suture material. For tunneling defects with bicortical bone destruction, it is advisable to treat the defect by means of resorbable membranes for guided tissue regeneration[7].

Postoperative controls and course

A single-tooth radiograph should be performed to document the procedure immediately after

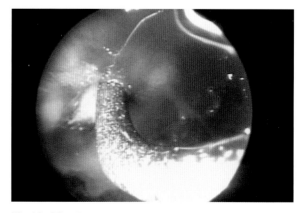

Fig 10-22 Endoscopic image of the retrograde preparation by piezosurgery.

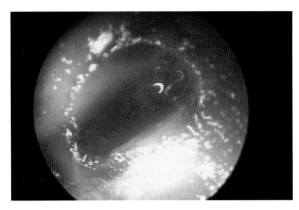

Fig 10-23   Endoscopic image of the mechanically cleared neo-apex shortly before it is decontaminated.

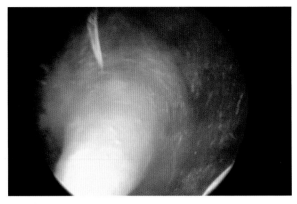

Fig 10-24   Endoscopic image of the absorbent points coated with EDTA for decontamination.

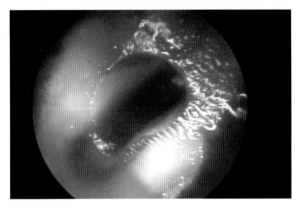

Fig 10-25   Endoscopic image after the neo-apex has been dried.

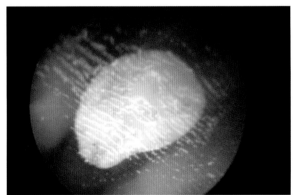

Fig 10-26   Endoscopic image after filling with HSC.

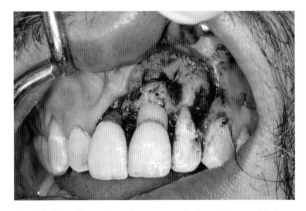

Fig 10-27   Situation after wound cleansing and irrigation with sterile isotonic saline prior to wound closure.

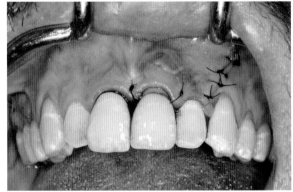

Fig 10-28   Interrupted sutures used to close the releasing incision, and vertical mattress sutures used for the papillae.

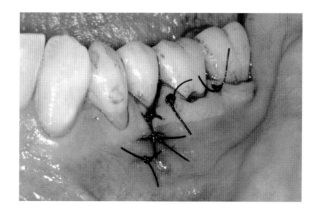

Fig 10-29 Situation after wound closure.

surgery or a few days later and should be used as a reference to check the course of progress and to assess the outcome (Figs 10-30 and 10-31). Recalls for surgical procedures usually take place on the second day postoperatively (Figs 10-32 and 10-33). During the check-up, the wound can be disinfected with 1% hydrogen peroxide or with povidone iodine solution. It is important to encourage patients to maintain their habitual hygiene measures after the procedure and to clean the wound area with a relatively soft toothbrush. The sutures are generally removed after a week (Figs 10-34 and 10-35). A clinical and radiographic check-up takes place 1 year after the apicoectomy (Figs 10-36 to 10-39). If the tooth is fitted with a provisional restoration, a clinical and radiographic check-up is recommended after 6 months. Freedom from clinical symptoms once the intervention-related complaints have subsided as well as radiographic consolidation define the success criteria for apicoectomies (Figs 10-40 and 10-41).

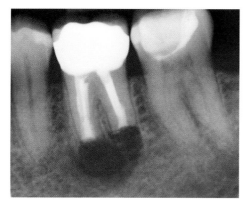
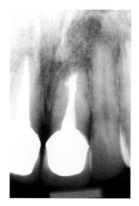

Figs 10-30 and 10-31 Single-tooth radiographs immediately after surgery.

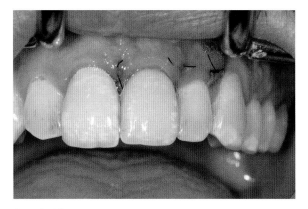

Fig 10-32   Recall 2 days after apicoectomy.

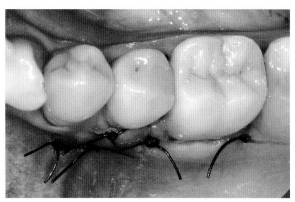

Fig 10-33   Slight plaque accumulation 2 days post-operatively.

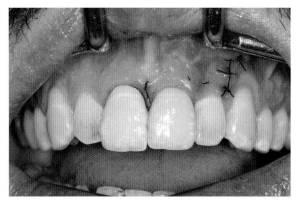

Fig 10-34   Recall after 1 week, at the time of suture removal.

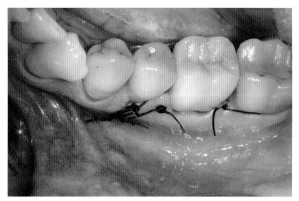

Fig 10-35   Situation 1 week after apicoectomy.

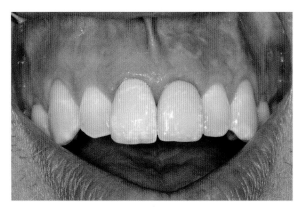

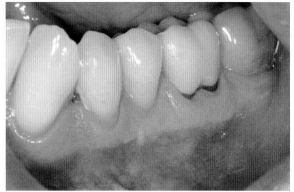

Figs 10-36 and 10-37   Clinical views 1 year after apicoectomy.

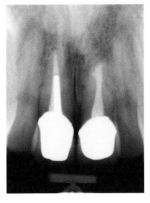 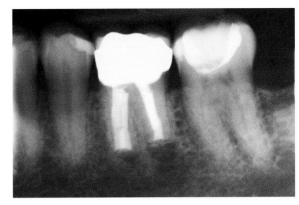

Figs 10-38 and 10-39 Control radiographs 1 year after apicoectomy.

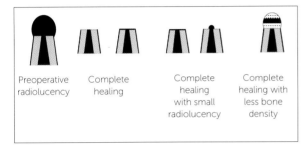

Fig 10-40 Possible radiographic findings assessed as treatment success 1 year after apicoectomy (adapted from Molven et al[3]).

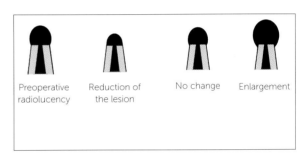

Fig 10-41 Possible radiographic findings assessed as treatment failure 1 year after apicoectomy (adapted from Molven et al[3]).

References

1. Kim S: Color Atlas of Microsurgery in Endodontics. Saunders, 2001.

2. Kraus RD, von Arx T, Gfeller D, Ducommun J, Jensen SS: Assessment of the nonoperated root after apical surgery of the other root in mandibular molars: a 5-year follow-up study. J Endod 2015;41:442–446.

3. Molven O, Halse A, Grung B: Observer strategy and the radiographic classification of healing after endodontic surgery. Int J Oral Maxillofac Surg 1987;16:432–439.

4. Ricucci D, Siqueira JF: Fate of the tissue in lateral canals and apical ramifications in response to pathologic conditions and treatment procedures. J Endod 2010;36:1–15.

5. Setzer FC, Kohli MR, Shah SB, Karabucak B, Kim S: Outcome of endodontic surgery: a meta-analysis of the literature – Part 2: Comparison of endodontic microsurgical techniques with and without the use of higher magnification. J Endod 2012;38:1–10.

6. Von Arx T, Peñarrocha M, Jensen S: Prognostic factors in apical surgery with root-end filling: a meta-analysis. J Endod 2010;36:957–973.

7. Von Arx T, AlSaeed M: The use of regenerative techniques in apical surgery: A literature review. Saudi Dent J 2011;23:13–127.

8. Von Arx T, Janner SF, Jensen SS, Bornstein MM: The resection angle in apical surgery: a CBCT assessment. Clin Oral Investig 2016;20: 2075–2082.

Tooth transplantation

11

Andreas Filippi

Nowadays, tooth transplantation is a highly reliable and integral part of oral surgery. The biologic processes following tooth transplantation (healing of the pulp and periodontium) are well documented scientifically and are described in standard textbooks on the subject[1,2]. Equally well documented are the risk factors for failure and how these factors can be influenced (pulp necrosis, infection-related root resorption, invasive cervical resorption, ankylosis)[3]. In principle, any tooth can be transplanted, but the most commonly transplanted teeth are third molars with immature roots and premolars. Strictly speaking, transplantation of first or second molars as well as primary canines should only be performed by very experienced clinicians[4] (Table 11-1). The prerequisites for successful treatment are the patient's cooperation, the correct timing of transplantation, the choice of a suitable transplant tooth in terms of size and shape, favorable maxillomandibular relationship conditions, adequate space in all dimensions, and sufficient keratinized (attached) gingival width in the recipient region. Transplantation of first molars or primary canines is possible from about 7 years of age, of second molars and premolars from around 10 years of age, and of third molars from roughly 15 years of age.

Indications

Tooth transplantation is now firmly established in dentistry as an alternative to prosthodontic, orthodontic or implantology treatments in the case of agenesis or premature loss of permanent teeth due to trauma or as a consequence of caries, marginal periodontitis or root resorption. Orthodontic, endodontic, traumatologic, periodontologic, and cariologic reasons thus determine whether tooth transplantation is indicated. The most common indications are first or second molars not worth preserving (mostly third molar transplantation) (Figs 11-1 to 11-20), absent mandibular second premolars (third molar or premolar transplantation) (Figs 11-21 to 11-50), and maxillary incisors lost due to trauma or not worth preserving (premolar or primary canine transplantation) (Videos 11-1 to 11-4).

Table 11-1   SAC classification of different autografts and corresponding recipient regions.

Tooth transplanted	Possible transplant location	SAC classification
Maxillary third molar	Maxillary molars (same quadrant)	S
	Mandibular premolars	A
	Contralateral maxillary molars	C
Mandibular third molar	Mandibular molars (same quadrant, contralateral)	S
	Mandibular premolars (possibly rotated 90 degrees)	A
	Maxillary molars (possibly rotated 90 degrees)	C
Maxillary primary canine	Maxillary incisors (possibly rotated 180 degrees)	C
Maxillary premolars	Other premolars	S
	Maxillary incisors (possibly rotated 90 degrees)	A–C
Mandibular premolars	Other premolars	S
	Maxillary incisors	A–C

S, straightforward; A, advanced; C, complex.

Contraindications

Tooth-preserving surgery is basically prohibited in patients with general medical problems such as planned heart valve replacement, antiresorptive therapies, immunosuppression, radiotherapy in the head and neck region, and severe psychiatric or degenerative central nervous system diseases. This applies equally to tooth transplantation.

As well as general medical contraindications and aspects of the risk–benefit assessment, which apply to all (elective) oral surgery procedures, poor compliance and advanced marginal periodontitis (as a matter of principle) as well as infections in the donor and recipient region are temporary contraindications for transplantation. In the Department of Oral Surgery in Basel, transplantations are generally only performed before jawbone and bodily growth is completed and ideally before root growth of the transplanted teeth is completed, hence at an age when implants are not yet possible (and will not be for some time).

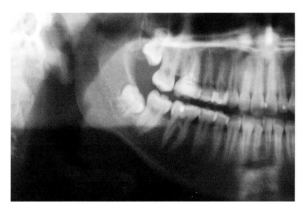

Fig 11-1 Pulp necrosis with acute apical periodontitis after multi-surface reconstruction of the maxillary right first molar in a 15-year-old patient.

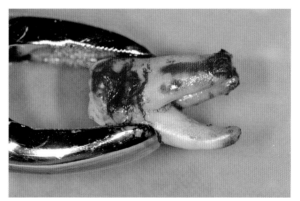

Fig 11-2 Removal of the molar, which could only be preserved at great expense and with considerable effort.

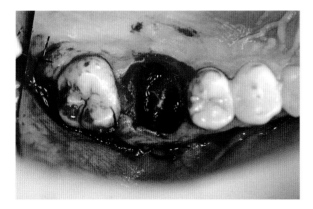

Fig 11-3 Recipient maxillary right first molar region before correction of the interdental septum and after removal of the transplant tooth (the maxillary right third molar).

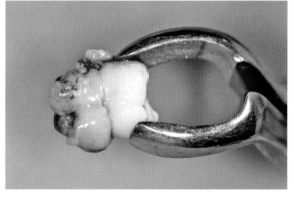

Fig 11-4 The transplant tooth shows an ideal crown-to-root ratio.

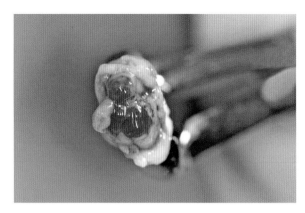

Fig 11-5   The transplant tooth also shows a wide-open apical foramen.

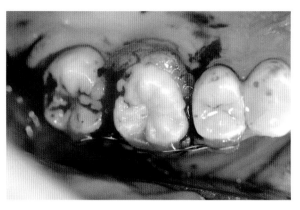

Fig 11-6   Situation after transplantation of the third molar in place of the first molar and splinting.

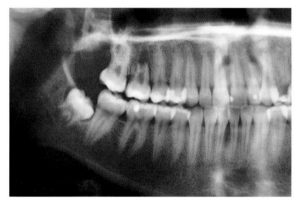

Fig 11-7   Control radiograph after transplantation of the third molar in the first molar region.

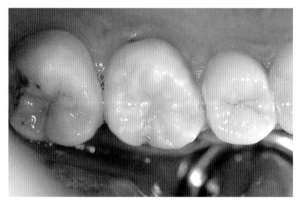

Fig 11-8   Clinical situation immediately after splint removal.

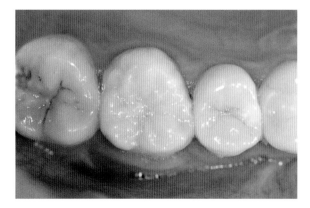

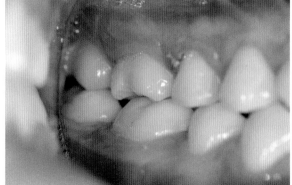

Figs 11-9 and 11-10   Occlusal and buccal views of the clinical situation 1 year later.

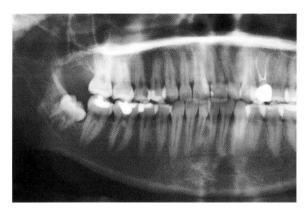

Fig 11-11 Control radiograph 1 year after transplantation showing vital pulp, completed root growth, and vital periodontium.

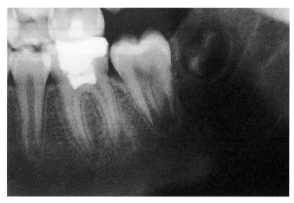

Fig 11-12 In a different case, the situation after pulpotomy and subsequent acute apical periodontitis of the mandibular left first molar in an 11-year-old patient.

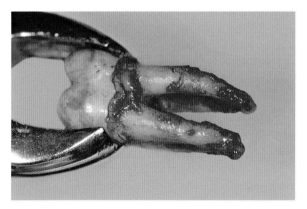

Fig 11-13 Situation after tissue-preserving extraction of the mandibular left first molar with apical inflammatory tissue.

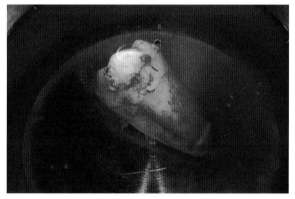

Fig 11-14 Situation after tissue-preserving extraction of the mandibular left second molar and storage in the medium from a tooth rescue box after the addition of NoResorb (Medcem).

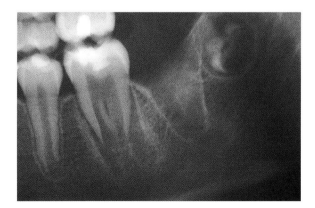

Fig 11-15 Radiograph after subsequent transplantation of the mandibular left second molar in the first molar region.

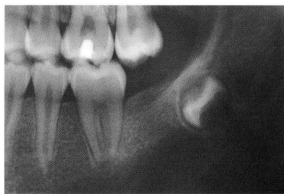

Fig 11-16 Control radiograph of the transplanted tooth 1 year postoperatively showing vital pulp (completed root growth) and vital periodontium.

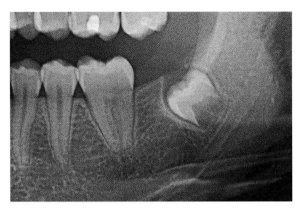

Fig 11-17 Control radiograph of the transplanted tooth and third molar 3 years postoperatively.

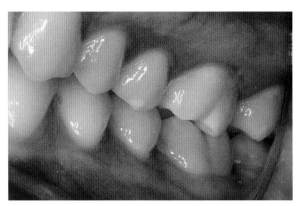

Fig 11-18 Buccal view of the situation 9 years postoperatively.

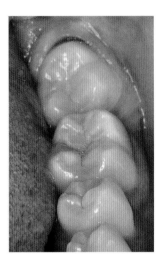

Fig 11-19 Occlusal view 9 years postoperatively. The third molar has spontaneously occupied the second molar position.

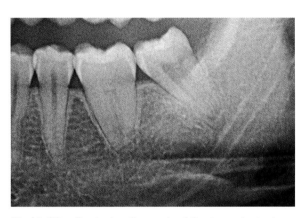

Fig 11-20 Control radiograph of the transplanted tooth 9 years postoperatively shows a perfect outcome with vital pulp and vital periodontium.

Step-by-step clinical procedure

For any tooth transplantation, the transplant tooth is removed in a manner that preserves as much tissue as possible (sharply cutting through the dentogingival seal of teeth that have already erupted) and immediately placed extraorally in a tooth rescue box (Dentosafe or Miradent SOS Tooth Box) (Video 11-1). Periodontal defects caused by the surgeon markedly worsen the prognosis of transplantation and lead to root resorption. The usual antiresorptive additive (i.e. antibiotic, corticosteroid) used in the area of tooth trauma is generally added to the organ

transplantation medium in the tooth rescue box. The transplant remains there for at least 10 minutes. The tooth that is not worth preserving (if it is still present) is also extracted in a tissue-preserving manner (Video 11-2), and the transplant bed in the recipient region is prepared without pressure using rotary instruments (Video 11-3). The ideal distance from root surface to the bony alveolar wall is about 0.5 to 1 mm; at the apex, the distance can be slightly larger without compromising the vital neighboring structures that are present (mental foramen, inferior alveolar nerve, lingual indentations of the mandible, floor of the maxillary sinus). Any kind of flap elevation should be avoided, if possible. The transplant tooth is transplanted in a pressure-free manner into the recipient region without the use of forceps or tweezers (Video 11-4) and fixed mesially and distally to a maximum of one neighboring tooth with a TTS splint (Medartis). In the process, the teeth are placed in occlusion. The occlusion is then checked and slightly corrected, if necessary. The splinting has an influence on the regeneration of the pulp and periodontium. Rigid immobilization increases the risk of ankylosis and has an adverse effect on revascularization of the pulp. In contrast to this, limited movements within the splinting encourage the survival of the pulp and reduce the risk of ankylosis. Furthermore, it is essential to ensure a tight dentogingival seal around the transplant.

Postoperative controls and course

Recalls are carried out after about 2 and 7 days, assuming healing progresses normally. A control radiograph of the transplant should also be performed within this period. This helps to confirm that the transplantation is correct and also serves as a reference image for monitoring the progress of root growth and revascularization of the pulp. Periodontal healing is usually completed within 4 to 8 weeks. The splint is normally removed if the percussion sound matches that of the adjacent teeth and significantly increased mobility is no longer discernible. Reconstruction (perhaps temporary at first) following transplantation into the anterior region can be performed shortly after removal of the splint. Further checks are generally carried out after 3 weeks, 3 months, 6 months, and 1 year. Revascularization of the pulp (with the apical foramen still wide open) can only be assessed on the basis of a control radiograph and not until 9 to 12 months. The most important single-tooth radiograph (in the same way as following traumatic dislocation

Video 11-1
Advanced infection-related root resorption of a maxillary left central incisor, agenesis of a mandibular right second premolar, and tissue-preserving transplant removal of a mandibular left second premolar.

Video 11-2
Tissue-preserving extraction of a maxillary left central incisor that is not worth preserving (infection-related root resorption, buccal fistula).

Video 11-3
Pressure-free preparation of the transplant bed under efficient cooling with sterile isotonic saline.

Video 11-4
Pressure-free transplantation of a mandibular left second premolar into the maxillary left central incisor region without the use of forceps. The emergence profile is determined by the surgeon.

of permanent teeth with the apex still open) is taken 3 weeks after the procedure. If there are signs of pulp necrosis-associated, infection-related root resorption, the tooth must be trephined immediately, and endodontic treatment must be initiated. Advancing root growth and/or obliteration of the pulp are signs of revascularization of the pulp. Pulp tests on transplanted teeth, in the same way as following severe dental trauma, are pointless and yield false negative results. The teeth can be orthodontically moved again 3 months post-transplantation.

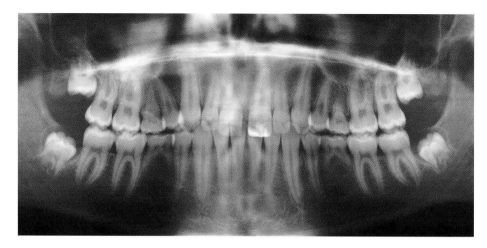

Fig 11-21
Agenesis of all second premolars in a 15-year-old patient. The primary maxillary second molars show hardly any root resorption.

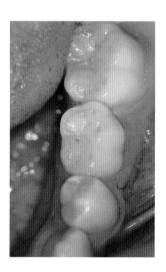

Fig 11-22   However, the primary mandibular left second molar is more mobile due to advanced root resorption. Planned treatment is transplantation of the maxillary third molars in place of the permanent mandibular second premolars.

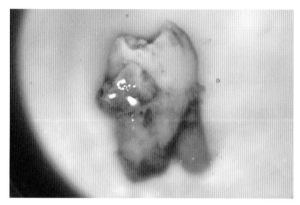

Fig 11-23   One of the two extracted maxillary third molars in the medium from a tooth rescue box after the addition of NoResorb.

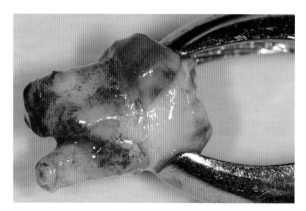

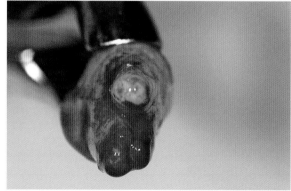

Figs 11-24 and 11-25   Good crown-to-root ratio and open apical foramina of the maxillary third molars.

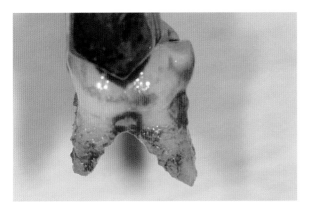

Fig 11-26 Tissue-preserving extraction of the persistent primary molars in the mandible.

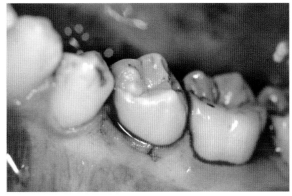

Fig 11-27 Transplantation of the maxillary left third molar in place of the mandibular left second premolar after adaptation of the socket.

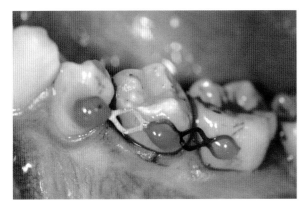

Fig 11-28 The transplant is rotated 180 degrees (buccal to lingual because this orientation is better for the tongue) and splinted in occlusion. The maxillary left third molar is shown here in place of the mandibular left second premolar.

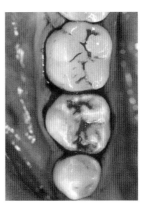

Figs 11-29 and 11-30 The maxillary right third molar in place of the mandibular right second premolar before and after splinting.

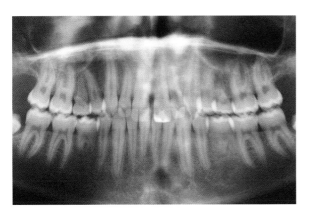

Fig 11-31 Postoperative control radiograph of the two transplants in the mandibular second premolar regions after splint removal.

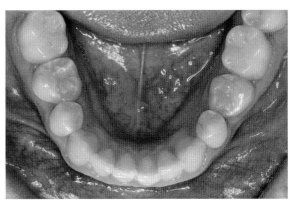

Fig 11-32 Situation 8 years postoperatively: occlusal view.

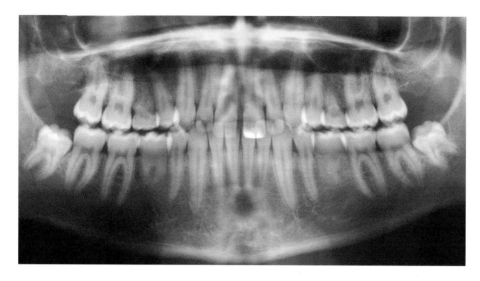

Fig 11-33 Control radiograph of the transplants after 8 years. Perfect outcome with vital pulp and vital periodontium.

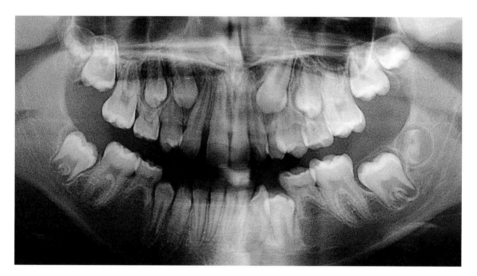

Fig 11-34 Agenesis of the mandibular second premolars (panoramic radiograph taken elsewhere). Planned interdisciplinary treatment is transplantation of the maxillary second premolars in place of the mandibular second premolars as well as orthodontic space closure in the maxilla.

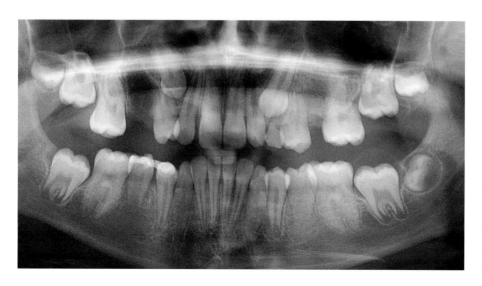

Fig 11-35 The maxillary second molars are inserted, rotated 90 degrees, after tissue-preserving extraction of the primary molars because of the much lower anatomical risk.

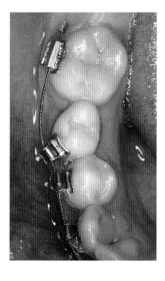
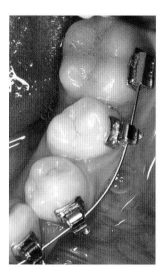

Figs 11-36 and 11-37
Start of orthodontic derotation 3 months post-transplantation on the right and left sides.

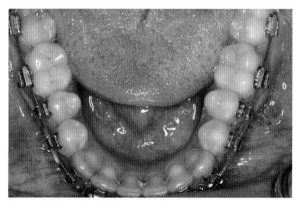
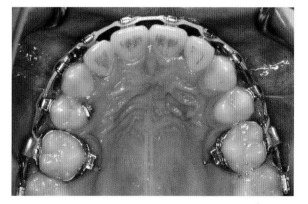

Figs 11-38 and 11-39 Situation 4 years postoperatively and shortly before the end of orthodontic treatment. The transplants are perfectly seated and the spaces are closed in both arches.

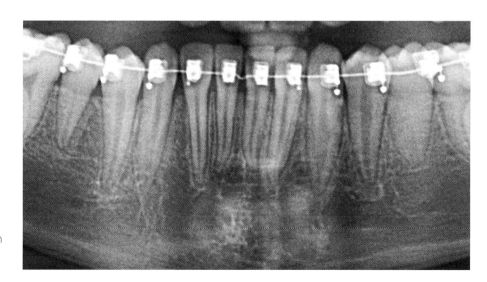

Fig 11-40 Control radiograph of the transplants after 4 years showing a perfect outcome, with vital pulp and vital periodontium.

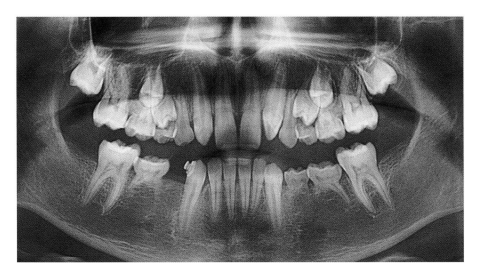

Fig 11-41 Complex case with multiple tooth agenesis, especially in the mandible, in a 15-year-old patient. Planned interdisciplinary treatment is transplantation of the maxillary second premolars in place of the mandibular second premolars, orthodontic space closure in the maxilla, and subsequently two implants in the mandibular first premolar regions.

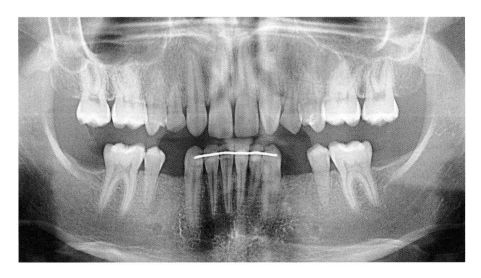

Fig 11-42 Control radiograph of the transplants 5 years postoperatively showing a perfect outcome, with vital pulp and vital periodontium.

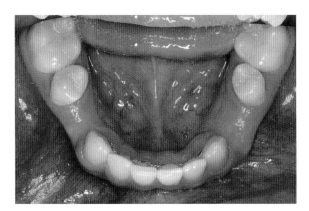

Fig 11-43 Clinical situation 5 years postoperatively. Implant placement will take place within the next few years.

Fig 11-44 Agenesis of the maxillary left first and second premolars as well as both the mandibular second premolars. Planned interdisciplinary treatment is transplantation of the maxillary right second premolar in place of the maxillary left second premolar, then orthodontic space closure in all four quadrants.

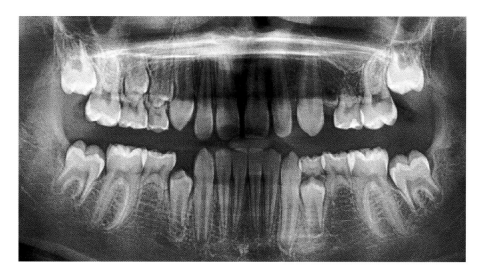

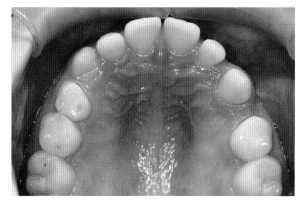

Fig 11-45   Preoperative occlusal view of the maxilla.

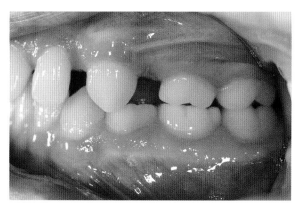

Fig 11-46   Preoperative left buccal view.

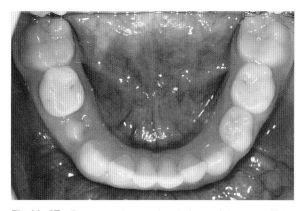

Fig 11-47   Preoperative occlusal view of the mandible.

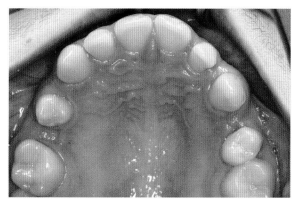

Fig 11-48   Clinical situation 6 months post-transplantation of the maxillary right second premolar in place of the maxillary left second premolar.

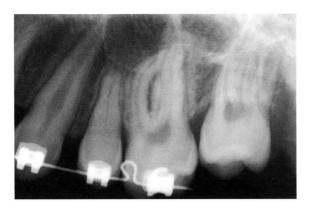

Fig 11-49 A few months later, the transplanted tooth is fully developed.

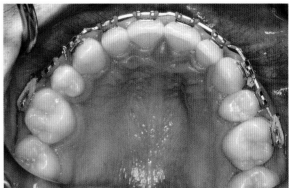

Fig 11-50 Clinical situation 2 years post-transplantation and shortly before the end of orthodontic therapy. The spaces in the maxilla are closed.

References

1. Filippi A: Zahntransplantation. Berlin: Quintessenz, 2009.

2. Filippi A, Kühl S: Moderne zahnerhaltende Chirurgie. Berlin: Quintessenz, 2018.

3. Filippi A: Vermeidung von Komplikationen nach Zahntransplantation. Quintessenz 2016;67: 1447–1454.

4. Mollen I, Bernhart T, Filippi A: Transplantation of teeth after traumatic tooth loss. ENDO 2014;8:301–307.

Recommended literature

Filippi A: Zahntransplantation. Quintessenz 2008;59: 497–504.

Intentional replantation

12

Andreas Filippi

Intentional replantation is an option when an affected tooth suffers from a disease in the root area and intraoral treatment is not feasible or possible from the dentist's or patient's perspective. Both parties decide that the tooth will be extracted with the option of trying to treat it outside the mouth (providing extraction has been carried out in a tissue-preserving manner), and then replanting it.

Indications

The most common indication for intentional replantation is apical periodontitis, when revision of a root canal treatment or an apicoectomy is not wanted or favored by the dentist and/or patient, and yet tooth loss has to be avoided.

The specific reasons for intentional replantation from the dentist's perspective can be many and varied. Examples include a root canal filling that is of a high quality, looks good on a single-tooth radiograph, and was performed by the same dentist; difficult intraoral access for an apicoectomy (e.g. mandibular second molar with an external oblique ridge of about 1-cm thickness before the buccal root surface can actually be seen, and frequent simultaneous lingual indentations in the mandible) (Fig 12-1); anatomically close neighboring structures (e.g. the mental foramen in the case of mandibular premolars, the maxillary sinus in the lateral maxilla, the palatine artery in the case of palatal roots of maxillary molars); and, needless to say, patients who are taking anticoagulants, are immunosuppressed or are of an advanced age and therefore cannot withstand any kind of strain and for whom elective procedures (such as an apicoectomy) are not indicated. In contrast to an apicoectomy, intentional replantation only creates a linear gingival wound – without sutures, without swelling, and with virtually no postoperative problems. In direct comparison, it is considerably more pleasant for the patient.

New crowns on affected teeth, unsuccessful previous apicoectomies (Figs 12-2 to 12-4), concerns about intraoperative and postoperative complications (particularly nerve lesions), postoperative pain, and financial considerations are reasons to favor intentional replantation from the patient's perspective.

A very different indication for intentional replantation is a crown-root fracture (Figs 12-5 and 12-6), which commonly affects the maxillary anterior (and hence single-rooted) teeth. Surgical crown lengthening in the esthetically visible area is not always possible, and orthodontic extrusion often does not function satisfactorily, tries the individual's patience over many weeks, and is rarely esthetically satisfactory or favorable at all because of the increasingly narrow emergence profile.

Contraindications

Intentional replantation is essentially out of the question for patients with general medical problems such as planned heart valve replacement, immunosuppression, radiotherapy in the head and neck region, and severe psychiatric or degenerative central nervous system diseases. It is also contraindicated if tooth roots basically can no longer be preserved (due to all kinds of advanced root resorption, crown-root fractures that end in a far subcrestal position, and longitudinal fractures) (Fig 12-7).

In principle, this technique is also contraindicated for root fractures (intra-alveolar transverse fractures) (Fig 12-8) because their prognosis is excellent even without invasive therapy.

When the risk versus benefit of extraoral tooth-preserving surgery is objectively assessed, the benefit must clearly outweigh the risk as a matter of principle.

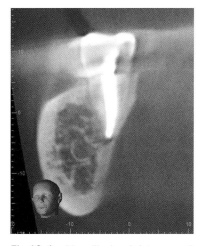

Fig 12-1 Mandibular right second molar on CBCT: Typical anatomical problems in a case of possible apicoectomy.

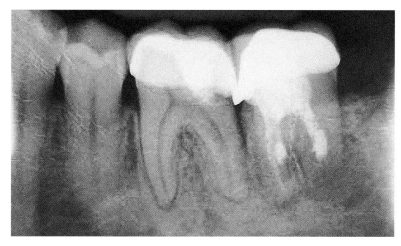

Fig 12-2 Recurrence of apical periodontitis after an apicoectomy was performed on the mandibular left second molar at another dental practice.

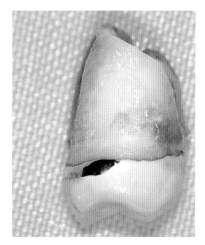

Fig 12-3 The extracted molar shows an unnecessary chamfer at resection.

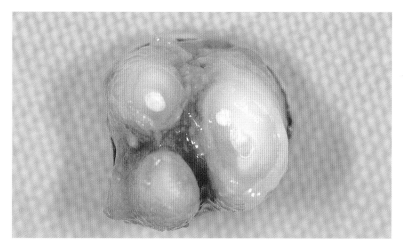

Fig 12-4 The extracted molar also shows a nonresected mesiolingual root tip.

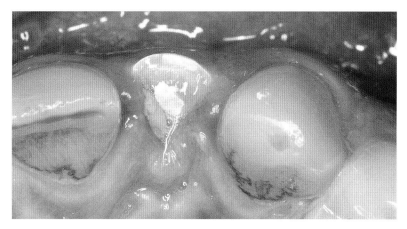

Fig 12-5 Typical crown-root fracture: The fracture ends subcrestally on the palatal side.

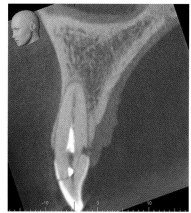

Fig 12-6 Typical crown-root fracture on CBCT.

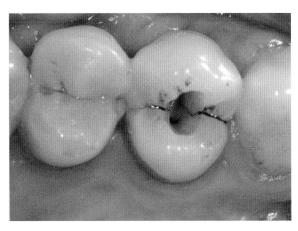

Fig 12-7 Longitudinal fracture of a maxillary premolar that cannot be treated by intentional replantation.

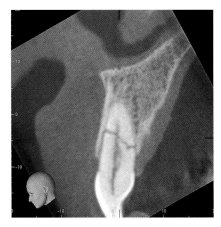

Fig 12-8 Typical root fracture that does not require invasive therapy.

Step-by-step clinical procedure

After appropriate local anesthesia, the procedure starts with an intrasulcular incision to sharply cut through the dentogingival seal (incised wound versus contused lacerated wound). Rapid and uncomplicated healing of this seal is crucial for postoperative periodontal progress. The incision should preferably be made with appropriate circular-cutting micro blades and not with crescent-shaped or pot-bellied scalpel blades (sizes 12 and 15). The tooth (or the root in the case of crown-root fractures) is removed while preserving as much tissue as possible and avoiding levering, tipping or luxating movements. The associated risk of cementum defects, eventual unnecessary ankylosis, root resorption, and tooth loss is too high. For single-rooted teeth, extraction is performed primarily with rotating movements; for multirooted teeth or root remnants, vertical, modern, tissue-preserving extraction techniques such as cow horn forceps or the Benex System (Meisinger) are used. The extraoral time must be kept as short as possible, and mechanical or chemical damage must not be inflicted on the root surface. During the treatment break, however brief, the tooth root is stored in a sterile multipurpose container with organ transplantation medium (e.g. from a tooth rescue box).

The extraoral treatment steps in a case of apical periodontitis are the same as those for a conventional apicoectomy (see Section 10) (Figs 12-9 to 12-41): Resect the root apex, stain with 2% methylene blue (to visualize loose areas of the orthograde root canal filling, dentinal cracks, and longitudinal fractures), perform retrograde ultrasound-driven cavity preparation, dry with short absorbent points, remove the smear layer with PrefGel® (Straumann), rinse and dry again, perform a retrograde filling with hydraulic silicate cement, and remove the filling excess. The entire extraoral treatment is of course performed under optical magnification (endoscope, microscope, strong magnifying glasses) in the same way as for apicoectomies. Immediately prior to replantation, the socket is briefly irrigated with sterile isotonic saline, thereby removing blood or coagulum. The clinician replants the tooth into its original position with their fingers, possibly after prior application of Emdogain® (Straumann) to the root surface if tooth extraction has not been performed in a

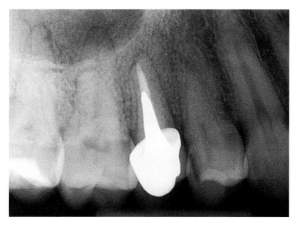

Fig 12-9 Preoperative radiographic situation after post insertion and placement of a new crown on the maxillary right second premolar with symptomatic apical periodontitis in a 32-year-old patient.

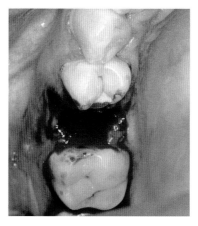

Fig 12-10 Situation after tissue-preserving extraction of the maxillary right second premolar.

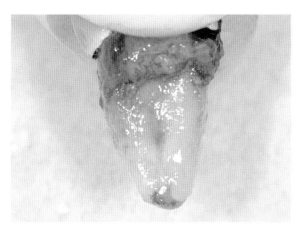

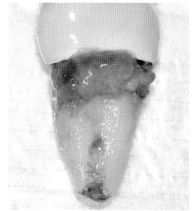

Figs 12-11 and 12-12 The tooth is held by the crown and checked for a possible longitudinal fracture after staining with 2% methylene blue.

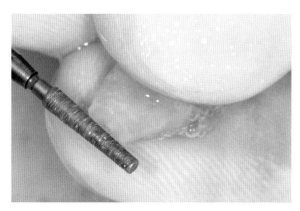

Fig 12-13 Extraoral resection of the root tip.

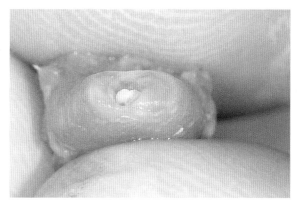

Fig 12-14 After extraoral preparation of a retrograde cavity.

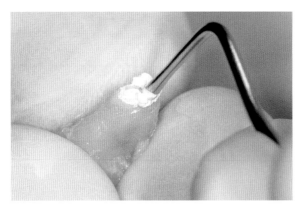

Fig 12-15   Retrograde filling with hydraulic silicate cement (Medcem MTA).

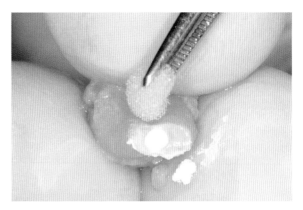

Fig 12-16   The excess is removed with sterile foam pellets.

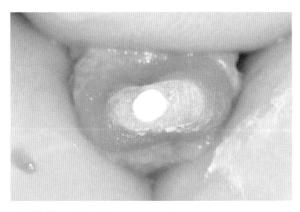

Fig 12-17   After the removal of the excess.

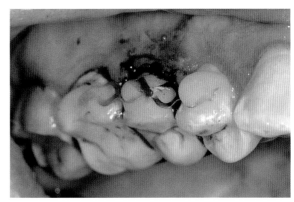

Fig 12-18   After replantation and splinting with a TTS splint (Medartis).

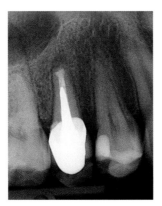

Fig 12-19   Radiographic situation immediately after replantation.

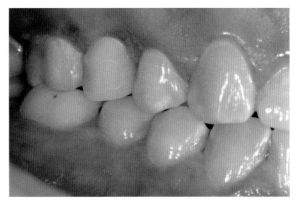

Fig 12-20   Clinically unremarkable situation 1 year later.

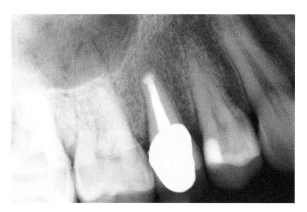

Fig 12-21   Correspondingly unremarkable radiographic findings 1 year later.

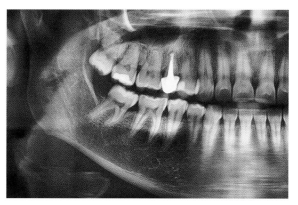

Fig 12-22   Unremarkable radiographic situation 4 years after intentional replantation.

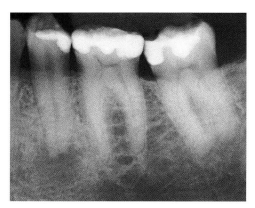

Fig 12-23   Pulp necrosis and apical periodontitis of the mandibular left second premolar in a 49-year-old patient.

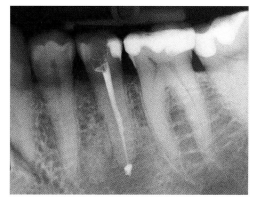

Fig 12-24   Root canal treatment of the mandibular left second premolar performed at another dental practice with some sealant filled beyond the apex.

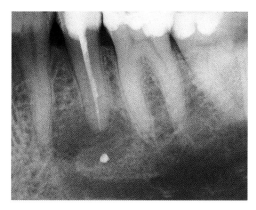

Fig 12-25   Caudal displacement of the foreign material with acute purulent infection and referral to the Department of Oral Surgery at the University Center for Dental Medicine Basel for an apicoectomy.

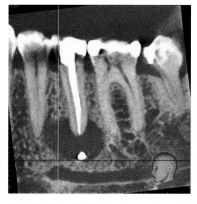

Fig 12-26   CBCT in the region of the mandibular left second premolar: Location of foreign body in relation to the superior edge of the mandibular canal. The patient declined to undergo an apicoectomy because of a certain risk of sensory impairment.

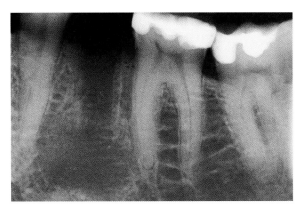

Fig 12-27   Control radiograph after tissue-preserving extraction of the mandibular left second premolar and removal of the foreign body solely by irrigation and aspiration.

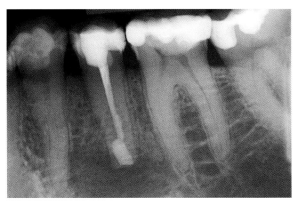

Fig 12-28   Control radiograph after extraoral apicoectomy, retrograde filling, intentional replantation, and splinting of the mandibular left second premolar.

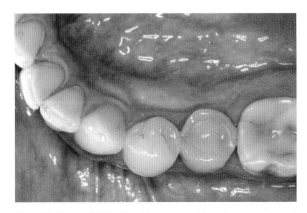

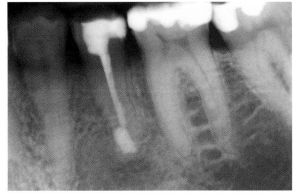

Figs 12-29 and 12-30   Unremarkable clinical and radiographic situation 2.5 years later.

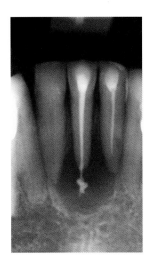

Fig 12-31   Acute apical infection due to massive overfilling of the mandibular right central incisor in a 68-year-old patient. The patient refused to undergo an apicoectomy.

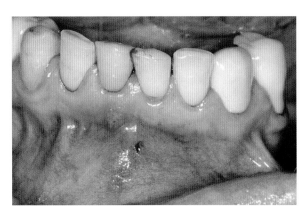

Fig 12-32   Buccally visible fistula in the mandibular right central incisor region.

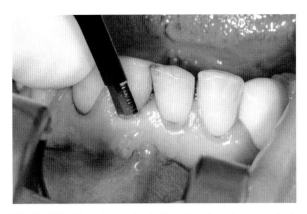

Fig 12-33   The dentogingival seal is sharply separated.

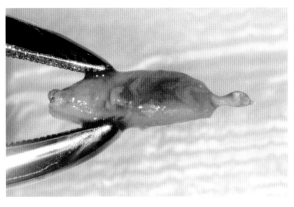

Fig 12-34   Situation after tissue-preserving extraction of the mandibular right central incisor.

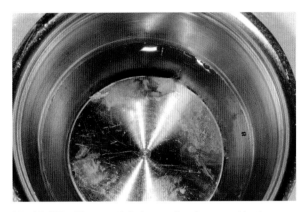

Fig 12-35   The tooth is immediately stored in the medium from a tooth rescue box.

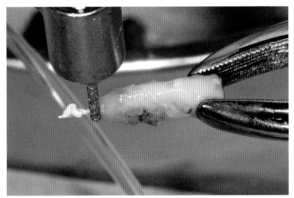

Fig 12-36   Extraoral resection of the root apex: interproximal view.

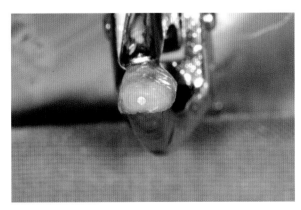

Fig 12-37   Extraoral resection of the root tip: apical view.

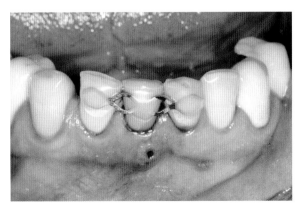

Fig 12-38   Situation after extraoral retrograde filling, intentional replantation, and splinting of the mandibular right central incisor.

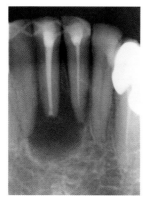 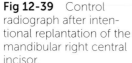 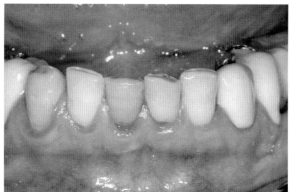 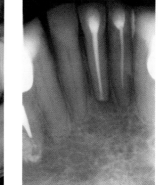

Fig 12-39   Control radiograph after intentional replantation of the mandibular right central incisor.

Figs 12-40 and 12-41   Completely unremarkable clinical and radiographic situation 3 years later.

very tissue-preserving manner. The other two pillars of antiresorptive regeneration-promoting therapy of avulsed teeth (topical and systemic antibiotics and topical steroids)[1] can be dispensed with because the preoperative situation is considerably better and pulp regeneration is not an issue – a great difference from avulsion and tooth transplantation (see Section 11). Papillary sutures are not usually necessary after a tissue-preserving procedure. The subsequent splinting does not differ from that following tooth trauma or transplantation: Condition the (buccal) enamel surface, aspirate and rinse off the etching gel after an appropriate exposure time, dry with an aspirator (not with an air syringe), apply bonding agent without blowing, light cure, and finally fix the TTS splint (Medartis) with light-body, tooth-colored composite with fluorescence. The latter is important to ensure enamel-preserving removal of the splint later[2]. The intentionally replanted tooth is fixed to the splint in its original position and hence in occlusion (with the patient biting). It is essential to avoid premature contacts or malposition. The splint encompasses a maximum of

one neighboring tooth mesial and distal to the replanted tooth. A postoperative control radiograph is taken shortly after the procedure. This helps to confirm that the replantation is correct and also serves as a reference image for recall appointments.

The pulp is often exposed after a crown-root fracture. This should be sealed on the day of the trauma, but intentional replantation should never take place on the day of the trauma. Whether the root canal filling should be carried out before or after intentional replantation must be discussed and decided on an individual basis. The extraoral treatment steps after a crown-root fracture (Figs 12-42 to 12-62) differ fundamentally from those described above. After tissue-preserving extraction of the root, the fracture surface is first inspected for other fractures or cracks by staining with 2% methylene blue. The tooth is then rotated 180 degrees axially (buccal to palatal) and replanted so that the entire fracture gap can be seen just outside the gingiva – a precondition for later crown preparation. This axial rotation improves not only the crown-to-root ratio but also the emergence

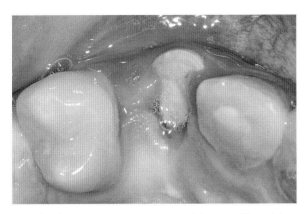

Fig 12-42 Crown-root fracture of the maxillary right canine in a 24-year-old patient.

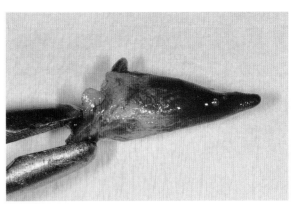

Fig 12-43 Interproximal view of the canine root after tissue-preserving extraction.

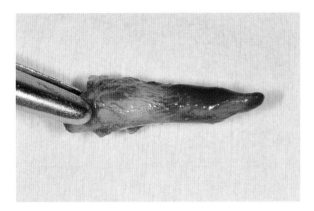

Fig 12-44 Buccal view of the root being held with forceps by the remaining enamel portion.

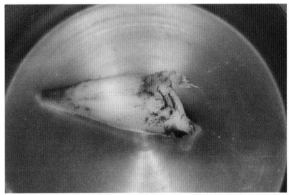

Fig 12-45 Root stored in the medium from a tooth rescue box during each treatment break.

profile, and hence the esthetic outcome at the end of the treatment because the palatal gingival contour lies up to 2 mm more incisally than the buccal contour. As a result of the rotation, the root does not have to be lifted so far out of the socket because in most crown-root fractures the fracture gap ends subcrestally on the palatal aspect and not on the buccal, mesial or distal aspects. The root is fixed in this new position with a TTS splint.

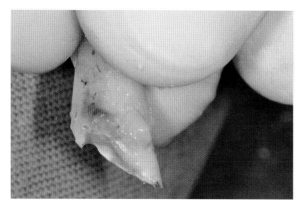

Fig 12-46   Fracture path of a crown-root fracture with the typical palatal subcrestal shoulder.

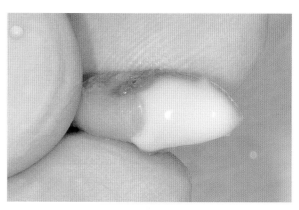

Fig 12-47   Adhesive sealing of the canal entrance for later root canal treatment.

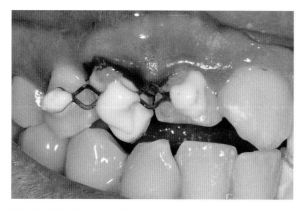

Fig 12-48   Replantation and splinting in supraposition after 180-degree axial rotation (crown-to-root ratio and emergence profile).

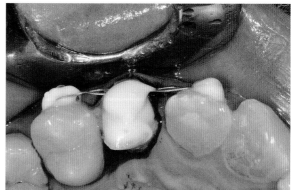

Fig 12-49   Axial occlusal view after intentional replantation.

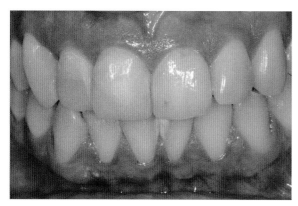

Fig 12-50   Situation 1.5 years later after composite reconstruction of the maxillary right canine.

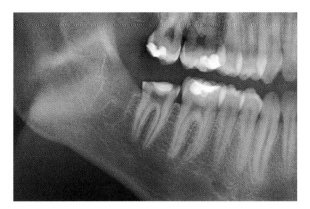

Fig 12-51 Radiographic situation of a crown-root fracture of the mandibular right second molar after surgical extraction of the adjacent third molar at another dental practice. Attempts at crown reconstruction were unsuccessful.

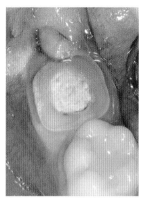

Fig 12-52 Clinical situation with a distally subgingival fracture path.

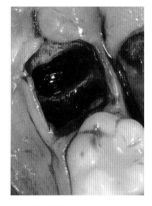

Fig 12-53 After tissue-preserving extraction of the mandibular right second molar (using cow horn forceps).

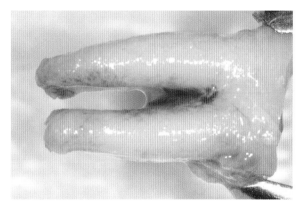

Fig 12-54 The extracted molar.

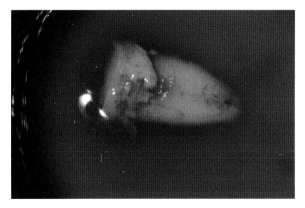

Fig 12-55 The molar placed in the medium from a tooth rescue box.

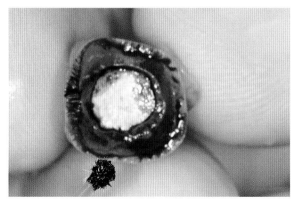

Fig 12-56 The tooth stained with 2% methylene blue to exclude more fractures.

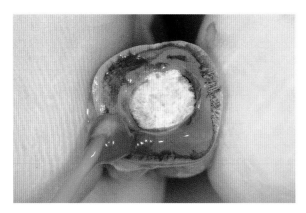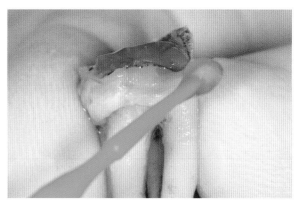

Figs 12-57 and 12-58 Occlusal and buccal views of the adhesive technique for subsequent splinting.

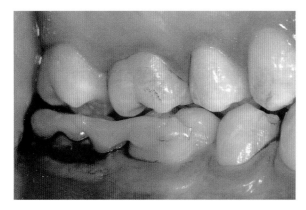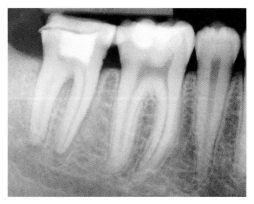

Fig 12-59 Situation after replantation in a 1-mm supraposition without axial rotation and splinting.

Fig 12-60 Radiographic situation immediately postoperatively: 1-mm supraposition.

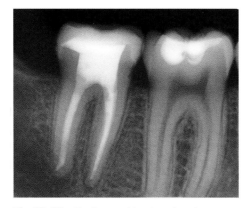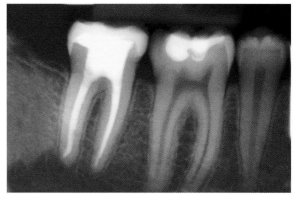

Fig 12-61 Radiographic situation 1 year later, after crown reconstruction and apical ossification.

Fig 12-62 Unremarkable radiographic situation 3 years after intentional replantation of the second molar.

Postoperative controls and course

Recalls are carried out after about 2 and 7 days, assuming healing progresses normally. The splint is usually removed if the percussion sound again matches that of the adjacent teeth and increased mobility is no longer discernible (normally after 2 to 4 weeks).

For teeth with crown-root fractures, buildup in the form of a long-term provisional restoration for about 1 year is carried out at this time. This not only aids visual acceptance by the patient in everyday life but also gives the interdental papillae enough time to assume their final form and position. Further recalls take place at increasing intervals (4 weeks, 3 months, 6 months, and 1 year). After 1 year, another control radiograph is taken and compared with the postoperative image. The periodontal space should be traceable throughout and comparable with the healthy neighboring teeth. Clinically, the tooth should not differ from the adjacent teeth in terms of percussion sound and mobility. For teeth with a crown-root fracture, the definitive fixed reconstruction (crown) is then fitted. The patient can then be switched to normal dental recall intervals.

Long-term clinical experience with intentional replantations is extremely good in the Basel Dental Trauma Center, where they are regularly performed for both of the above-mentioned indications. They have become routine practice, and the extraoral time can consequently be kept short (for apical periodontitis, < 5 minutes; for crown-root fractures, < 1 minute). This is only possible with well-coordinated, experienced teams and has an influence on periodontal healing despite the constant immersion in organ transplantation medium from a tooth rescue box. Before intentional replantation, patients should always be told about the possibility of a tooth fracture during extraction. However, this risk can be significantly reduced by the use of modern extraction techniques compared with conventional tooth extraction. In principle, all replanted teeth can ankylose, but this rarely happens because of the tissue-preserving procedure described above. The average age of the patients concerned is usually much higher than for tooth transplantations (apical periodontitis, > 30 years; crown-root fracture, > 20 years) so that ankylosis would not lead to rapid tooth loss (see Section 13) – quite the opposite of tooth transplantation. If intentional replantation has been performed instead of an apicoectomy, recurrences of apical periodontitis are possible but very unlikely if the procedure is done correctly. It is significantly easier to view the resection surface and make the associated diagnosis than with an intraoral approach. Clearly, the same also applies to retrograde fillings when magnifying aids are used.

References

1.   Pohl Y, Filippi A, Kirschner H: Results after replantation of avulsed permanent teeth. II. Periodontal healing and the role of physiologic storage and antiresorptive-regenerative therapy (ART). Dent Traumatol 2005;21:93–101.

2.   Saccardin F, Ortiz V, Dettwiler C, Connert T, Filippi A: Removal of composite-bonded trauma splints using the Fluorescence-aided Identification Technique (FIT). Quintessence Int 2019;50:456–460.

Recommended literature

Filippi A, von Arx T, Lussi A: Comfort and discomfort of dental trauma splints – a comparison of a new device (TTS) with three commonly used splinting techniques. Dent Traumatol 2002;18:275–280.

Filippi A: Reimplantation nach Trauma: Einfluss der Schienung auf die Zahnbeweglichkeit. Z Zahnärztl Implantol 2000;16:8–10.

Joos M, Filippi A: Intentionelle Replantation statt Wurzelspitzenresektion. Quintessenz 2018;69:52–57.

12 Intentional replantation

Krastl G, Weiger R, Filippi A: Grenzfälle der Zahn-erhaltung: Intraalveoläre Transplantation und intentionelle Replantation im Frontzahngebiet. Zahnmedizin Up2date 2015;9:15–30.

Mukaddam K, Filippi A: Intentionelle Replantation als Alternative zur chirurgischen Kronen-verlängerung. Quintessenz 2019;70:88–94.

Von Arx T, Filippi A, Lussi A: Comparison of a new dental trauma splint device (TTS) with three commonly used splinting techniques. Dent Traumatol 2001;17:266–274.

Transreplantation

13

Andreas Filippi

The term *transreplantation* is rather clumsy and has been repeatedly debated, but, as yet, no other term has prevailed, and an increasing number of publications to date use this term. The prefix "trans" describes the fact that, depending on the case, the tooth is replanted into a different position within its socket; this is actually exactly the same as for intentional replantation of teeth with a crown-root fracture. Essentially, transreplantation is merely intentional replantation but with an entirely different indication.

Indications

The most important indication for transreplantation is terminal marginal periodontitis, which is associated with probing depths in the two-digit range, severe loosening, elongation, and/or malpositioning of the affected tooth. For both the dentist and patient, it is clear that the tooth has to be extracted because the patient's quality of life is greatly reduced: the tooth threatens to fall out, can no longer be used functionally, and is constantly subject to local infections. The problem following tooth extraction is ongoing treatment of the resulting space, especially in an esthetically visible area. Due to considerable local bone loss, implants are not feasible or only with major surgical effort and financial expense, while the neighboring teeth are rarely suitable periodontally to serve as abutments for a fixed tooth-supported reconstruction. The indication for transreplantation should be confined to single teeth.

An alternative indication for transreplantation is avulsed teeth that are only discovered days or weeks after trauma-induced tooth loss and are to be preserved despite an epithelialized or even (partially) ossified socket. Transreplantations should usually only be performed in adults, and long after jaw and bodily growth is completed.

Contraindications

Possible contraindications arise solely from general medical problems or from the fact that the patient will not consent to an attempt at extraoral surgical tooth preservation.

Step-by-step clinical procedure

If transreplantation is performed because of terminal marginal periodontitis (Figs 13-1 to 13-36), an intrasulcular incision is made after appropriate local anesthesia. The greatly loosened tooth is generally extracted. No allowance needs to be made for the virtually nonexistent vital periodontal cells. As a rule, substantial marginal parts of the socket are already lined with epithelium. This epithelium must be entirely removed, and the underlying bone must be exposed. First, an intrasulcular incision is made, which should roughly coincide with the diameter and shape of the tooth that has just been extracted. Thereafter, the socket is deepithelialized in the apical direction.

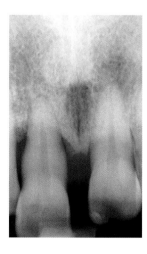

Fig 13-1 Radiograph showing terminal marginal periodontitis of the maxillary right central incisor in a 46-year-old patient with a midline diastema after several periodontal attempts at preserving the tooth.

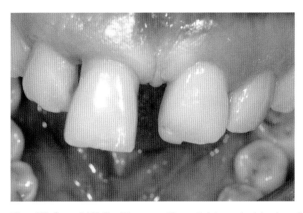 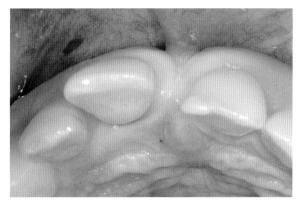

Figs 13-2 and 13-3   The maxillary right central incisor is extruded, severely loosened, and inclined buccally.

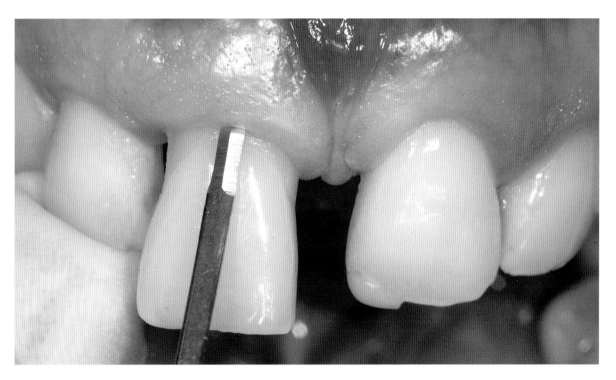

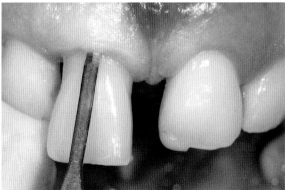 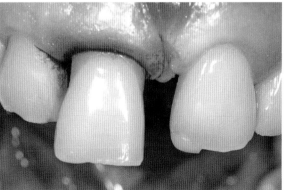

Figs 13-4 to 13-6   An intrasulcular incision is made with circular cutting micro scalpels to completely detach the dentogingival seal.

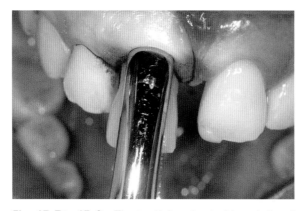
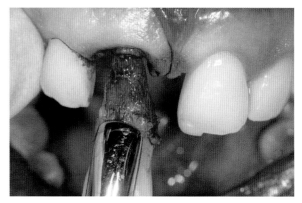

Figs 13-7 to 13-9   The tooth is extracted by rotating it and carefully lifting it out of the socket.

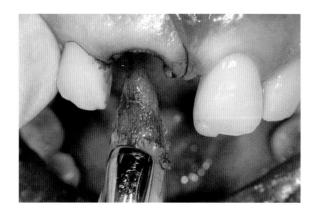
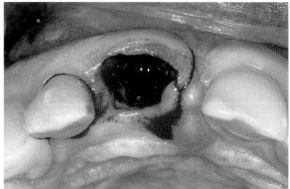

Fig 13-10   Occlusal view of the empty socket.

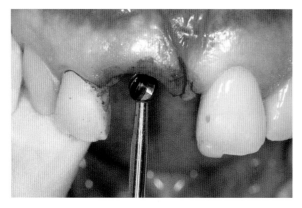
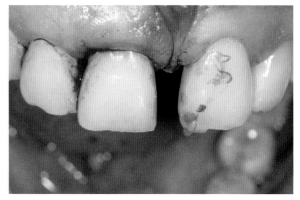

Figs 13-11 and 13-12   The socket is carefully deepened until the extruded tooth can be brought into its original position.

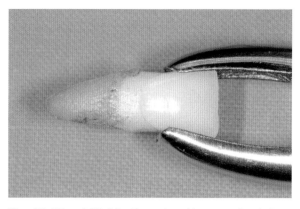 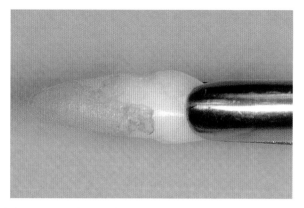

Figs 13-13 and 13-14 Buccal and interproximal views of the extracted central incisor.

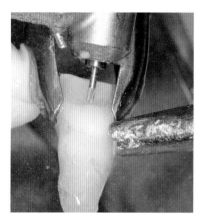 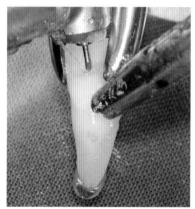 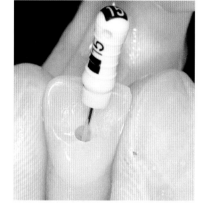

Figs 13-15 and 13-16 Extraoral trephination of the tooth, during which the tooth is held with forceps by the crown.

Fig 13-17 Extirpation of the pulp.

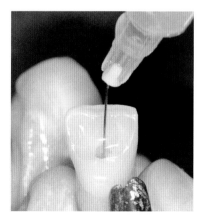 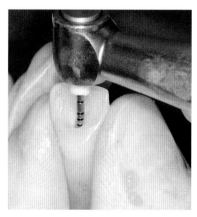 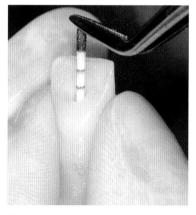

Fig 13-18 Disinfectant and tissue-dissolving rinses of the root canal.

Fig 13-19 Preparation of the root canal.

Fig 13-20 Drying with absorbent paper points.

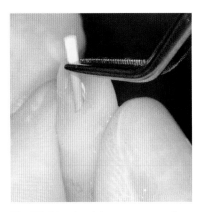

Fig 13-21   Applying gutta-percha point and sealant.

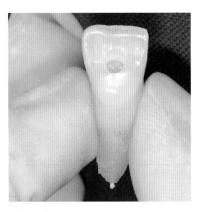

Fig 13-22   Situation after clearing gutta-percha and sealant remnants from the coronal pulp.

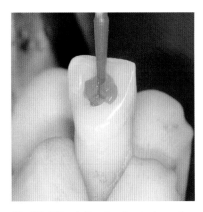

Fig 13-23   Adhesive technique for sealing the trephination opening palatally.

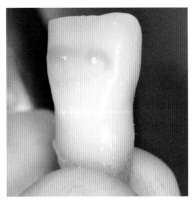

Fig 13-24   At the same time, adhesive is applied buccally for fixing the splint.

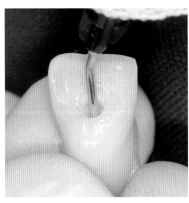

Fig 13-25   Sealing the trephination opening with composite.

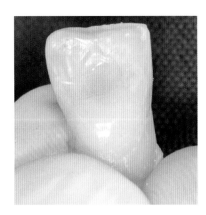

Fig 13-26   The excess is removed and the surface is polished.

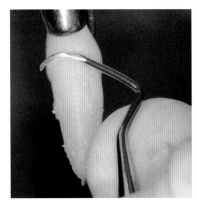

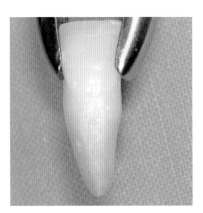

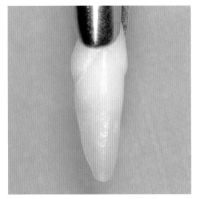

Figs 13-27 to 13-29   Thorough mechanical removal of the entire necrotic residual periodontal ligament and excess apical filling material until the root surface shines on all sides.

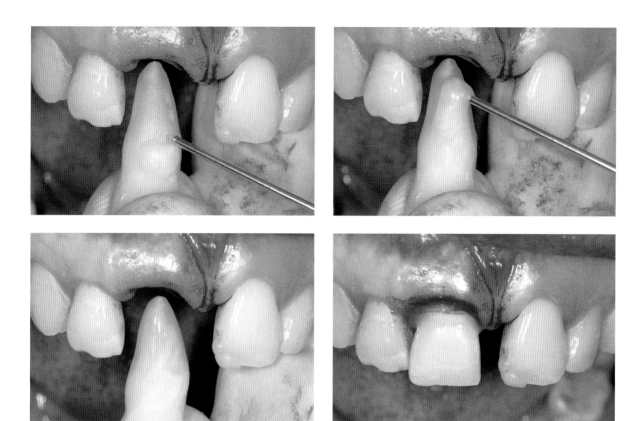

Figs 13-30 to 13-33 Immediately before replantation, after drying the root with an aspirator, Emdogain® (Straumann) is applied to the entire root surface and the tooth is replanted in its original position.

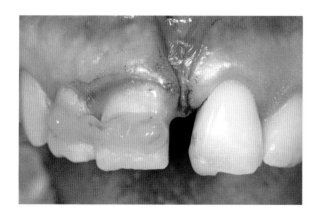

Fig 13-34 Rigid splinting with a TTS splint (Medartis).

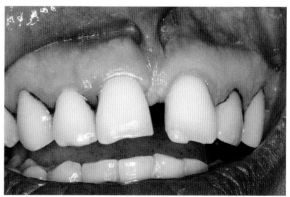

Fig 13-35 After 18 months, a tooth without increased mobility (ankylosis) and with normal probing depths is observed clinically. The patient is very satisfied (image courtesy of Dr Magali Müller).

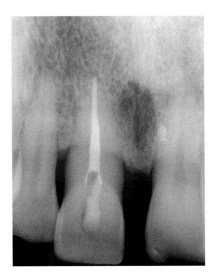

Fig 13-36   Radiographically unremarkable situation of ankylosed maxillary right central incisor after 18 months. Hardly any bone remodeling can be seen (radiograph courtesy of Dr Magali Müller).

If transreplantation is performed because of avulsion with greatly delayed tooth rescue, a completely new socket needs to be created (Figs 13-37 to 13-59). After the appropriate incision on the alveolar ridge, the underlying bone is exposed, and possible granulation or connective tissue is mechanically removed. Once again, it is important to ensure complete exposure of the bone.

If the tooth does not yet have a sufficient root canal filling (which applies to nearly all teeth that are considered for transreplantation), the tooth is held by the crown with anterior dental forceps interproximally and is trephined extraorally. The pulp that has been torn apically by the tooth extraction is extirpated, the root canal is machine-prepared and then irrigated according to the established conventional protocols, and the root canal is filled as tightly as possible. Excess filling material in the area of the apex is then removed under direct vision. Teeth that have

been stored extraorally under nonphysiologic conditions for an extended period undergo an extraoral apicoectomy purely for microbiologic reasons (resect about 3 mm of the root apex with conical or cylindrical rotary instruments, perform retrograde ultrasound-driven cavity preparation, dry with short absorbent paper points, remove the smear layer with PrefGel® [Straumann], irrigate and dry again, perform a retrograde filling with hydraulic silicate cement, and remove excess filling material; see Section 10). The use of magnifying aids improves the treatment. The coronal pulp is cleared of gutta-percha remnants and sealed with composite. This is followed by removal of excess material and polishing. During the acid-etching technique required at this stage, the bonding surface can and should be prepared immediately for eventual splinting. The next step is to denude the entire root surface mechanically with periodontal curettes or scalers; all the remaining necrotic periodontal ligament as well as all types of biofilm must be removed. If the tooth was preoperatively elongated, the socket is deepened in the apical area with rotary instruments under cooling with sterile isotonic saline. The same is done if the socket is partially ossified after delayed tooth rescue. At the end of socket preparation, the tooth must be replantable in its original position without pressure. The tooth is taken out again, rinsed off with saline, and its root surface dried with an aspirator. Emdogain® is then applied to the root surface without prior conditioning with PrefGel®, and the tooth is replanted in its original position and fixed with a TTS splint. Papillary sutures may be necessary; it is essential to aim for a tight dentogingival seal. The splinting employed does not differ from that used following dental trauma, tooth transplantation or intentional replantation. Postoperative antibiotic administration is not indicated in the case of previous terminal marginal periodontitis but is certainly required if tooth rescue has been greatly delayed.

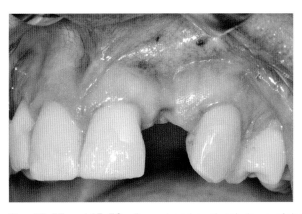 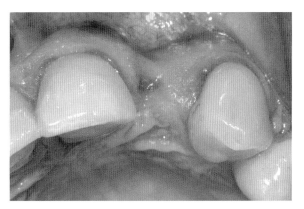

Figs 13-37 and 13-38 Buccal and occlusal views of the clinical situation 4 weeks after trauma-induced tooth loss in a 50-year-old patient. The tooth could not be found.

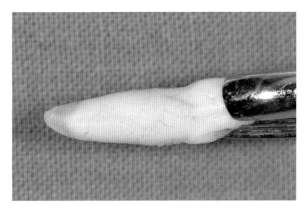 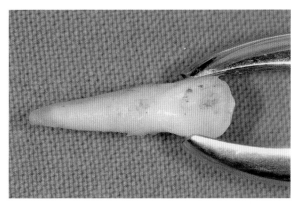

Figs 13-39 and 13-40 Four weeks after the accident, the tooth was found by chance in a roadside ditch, dirty and contaminated.

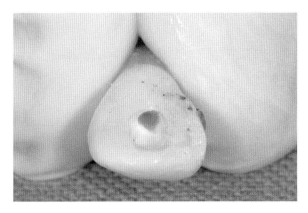 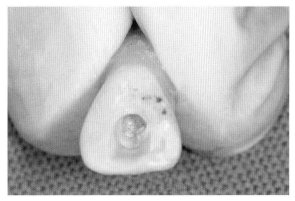

Fig 13-41 Extraoral trephination, pulp extirpation, and preparation of the root canal.

Fig 13-42 Filling the root canal and removal of sealant and gutta-percha from the coronal pulp.

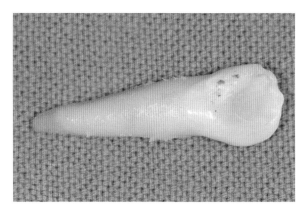

Fig 13-43   Adhesive sealing of the trephination opening.

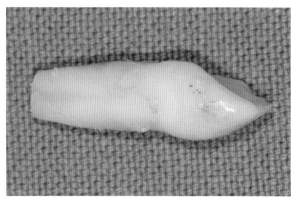

Fig 13-44   Extraoral apicoectomy.

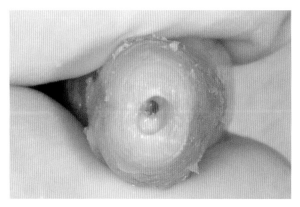

Fig 13-45   Retrograde cavity preparation.

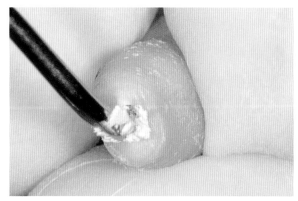

Fig 13-46   Retrograde filling with hydraulic silicate cement (Medcem MTA).

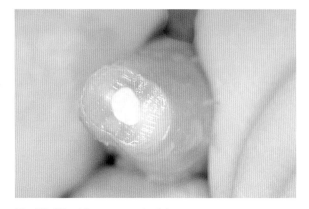

Fig 13-47   After removal of the excess.

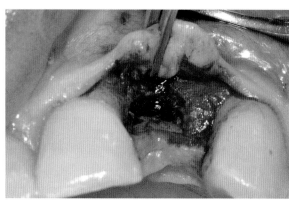

Fig 13-48   Situation after flap reflection: Loss of the buccal wall; the former socket has to be recreated.

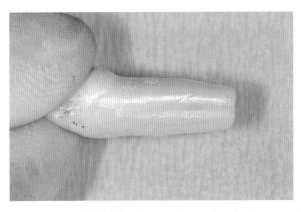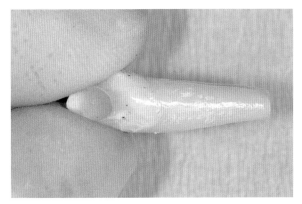

Figs 13-49 and 13-50   Thorough mechanical removal of the entire necrotic residual periodontal ligament until the root surface shines on all sides.

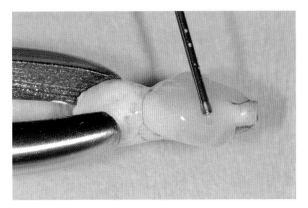

Fig 13-51   Extraoral application of Emdogain®.

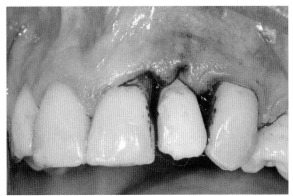

Fig 13-52   Replantation of the tooth in its original position.

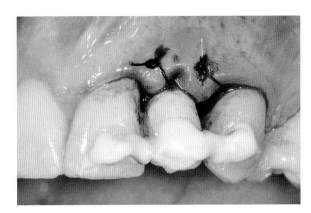

Fig 13-53   Rigid splinting.

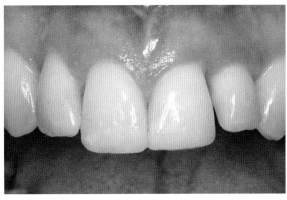

Fig 13-54   After 2 years, a tooth without increased mobility (ankylosis) and with normal probing depths is observed clinically. The patient is very satisfied.

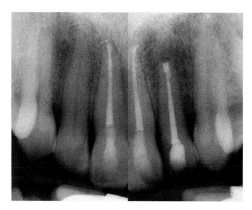

Fig 13-55   Radiographically unremarkable situation of ankylosed maxillary left lateral incisor after 2 years. Hardly any bone remodeling is noticeable.

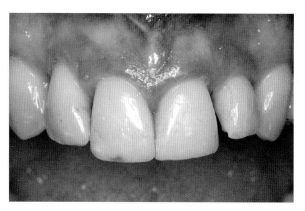

Fig 13-56   Clinical situation 7 years after transreplantation. The patient is very satisfied.

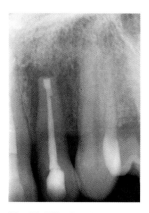

Fig 13-57   Radiographic situation 7 years after transreplantation. There is slight remodeling in the midroot area.

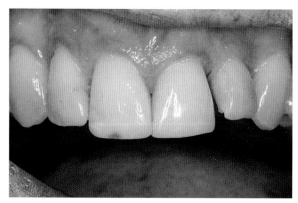

Fig 13-58   Clinical situation 9 years after transreplantation. The patient is still very satisfied.

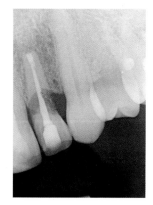

Fig 13-59   Radiographic situation 9 years after transreplantation. Distinct remodeling of the root. Further restoration work will be required in the foreseeable future.

Postoperative controls and course

Recalls are carried out after about 2 and 7 days, assuming healing progresses normally. The splint is normally removed when there is an increased metallic percussion sound. This can take a few weeks, depending on the preoperative situation, and can easily be checked within the splint setup because the TTS splint is flexible. No postoperative complications are to be expected within the first few months after the procedure, with the exception of possible wound infection.

Postoperative invasive cervical resorption was repeatedly reported in earlier publications. They can obviously be avoided by the application of Emdogain® immediately prior to transreplantation. The scientific evidence for this treatment step is minimal but, based on clinical experience nowadays, there is no longer invasive cervical resorption after transreplantation as a result of the described procedure.

Postoperatively, increased probing depths are also not observed in the case of teeth with terminal periodontal disease, provided a good dentogingival seal is achieved intraoperatively and is maintained by the patient through perfect local plaque control within the first week.

Depending on the actual preoperative situation and the patient's age, radiographically visible root remodeling processes may be observed at an early stage, but these usually have no clinical relevance for many years[1]. After bony incorporation has taken place in the sense of ankylosis, the recall intervals can be reduced to once or twice a year and are the same as for routine dental check-ups. If the root is remodeled largely into bone years later, further treatment can be discussed and planned with the patient.

The preoperative situation in these cases is periodontally hopeless. Therefore, the objective should be bony incorporation of the tooth (ankylosis), which is achieved in nearly all cases with the described procedure and when performed by a clinician with relevant experience of extraoral tooth-preserving surgery.

For adults, this means they can keep their tooth for several years even though it was hopelessly diseased or already lost. If more or less complete remodeling of the root into bone has occurred, decoronation (see Section 8) with subsequent implant placement should be carried out or at least considered. The replanted tooth rebuilds the lost bone in the case of terminal marginal periodontitis with two-digit probing depths and/or elongation. Long-term clinical experience with transreplantation is extremely good at the Basel Dental Trauma Center.

Reference

1. Andersson L, Bodin I, Sorensen S: Progression of root resorption following replantation of human teeth after extended extraoral storage. Endod Dent Traumatol 1989;5:38–47.

Recommended literature

Filippi A, Kühl S: Moderne zahnerhaltende Chirurgie. Berlin: Quintessenz, 2018.

Filippi A, von Arx T, Lussi A: Comfort and discomfort of dental trauma splints – a comparison of a new device (TTS) with three commonly used splinting techniques. Dent Traumatol 2002;18:275–280.

Filippi A: Reimplantation nach Trauma: Einfluss der Schienung auf die Zahnbeweglichkeit. Z Zahnärztl Implantol 2000;16:8–10.

Pohl Y, Filippi A, Kirschner H: Results after replantation of avulsed permanent teeth. II. Periodontal healing and the role of physiologic storage and antiresorptive-regenerative therapy (ART). Dent Traumatol 2005;21:93–101.

Pohl Y, Hiedl T: Transreplantation. In: Filippi A (Hrsg): Zahntransplantation. Berlin: Quintessenz, 2009.

Solakoglu Ö, Filippi A: Die Transreplantation – eine Alternative für parodontal hoffnungslose Zähne. Quintessenz 2014;65:1395–1402.

Solakoglu Ö, Filippi A: Transreplantation: An alternative for periodontally hopeless teeth. Quintessence Int 2017;48:287–293.

Von Arx T, Filippi A, Lussi A: Comparison of a new dental trauma splint device (TTS) with three commonly used splinting techniques. Dent Traumatol 2001;17:266–274.

Vestibuloplasty and apically repositioned flap

14

Mathieu Gass, Tobias Fretwurst, Katja Nelson

Indications

Vestibuloplasty serves to improve the denture-supporting area and is considered a method of preprosthetic surgery. In the era of implant dentistry, it is mainly performed in combination with implant treatments. Assessment of alveolar ridge height as well as the quantity and localization of attached and unattached gingiva around the implant will determine whether a vestibuloplasty or an apically repositioned flap is indicated.

An apically repositioned flap is a mucoperiosteal flap that is advanced in an apical direction. This is used in periodontal surgery for reducing pockets or for surgical crown lengthening. In implant surgery, however, a mucosal flap is elevated and serves to widen the peri-implant attached gingiva. An apically repositioned flap can be carried out if there is sufficient alveolar ridge height and an adequate width of attached gingiva.

In a situation where the alveolar ridge height is not sufficient and the transition to the vestibule is flat, alveolar ridge augmentation is required.

This can be subdivided into relative ridge augmentation (deepening the vestibule) and absolute ridge augmentation (building up the alveolar process). Vestibuloplasty denotes relative ridge augmentation and is performed by advancing a mucosal flap apically. This is carried out in combination with secondary epithelialization of the exposed periosteal area or by coverage with a free mucosal or skin graft. Nowadays, vestibuloplasty is mainly performed in combination with a free mucosal graft (see Section 15). Deepening of the vestibule can also be performed using the Obwegeser submucous technique.

Specific risks

Vestibuloplasty and apically repositioned flaps can be employed in both the maxilla and mandible, provided there is an adequate available width of attached gingiva. Damage to the mental nerve is a specific risk in the mandible. To avoid injury to the mental nerve, it is advisable to raise the mucosal flap with blunt scissors.

Apically repositioned flap

Step-by-step clinical procedure

The surgical technique in the presence of implants is described below.

There should be a minimum of 2 mm of attached gingiva around the implant to guarantee long-term implant success. This is particularly important in view of structural differences between the natural tooth and an implant (e.g. lack of periodontal ligament) because plaque

accumulation and microbial invasion will make the peri-implant tissue more susceptible to inflammation and bone loss. Prevention with an adequate width of attached gingiva is therefore desirable.

Given adequate ridge height and width of attached gingiva, the apically repositioned flap can be used when uncovering implants (Figs 14-1 to 14-14). Firstly, appropriate local anesthetic must be administered at the surgical site. This should guarantee an adequate duration of action and minimal intraoperative bleeding (with adrenaline/epinephrine 1:100,000). A panoramic radiograph provides information about the implant regions (Fig 14-1). If the vestibular shoulder of the implant is less than 2 mm from the mucogingival border, an apically repositioned flap becomes necessary (Fig 14-2).

The incision for implant exposure is made into the attached gingiva 2 to 4 mm from the mucogingival border. An apically repositioned

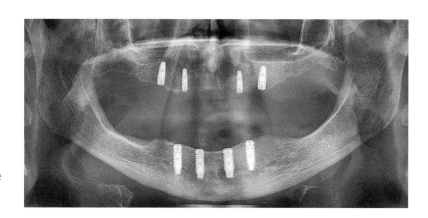

Fig 14-1 Panoramic radiograph after implant placement in the maxillary first molar regions and canine positions and mandibular second premolar regions and canine positions (SICtapered implants in the maxilla and SICace implants in the mandible, SIC Invent).

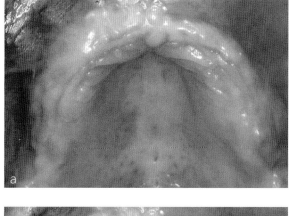

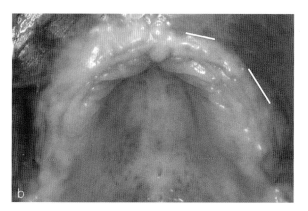

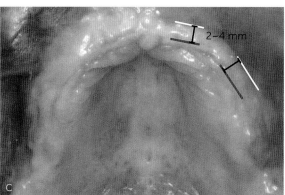

2–4 mm

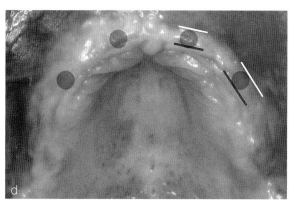

Fig 14-2 Initial situation after implant placement (a). The white line represents the transition between the attached and unattached gingiva (mucogingival border) (b). For uncovering, the same incision path is followed as that already used for implant placement (red line) (c). This incision is made a minimum of 2 mm, preferably 4 mm, from the mucogingival border. The illustrated representation of the implants (gray circles) shows that an apically repositioned flap is needed to generate attached gingiva buccal to the implants and is possible without further scar formation via the incision path already intended for implant placement (d).

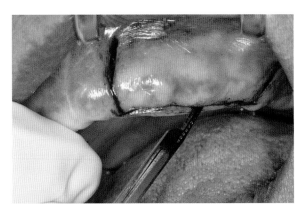

Fig 14-3   The incision is made crestally in the attached gingiva with a 15C scalpel blade to dissect a mucosal flap. The vertical releasing incision is extended mesially and distally into the unattached mucosa. Guidance of the scalpel should always be supported (here on the edentulous jaw; alternatively on the teeth).

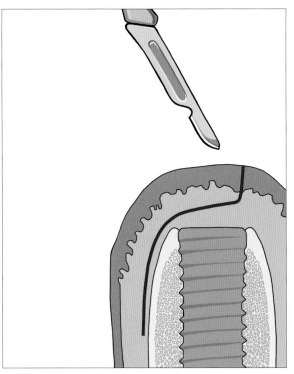

Fig 14-4   Diagram of the incision path for raising a mucosal flap (blue line). After the crestal incision, dissection runs parallel to the bone contour or periosteum.

flap is a mucosal flap. As well as the crestal incision, vertical releasing incisions are made mesially and distally, which are extended into the unattached mucosa, resulting in a trapezoidal flap. This extension of the incision is important for mobilizing the mucosal flap because adequate mobilization is only possible if the incision extends into the unattached mucosa (Fig 14-3).

It is important to ensure that the incision only cuts through the mucosa and stops at the periosteum in order to avoid dissecting a full-thickness mucoperiosteal flap (Fig 14-4). After the incision, the scalpel is reoriented so that the blade for dissecting the mucosal flap is always held and guided parallel to the bone contour. In this case, parallel means that the surface of the scalpel blade follows the curvature of the bone (Figs 14-4 and 14-5a). Continuous dissection in this layer should be ensured (Fig 14-5b). When raising the flap, it is important to maintain

visibility to allow continuous dissection in the desired layer and to avoid perforation of the flap (Fig 14-6). Any thinning of the mucosa can lead to perforation of the gingiva; this is more likely to be an intraoperative risk if the patient has a thin gingival phenotype. Any removal of the periosteum should be avoided. If a periosteal perforation does occur, the exposed bone should be covered with soft tissue. Care should be taken to ensure blunt retraction of the mucosal flap with closed surgical forceps. In this way, injury to the tissue at the flap border can be avoided (Fig 14-6).

After mobilization and apical displacement of the mucosal flap (Fig 14-7), the surgeon should check whether the remaining tissue (periosteum) vestibular to the implant shoulder is mobile. This can be done by trying to move the tissue back and forth with a blunt instrument. The remaining tissue around the implant must

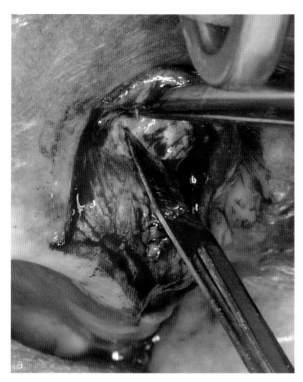 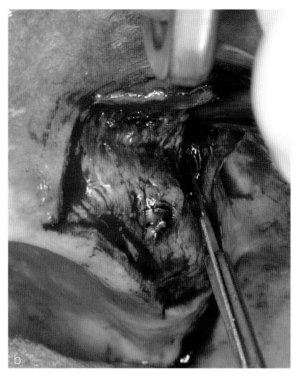

Fig 14-5 (a and b) The scalpel blade is aligned parallel to the bone in order to avoid thinning and perforation of the flap. Adequate dissection must be performed in the mesiodistal and apical directions in the area of the vestibule so that the attached gingiva located at the flap border can be advanced and fixed buccal to the implant.

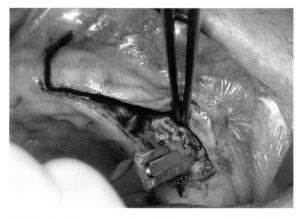

Fig 14-6 Blunt retraction of the mucosal flap with closed surgical forceps in order to avoid injuring the flap border. The incision for mucosal flap elevation is made parallel to the bone contour. It is important to dissect in the appropriate layer (directly above the periosteum) so that the mucosal flap created is not too thin and yet enough periosteum/connective tissue is left around the implants. Initial entry into the correct layer allows rapid dissection. Caution: If the mucosal flap is too thin, there is a risk of perforating the flap and leaving mobile mucosal tissue buccally.

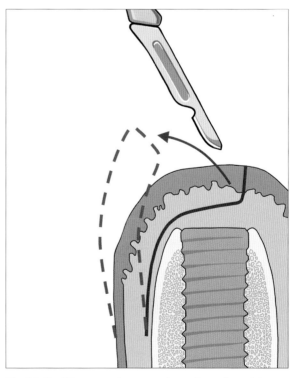

Fig 14-7 Diagram of correct tissue layer for raising a mucosal flap.

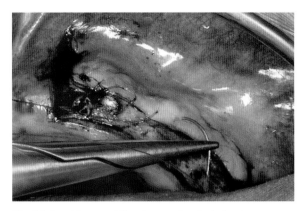

Fig 14-8   After mobilization and apical displacement of the mucosal flap, the flap border is sutured to the periosteum using a micro needle holder and a suitable resorbable suture material in a continuous technique.

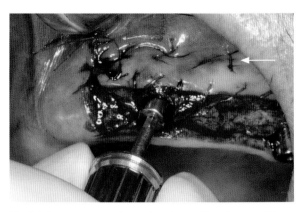

Fig 14-9   Horizontal suturing (arrow) is also used in the vestibule for fixation of the mucosal flap to the periosteum. After flap fixation, the cover screws are removed and the gingival former is inserted.

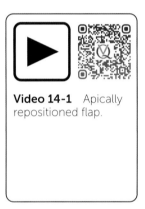

Video 14-1   Apically repositioned flap.

not permit any movement. If this is not the case, it is because the tissue layer was not sufficiently thinned and there are still mobile submucosal structures (attachments) present on the periosteum. In this case, renewed dissection into a deeper layer must be carried out. This "re-dissection" can be avoided with a little practice by initially locating the correct layer.

Fixation of the apically repositioned mucosal flap is carried out with resorbable suture material (5-0). The flap border must be fixed immovably to the periosteum (Fig 14-8). Interrupted or continuous sutures can be chosen for fixation. Another suture for fixing the flap to the periosteum should be placed at the transition

of the mucogingival border or in the vestibule (Fig 14-9). The mobility of the flap border is then checked again. The fixed, displaced part of the mucosal flap must not exhibit any peri-implant movement.

After fixation of the apically repositioned flap, the cover screws are removed and the gingival former is inserted. The gingival former can also be placed before flap fixation, but it makes suturing more difficult (Fig 14-9, Video 14-1).

If there is slight bleeding, electrocoagulation should be avoided because it will impair wound healing; instead, it is advisable to apply a hemostat (e.g. Tabotamp, Ethicon) after suturing is completed. Edentulous patients require

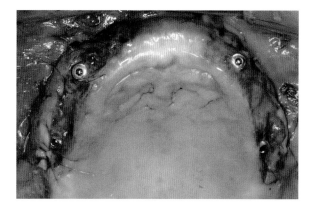

Fig 14-10 Clinical check-up on the first day postoperatively. There are already early signs of non-irritated granulation on the exposed periosteum. The interim prosthesis is ground out intraoperatively and permanently soft relined (Soft-Liner) and the wounds are covered with Tabotamp. The Tabotamp is removed on the first day postoperatively, and wound cleansing is carried out with mucous membrane antiseptic.

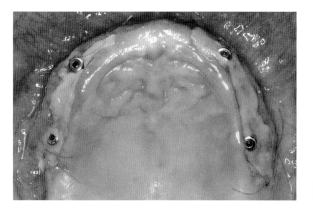

Fig 14-11 Clinical check-up 7 days postoperatively. There is stage-appropriate wound healing with fibrin coating in the wound area.

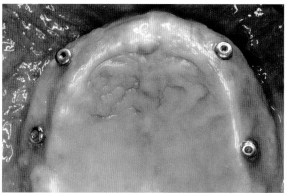

Fig 14-12 Clinical check-up 3 weeks postoperatively. There is sufficient attached gingiva around the four implants.

permanent soft relining (e.g. Soft-Liner, GC Europe) of the ground-out replacement tooth and its immediate insertion for wound coverage. This can also minimize the risk of bleeding.

Postoperative controls and course

Clinical recalls can take place on the first and seventh postoperative days. There are already early signs of non-irritated granulation on the exposed periosteum on the first postoperative day (Fig 14-10). The hemostat applied the day before can be removed, and the wound can be treated with an antiseptic (e.g. Braunol mucous membrane antiseptic, B. Braun).

The clinical check-up after 7 days shows stage-appropriate wound healing with fibrin coating in the wound area. Suture removal does not take place in order to minimize recurrence in terms of shrinkage of the achieved width. Instead, the suture material is left to resorb by itself (Fig 14-11). Three weeks postoperatively, there should be complete granulation of the periosteal wound and hence a stable outcome with sufficient attached gingiva (Fig 14-12). In the case study presented here, an implant-supported bar restoration was carried out (Figs 14-13 and 14-14).

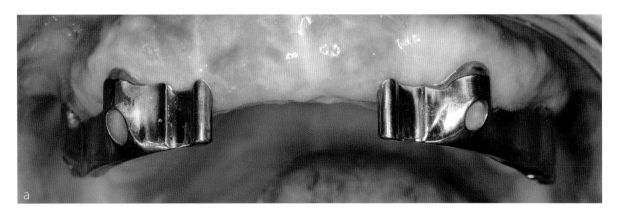

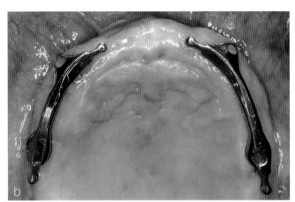

Fig 14-13 (a and b)   Final images with implant-supported bar restoration.

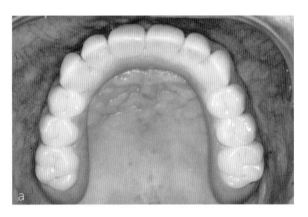

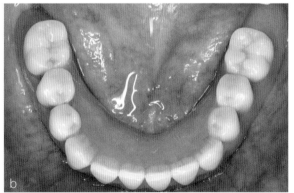

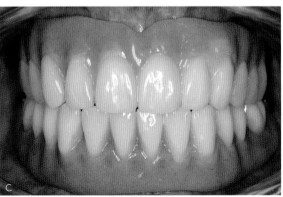

Fig 14-14 (a to c)   Final prosthodontic work in situ (images courtesy of Dr Stefano Pieralli, Department of Prosthodontics, Charité—Universitätsmedizin Berlin).

Vestibuloplasty

In a situation where the height of the alveolar ridge is inadequate or the vestibule is at the same height, relative ridge augmentation in terms of a vestibuloplasty is required (Fig 14-15). The objectives are both to visualize the alveolar ridge and to preserve the attached gingiva around the implants by surgically lowering the vestibule and/ or the floor of the mouth. The procedure follows implant placement during the uncovering of the implants (Fig 14-16). At implant placement, an impression should be taken of the implants so that an implant-supported acrylic splint can be inserted to cover the wound and secure the regenerated vestibule.

Step-by-step clinical procedure

Dissection for a vestibuloplasty follows the surgical technique described for an apically repositioned flap, ensuring that dissection of the mucosal flap always leaves the periosteum on the bone (Fig 14-17). The case study presented here shows a situation after resection of a squamous cell carcinoma in the anterior left mandible with primary wound closure (Fig 14-16). After displacement of the tissue into the floor of the mouth and the vestibule, the mucosal flap is first sutured to the periosteum. Then, a

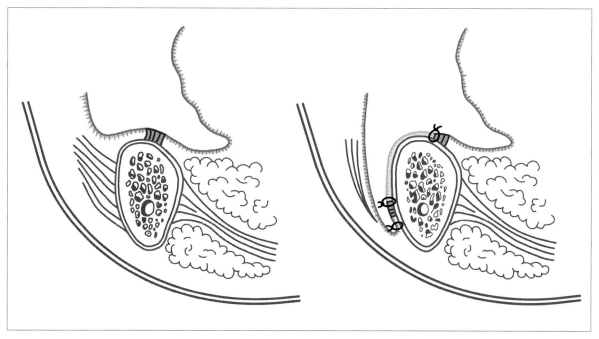

Fig 14-15   Diagram of a vestibuloplasty in the mandible. When raising the mucosal flap (orange), bear in mind that the periosteum (blue) must be left on the bone. The incision is made centrally through the attached gingiva (red), and the tissue is displaced in the vestibular direction and also lingually, if necessary. The graft (yellow) is placed and sutured to the mucosa and to the periosteum. The deep anchoring suture in the vestibule with fixation to the periosteum helps to minimize mobility during the healing period.

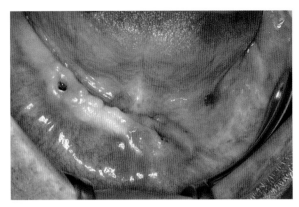

Fig 14-16 Situation after resection of a squamous cell carcinoma in the anterior left mandible with primary wound closure and implant placement without bone augmentation. The lack of attached gingiva is clearly seen.

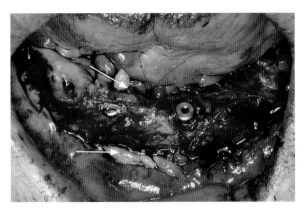

Fig 14-17 After a mucosal flap is raised, it is sutured to the periosteum (arrows) on the lingual and vestibular aspects with a continuous resorbable suture material (5-0) to create a new vestibule. The periosteum is left on the bone.

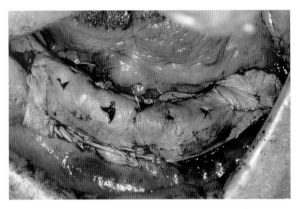

Fig 14-18 Placement of a split-thickness graft (0.4-mm thick) harvested from the thigh with a dermatome, which is fixed to the periosteum with resorbable suture material (5-0).

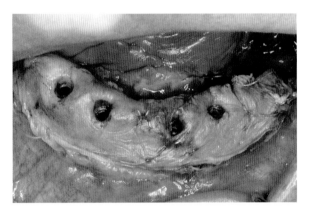

Fig 14-19 Clinical situation 1 week postoperatively.

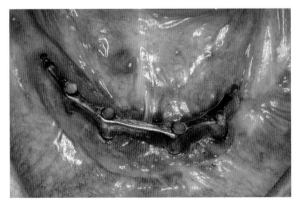

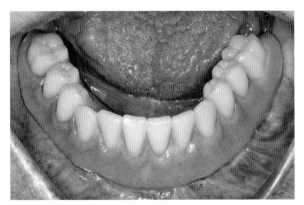

Figs 14-20 and 14-21 Clinical views 1.5 years after placement of the restoration (Prosthodontics by Dr A. Trinkner, Department of Prosthodontics, University of Freiburg).

split-thickness graft harvested from the thigh (0.4-mm thick) is laid onto the periosteum and fixed with continuous sutures (Fig 14-18). The acrylic splint is intraoperatively adapted (e.g. Coe-Pack, GC Europe) and can be fixed to either the residual dentition or to the implants

to guarantee secure fixation. A closed wound surface and contouring of the vestibule can be seen 1 week postoperatively (Fig 14-19). At the follow-up 1.5 years after insertion of the restoration, the soft tissue conditions are stable (Figs 14-20 and 14-21).

Recommended literature

Brito C, Tenenbaum HC, Wong BK, Schmitt C, Nogueira-Filho G: Is keratinized mucosa indispensable to maintain peri-implant health? A systematic review of the literature. J Biomed Mater Res B Appl Biomater 2014;102:643–650.

Buyukozdemir Askin S, Berker E, Akincibay H, Uysal S, Erman B, Tezcan İ, Karabulut E: Necessity of keratinized tissues for dental implants: a clinical, immunological, and radiographic study. Clin Implant Dent Relat Res 2015;17:1–12.

Chung DM, Oh TJ, Shotwell JL, Misch CE, Wang HL: Significance of keratinized mucosa in maintenance of dental implants with different surfaces. J Periodontol 2006;77:1410–1420.

Heberer S, Nelson K: Clinical evaluation of a modified method of vestibuloplasty using an implant-retained splint. J Oral Maxillofac Surg 2009;67: 624–629.

Ladwein C, Schmelzeisen R, Nelson K, Fluegge TV, Fretwurst T: Is the presence of keratinized mucosa associated with periimplant tissue health? A clinical cross-sectional analysis. Int J Implant Dent 2015;1:11.

Lin GH, Chan HL, Wang HL: The significance of keratinized mucosa on implant health: a systematic review. J Periodontol 2013;84:1755–1767.

Thoma DS, Naenni N, Figuero E, Hämmerle CHF, Schwarz F, Jung RE, Sanz-Sánchez I: Effects of soft tissue augmentation procedures on peri-implant health or disease: A systematic review and meta-analysis. Clin Oral Implants Res 2018;29(Suppl 15):32–49.

Thoma DS, Buranawat B, Hämmerle CH, Held U, Jung RE: Efficacy of soft tissue augmentation around dental implants and in partially edentulous areas: a systematic review. J Clin Periodontol 2014;41(Suppl 15):77–91.

Autologous soft tissue grafts

15

Henrik Dommisch, Frank Peter Strietzel

All the techniques used to harvest autologous grafts genuinely enhance the range of possibilities in medicine. Autologous soft tissue grafts offer a number of biologic advantages[31]. These include not only the obvious advantages of immunologic acceptance in the recipient region and the associated good incorporation of grafts. In the case of oral soft tissue grafts, the advantages also lie in their histologic and structural similarities with the recipient region. This means that, due to connective tissue augmentation, the shape, color, and structure of the augmented area is identical to the adjacent tissue[8,15].

Harvesting of a free mucosal graft is a surgical technique that involves obtaining a full-thickness epithelial tissue segment, including epithelium and connective tissue, from the palatal mucosa (fibroepithelial mucosa). The purpose of this grafting technique is primarily to transplant a full-thickness free gingival graft to the recipient region, to increase the area of keratinization, to augment the soft tissue, and to increase the gingival thickness in that region[27].

Harvesting of autologous connective tissue is another surgical technique that involves the anatomical region of the palate as the donor region. A number of techniques are available for harvesting connective tissue, which take into account the relevant anatomical variations of the palatal mucosa. Grafting of connective tissue can have a variety of objectives. On the one hand, the grafted tissue helps to increase volume in the recipient region, and, on the other hand, connective tissue augmentation helps to widen the vestibular keratinized gingiva[17].

Aspects of the different indications through the practical clinical procedures for autologous soft tissue grafts are examined in detail in this section.

Indications for harvesting a free mucosal graft

Transplantation of a free mucosal graft is considered if the keratinized gingiva is to be widened and thickened. In some cases, a free mucosal graft can be used to completely build up keratinized tissue. In mucosal areas around dental implants, there may be an absolute absence of keratinized epithelial tissue. Therefore, in recent decades, the range of indications for free mucosal grafts has expanded accordingly, and they can be used for soft tissue augmentation in the context of vestibuloplasty (see Section 14), preprosthetic soft tissue rehabilitation, implant therapy (e.g. as a so-called mucosal patch in the course of ridge preservation), and treatment of peri-implantitis[12,14,26,27,31]. In addition, augmentation of peri-implant mucosa in the absence of keratinized mucosa can be obtained with the aid of a graft harvested from the palatal mucosa with fully or partially keratinized areas. Thus, the peri-implant mucosa can be augmented with respect to peri-implant tissue volume. Partially keratinized mucosal grafts are used for the purpose of recession coverage in the case of peri-implant soft tissue defects.

In periodontology, grafting of free mucosa is indicated during the coverage of vestibular recessions. However, this indication area has narrowed considerably recently because a color discrepancy between the graft and recipient tissue can often result, and techniques such as connective tissue grafts or the application of collagen matrices demonstrate clinically excellent results after recession coverage.

Indications for harvesting a connective tissue graft

Autologous connective tissue grafts from the palatal mucosa have a wide spectrum of variable indications[24]. They are used for the augmentation of vestibular soft tissue in terms of thickening the vestibular mucosa, with the aim of increasing the width of keratinized gingiva. In this context, the grafting of connective tissue is indicated for covering gingival or mucosal recessions around teeth and implants, correction of peri-implant mucosa, soft tissue thickening prior to orthodontic treatment, preprosthetic augmentation, reconstruction of the alveolar ridge following extraction defects, papilla reconstruction, and coverage of dehiscences in the context of ridge preservation measures[7,8,10,15,17,21,31,32].

When there is an indication for autologous soft tissue grafts, it is always important that the practical procedure, preconditions, postoperative care or behavior, and also the possible risks and complications associated with the procedure are fully explained to the patient. In this context, treatment alternatives should always be offered, and the considerations associated with two intraoral surgical sites should be explained in detail. The use of collagen matrices (xenogeneic material) is one treatment alternative for both graft types. The postoperative results are equally acceptable but, in many cases, inferior to autologous grafts[3,9,11]. The advantage of these matrices is that the second intraoral procedure on the palate, and hence the associated complications, can be avoided[4,19].

Contraindications

Patients with an increased general medical risk profile are among the absolute contraindications. This includes patients with hereditary and acquired forms of hemorrhagic diathesis, immunosuppressed patients or those receiving immunosuppressant treatment, intraoral malignant changes (including potentially malignant oral lesions such as forms of leukoplakia and erythroplakia), concurrent chemotherapy,

previous radiotherapy in the head and neck region, a known history of wound healing difficulties, and manifestations of autoimmune forms of disease (e.g. pemphigus, bullous mucosal pemphigoid, various forms of oral lichen planus) as well as those who do not provide consent. It is unclear what influence different approaches to antiresorptive therapy (e.g. oral or intravenous bisphosphonates) have on soft tissue healing when the underlying bone is not exposed. Therefore, autologous soft tissue grafts should not be performed as an elective intraoral intervention in patients undergoing antiresorptive treatment.

There are a number of other contraindications, but, after the appropriate intervention, these may be of a temporary nature[24]. One significant aspect relates to the patient's individual oral hygiene. It is crucial that patients are capable of practicing optimal oral hygiene. This is not only regarded as a preoperative requirement for maintaining a healthy mucosa and gingiva, but it also relates to the oral hygiene that is required perioperatively and postoperatively.

In this regard, inflammatory changes (plaque-associated: untreated gingivitis and periodontitis; non-plaque–associated: specific infections of the oral mucosa) are contraindications and must be treated in advance. In the presence of inflammatory lesions following mechanical, thermal or chemical trauma to the palatal mucosa, surgery should not be planned until these lesions have completely healed. Inadequate restorations (especially in cervical areas) interfere with optimal oral hygiene, among other things, and are plaque retentive. These should be properly corrected or replaced, if necessary, before graft surgery is planned.

Other temporary contraindications relate to the patient's general health. For instance, infectious diseases (e.g. seasonal colds and flu), acute herpes infections (including labial herpes, herpes zoster, and recurrent intraoral herpes), and diseases otherwise impairing general well-being are considered temporary exclusion criteria for intraoral surgical procedures.

Systemic diseases such as diabetes mellitus and hypertension require appropriate drug treatment. Care should also be taken to ensure that optimal glycemic control (HbA$_{1c}$ value) is achieved in patients with diabetes (note that there is a prevalence of periodontitis in patients with diabetes). In patients with hypertension (for whom caution is advised regarding use of local anesthesia with adrenaline/epinephrine), their medication should similarly ensure therapeutically optimal blood pressure control.

Patients should always be asked for their current HbA$_{1c}$ level and their up-to-date blood pressure measurements before the start of treatment.

Females of childbearing age should be asked about the possibility of being or becoming pregnant. An existing pregnancy and subsequent breastfeeding are temporary contraindications.

Requirements for the donor region

Essentially, the palatal mucosa as the donor region should be completely healthy and free of irritations. Areas of the palatal mucosa that are as smooth and even as possible should be chosen for harvesting a **free mucosal graft**. It is not advisable to remove mucosa in the region of the palatine rugae. The ideal harvesting site is the area of the palatal mucosa distal to the maxillary canine through the mesial region of the maxillary first molar[28] (Fig 15-1). In this area, the mucosa is usually uniformly flat so that this tissue is able to integrate well into the recipient bed after grafting. In most cases, there is an adequate thickness of palatal mucosa available. Care must be taken to ensure that harvesting of the palatal mucosa is not accompanied by injury or removal of the periosteum.

Before **connective tissue** is harvested, as part of treatment planning, the tissue should be assessed and possibly measured to determine palatal mucosal thickness. The measuring can be carried out with a sterile Kerr endodontic file (ISO 10 or ISO 15) after the tissue has been treated with surface anesthetic. The stopper on the file is advanced in the direction of the instrument tip, and the file is inserted perpendicular to the surface of the mucosa like a puncture needle. The stopper is pushed along the file, so that the distance between the instrument tip and the stopper indicates the thickness of the mucosa. This measurement should be repeated at several points so that the mucosal thickness in relation to the eventual graft dimension is known[22].

Essentially, two regions on the palate are suitable for harvesting a **connective tissue graft**: the area distal to the maxillary canine through the mesial region of the maxillary first molar, and the tuberosity area distal to the maxillary second molar[28]. In most cases, the retromolar tissue of the tuberosity region offers sufficient thickness. However, the limitation of this harvesting site is its length. Although connective tissue of sufficient thickness can often be obtained here, for the most part the graft will be no longer than 10 mm. Since harvesting connective tissue in the tuberosity area also involves removing a narrow border of keratinized gingiva, it is essential to ensure that this area exhibits a sufficient width of keratinization (be aware that the more distal the location, the narrower the area of attached keratinized gingiva will be).

The described harvesting site on the hard palate should offer sufficiently thick mucosa, measuring at least 2 mm.

Thick palatal mucosa (≥ 2.5 mm) enables dental surgeons to perform different operating techniques for harvesting connective tissue. A connective tissue graft approximately 15 to 20 mm in length can be obtained, depending on individual anatomy.

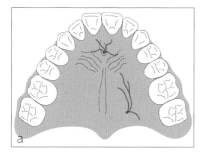 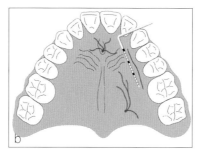 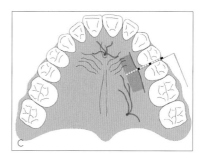

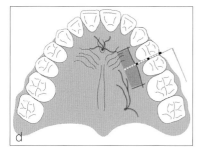 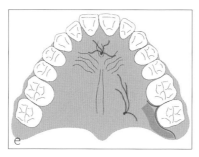 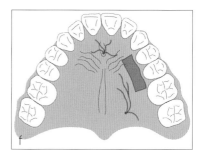

Fig 15-1 Schematic diagram of the anatomy in the palatal area. Both the free mucosal graft and the connective tissue graft are usually harvested from regions of the hard palate between the canine and the first molar or from the area of the retromolar tuberosity. Particular anatomical landmarks are the neurovascular bundle with the associated exit points of the incisive foramen and greater palatine foramen. Satisfactory knowledge of the regular paths of the neurovascular bundle is absolutely essential for surgical procedures on the hard palate. (a) Path of the nasopalatine artery and the greater palatine artery. (b) The dimensions of the graft being harvested can be measured with the aid of a periodontal probe (PCP UNC-15). The probe can additionally be used to help guide the scalpel blade like a ruler. This technique increases dissecting safety and enables the operator to assess graft dimension correctly. (c to f) Diagrams of the incision path for: the single incision technique (c), the trap-door technique (d), harvesting connective tissue at the tuberosity (e), and harvesting a free mucosal graft or a full-thickness connective tissue graft (f).

Attention should also be paid to the shape of the palatal arch. This can be very high and steep but can also be very shallow. Particularly shallow palatal arches can make surgical access more difficult in terms of correct angulation of the scalpel blade. Furthermore, shallower palatal arches often have thinner mucous membrane than high arches.

Specific risks

The risks can be divided into three basic categories: intraoperative risks, perioperative risks, and postoperative risks.

Intraoperative risks

The two types of grafts (free mucosal and connective tissue) differ in terms of surgical depth.

Hence, different risks are associated with these grafting techniques. Generally, the anatomy of the hard and soft palate must be taken into account for both types. The anterior region is the location of the neurovascular bundle, which emerges from the incisive foramen and supplies the anterior region of the hard palate on the left and right sides. This is why the incision path generally should not extend beyond the distopalatal region of the canine in the mesial direction in order to prevent arterial bleeding from the incisive artery (see Fig 15-1). The neurovascular bundle exits bilaterally in the posterior region of the hard palate or at the junction of the hard and soft palate through the Foramen palatinus major. The incision should not extend beyond the mesial aspect of the first molar in order to protect the greater palatine artery in the distal area. Nevertheless, there is a risk of arterial bleeding because of the surgical depth[28]. As subepithelial connective tissue is harvested in most techniques, arterial branches or even anastomoses may be injured. Arterial bleeding requires stringent and coordinated handling. In the event of an arterial bleed, the bleeding vessels should be identified and tied off with appropriate suture material. Alternatively, the vessel can be obliterated by electrocoagulation. The dental technician should in any case fabricate a palatal protector prior to the surgical procedure. This allows for wound care in the sense of a pressure dressing. The diagram in Fig 15-1 plots the paths of the major vessels in the area of the hard palate.

Other intraoperative risks in the area of the donor site can be perforation of the mucosa and damage to adjacent anatomical structures.

There are various risks in the area of the recipient bed, depending on its localization. In the mandible, special attention should be paid to the bilateral localization of the mental foramen (exit point of the mental nerve, mental artery, and mental vein). Substantial arterial bleeds can also occur in this region, which, as described above, require structured and practical emergency management. To avoid this complication, the anatomy should be carefully studied in advance, and, if necessary, the mental foramen together with neurovascular bundle should be visualized.

Perioperative risks

The dimension of the flap in the recipient bed is crucial. It is important to ensure good perfusion of the flap here. Underperfusion due to poor width at the flap base or perforations of the flap can lead to considerable wound healing difficulty and associated necrosis in the recipient bed. Necrosis of papilla apices (e.g. in the coronally advanced flap technique) are very frequently observed. The suturing technique can be another cause of necrosis in the recipient

bed. If wound closure is too tight because of an incorrect suturing technique, this may result in the strangulation of flap areas, which can greatly compromise perfusion of the flap.

Necrosis can also occur in the donor region. While tissue necrosis is rare when employing a free mucosal graft technique, necrosis is more commonly associated with subepithelial harvesting of connective tissue grafts. An adequate thickness of epithelial cover (≥ 1 mm) can minimize the probability of necrosis of the palatal mucosa. In the case of connective tissue grafts, harvesting of a full-thickness graft (secondary de-epithelialization) can be associated with less pain[34].

Application of local anesthetic may be another cause of necrosis of the mucosa. As a result of the firm structure and composition of the palatal mucosa, application of appropriate pressure and the volume of local anesthetic administered can cause mucosal necrosis as well as considerable pain. In this context, it is also worth mentioning what is known as a syringe abscess.

Postoperative risks

In the postoperative course, infections and mechanical, thermal, and chemical influences can cause wound healing complications. Wound healing complications for immunologic reasons are serious, which is why these procedures should be avoided in patients with a known history of reduced immunocompetence (see above under Contraindications). In this context, wound healing complications can prevent the graft from becoming incorporated into the recipient bed. This risk also exists if the recipient bed is underperfused or the graft bed is not vascularized (e.g. extensively exposed tooth or implant surface). Postoperative recession can be a consequence of wound healing complications in smaller areas in the region of the marginal mucosa or gingiva. A strict postoperative regimen and clear advice on safety can minimize the risk of wound healing complications.

Injury and possibly removal of the periosteum can result in postoperative pain in the recipient or donor region[6,30]. The possibility of significant postoperative swelling should also be mentioned. This may be part of the reactive hyperemia after the relative ischemia caused by the local anesthetic and can thus contribute to the symptoms experienced. Good postoperative cooling of the region and the use of local anesthetic with low concentrations of adrenaline/epinephrine can minimize the risk.

Postoperative bleeding can occur in both surgical sites. Good emergency management (emergency service, palatal protector, sterile swabs) and appropriate patient education regarding perioperative and postoperative behavior are crucial.

In addition, longer-term or permanent anesthesia or paresthesia can occur after a nerve block and infiltration anesthesia, but also after injury to nerve endings.

Step-by-step clinical procedure

Local anesthesia in the donor region usually involves two nerve blocks at the nasopalatine nerve and Nervus palatinus major. To avoid possible neuronal anastomoses, vestibular nerve blocks should be carried out in the tooth regions where the graft is being harvested, and palatal nerve blocks should be used directly in the donor region. Application of local anesthetic to the palate only permits small volumes per puncture site ($\approx$ 0.1 mL; be mindful of the danger of necrosis).

In the recipient region, nerve blocks (inferior alveolar nerve, mental nerve, buccal nerve) and regional infiltration anesthesia are required in the mandible. The latter applies to both the maxilla and mandible. As a rule, the local anesthetic should be infiltrated in an overlapping manner in order to block neuronal anastomoses.

Articaine with adrenaline/epinephrine additive is generally used. The exception is patients who cannot tolerate articaine or cannot receive epinephrine for general medical reasons. The epinephrine concentration should be taken into account as a matter of principle. In the recipient region, a concentration of 1:200,000 is recommended because this dosage weakens the degree of reactive hyperemia, and swelling is less pronounced. However, the procedure should be time-limited because the duration of action is correspondingly short. In the donor region, an epinephrine concentration of 1:100,000 can be useful. The very small volumes can thus be compensated and hence the duration of action of the local anesthetic can be lengthened. An additional advantage of the higher concentration of epinephrine is that transient ischemia (or underperfusion) is achieved at the surgical site. Especially when harvesting connective tissue, this creates better intraoperative visibility. The connective tissue on the palate is very well perfused so that oozing of blood is difficult to distinguish from minor arterial bleeding. In addition, the visibility of the surgical site in relation to scalpel guidance and connective tissue dissection is reduced. It can be helpful to choose a rather higher dosage of vasoconstrictor additive in the local anesthetic.

The clinical procedure for grafting free mucosa or connective tissue can be broken down into **five phases**:
1. Preparatory phase,
2. Dissection of the recipient bed,
3. Harvesting of the graft and wound care at the donor site on the palate,
4. Integration of the graft into the recipient bed and wound closure,
5. Follow-up phase.

Before planning the surgical intervention, the aspects covered below should be considered as absolute prerequisites.

Prerequisites for surgical intervention

- Medical history (general medical, dental, and periodontal history).
- Record of clinical, and, if applicable, radiographic findings (extraoral and intraoral findings, functional findings, periodontal findings).
- Photographs of the preoperative situation (intraoral photographic status comprising five images [frontal aspect, right lateral aspect, left lateral aspect, maxillary arch, and mandibular arch], detailed images of the clinical findings).
- Diagnosis[13].
- Suitability for treatment.
- Patient information, instruction, and motivation to achieve optimal oral hygiene.
- Professional mechanical plaque removal.
- Explanation to the patient of advantages, disadvantages, risks, and alternatives to the planned procedure and concerning local anesthesia as well as the expected treatment costs (at least 24 hours before the planned procedure).
- Impression of the maxilla (e.g. with alginate) to fabricate a palatal protector.
- Planning the surgical procedure on a model or with the aid of clinical photographs.

The five phases mentioned above are outlined below step by step.

1. Preparatory phase

- Prepare the surgical armamentarium (including sterile surgical light handles).
- Disinfect the oral cavity (e.g. with 0.2% chlorhexidine mouthwash for 1 minute).
- Disinfect the perioral skin areas and lips (e.g. iodine solution).
- Deliver local anesthesia in the area of the recipient bed (local anesthesia in the donor region can be performed in Phase 3).

- Apply sterile drapes to the patient, including the use of a fenestrated drape to cover the face and hair.
- Position the patient.

2. Dissection of the recipient bed

- Check the local anesthesia.
- Possibly take periodontal measurements prior to incision.
- Note: During dissection of the soft tissue, diamond-coated anatomical micro forceps should be used so that the integrity of the epithelium is not compromised.

Preparation to receive a free mucosal graft to widen the keratinized gingiva or mucosa (Figs 15-2 to 15-4 and 15-5a to 15-5dd)

- Vestibular incision approximately 1 mm coronal to the mucogingival border line if a narrow area of keratinized tissue is present.
- Alternatively: vestibular incision along the mucogingival border line.
- Raise a mucosal flap in the apical direction while sparing the periosteum (be mindful of the neurovascular bundle in the area of the mental foramen).
- Apical repositioning and fixation of the alveolar mucosa to the periosteum with 6-0 monofilament suture material. (Note: The dimension of the graft should be chosen so that there is no tissue overlapping. Care should also be taken to ensure that the alveolar mucosa is fixed far enough apically.)
- Measure the graft bed with a periodontal probe, and, if appropriate, transfer the graft dimensions to sterile foil, which is later used on the palate as orientation for the incision path.
- Cover the graft bed with sterile gauze soaked in sterile 0.9% NaCl solution. (Note: Throughout the duration of the surgery, make sure that the soft tissue is kept moist enough with sterile 0.9% NaCl solution.

The surgical aspirator can easily dry out the mucosa, and this should always be avoided.)

- Continue with Phase 3.

Preparation to receive a connective tissue graft (Figs 15-5ee to 15-5ii and 15-6 to 15-15)

A number of different techniques for individual indications are available for preparing the graft bed to receive a connective tissue graft. These are examined in more detail in Section 16.

- Mucosal flap formation using a tunnel dissection (tunnel technique).
- Combined flap elevation as a mucosal-mucoperiosteal-mucosal flap for coronal displacement of the mucosa (known as a coronally repositioned or advanced flap).
- Elevate a mucosal flap using a pocket technique in edentulous jaw segments.
- Measure the graft bed with a periodontal probe.
- Cover the graft bed with sterile gauze soaked in sterile 0.9% NaCl solution. (Note: Throughout the duration of the surgery, make sure that the soft tissue is kept sufficiently moist with sterile 0.9% NaCl solution. The surgical aspirator can easily dry out the mucosa, and this should always be avoided.)
- Continue with Phase 3.

3. Harvesting of the graft and wound care at the donor site on the palate

- Deliver local anesthesia at the donor region.
- Measure the graft dimensions with a periodontal probe or application of the previously contoured sterile foil (see Fig 15-4d).
- Note: During dissection of the soft tissue on the palate, diamond-coated anatomical or surgical micro forceps can be used.

Harvesting the free mucosal graft and wound care (Figs 15-3 and 15-4)

- Incise along the marking or the foil to a cutting depth of approximately 1.5 mm. (Note: To avoid arterial bleeding, the harvesting should be performed in the region distal to the maxillary canine to mesial to the first molar.)
- Subepithelial dissection in one layer (1.5 mm subepithelial), starting from the mesial incision margin.
- Extraoral storage on a sterile board and cover with a sterile swab soaked in sterile 0.9% NaCl solution.
- Epithelial wound care (secondary wound healing) with Histoacryl glue or a xenogeneic collagen fleece.

Harvesting the connective tissue graft (Figs 15-6, 15-8, 15-10, 15-14, and 15-15)

Single-incision technique

Subepithelial harvesting of the connective tissue via a single surface incision[16,18].

- First cut: Horizontal and 2 mm apical to the marginal gingiva.
- Second cut: Parallel to the epithelial surface to a depth corresponding to the eventual graft dimension. (Note: The epithelial layer should be maintained at a minimum thickness of 1 mm. Take care to avoid perforation of the palatal mucosa.)
- Third cut: Parallel to the second incision supraperiosteally, if possible. (Note: If the periosteum is also removed, the dimension of the graft may turn out to be smaller after harvesting. In this case, the periosteum on the underside of the graft should be carefully slit under appropriate optical magnification.)
- Fourth and fifth cuts: Vertical mesial and distal subepithelial incision.
- Fifth cut: Incise at the basal surface of the graft. (Note: The graft should now be held

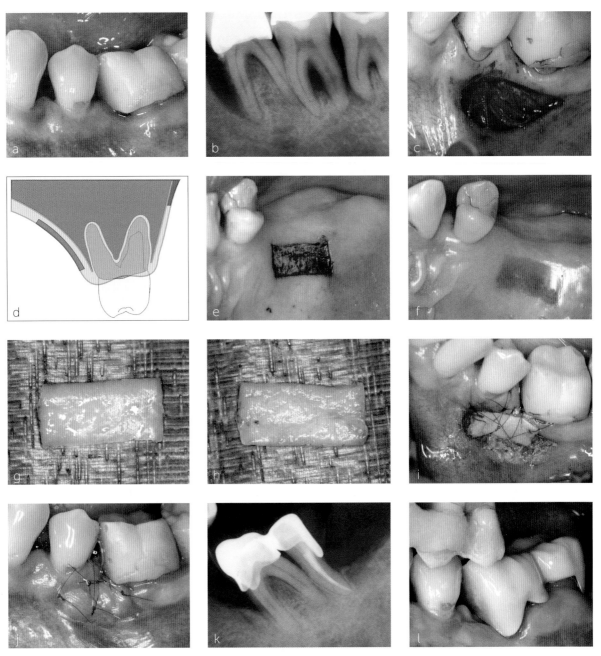

Fig 15-2   Free mucosal graft to widen the keratinized gingiva before periodontal regeneration of a deep infra-alveolar bony pocket. (a) Preoperative situation with very narrow keratinized gingiva in the area of the bone defect. (b) Radiograph showing the infra-alveolar bone defect mesial to the mandibular left first molar; additional horizontal bone defect at the adjacent second and third molars with grade 3 furcation involvement. (c) Incision and dissection of the mucosal flap. (d) Schematic diagram of the graft dimensions and surgical depth. (e) Situation after graft harvesting, with clearly visible subepithelial connective tissue. (f) Healing progress 2 weeks after graft harvesting. Immediately after the procedure, a palatal protector made of transparent plastic is adapted and given to the patient (protector to be inserted in the event of bleeding and/or while eating). (g) Epithelial surface of the graft. (h) Underside of the graft (note that it is free of fatty and glandular tissue). (i) Fixation of the graft with interrupted sutures in the coronal portion and crossover external mattress sutures. (j) Situation after 2 weeks of healing (before suture removal). (k) Radiograph showing the mandibular left first and second molars after hemisection and regenerative surgical procedure mesial to the first molar (after application of enamel matrix protein [Emdogain®, Straumann]; regeneration to 55% of the root surface). (l) Situation 1 year after regenerative procedure and prosthetic restoration.

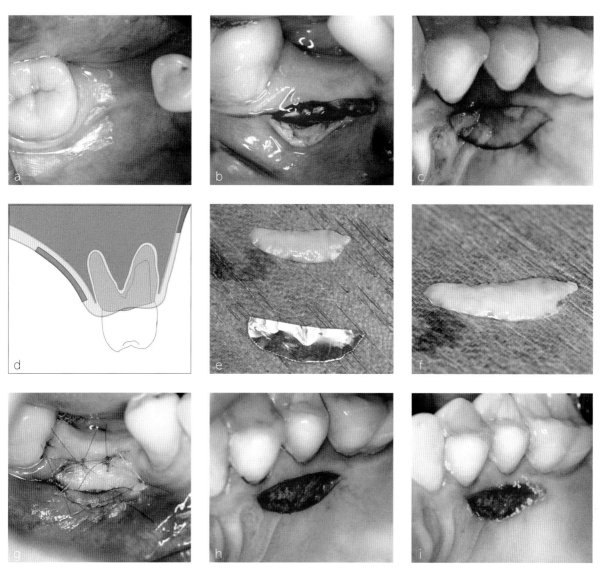

Fig 15-3 Free mucosal graft to widen the keratinized gingiva prior to implant placement in the mandibular right first molar region. (a) Preoperative situation with highly radiating alveolar mucosa in the mandibular right first molar region. (b) Incision before mucosal flap elevation in the way of a vestibuloplasty. (c) Incision path on the palate from distal to the maxillary left canine until mesial to the left first molar after transfer of graft dimensions using sterile foil. (d) Schematic diagram of graft dimensions and surgical depth. (e) Graft in relation to the template. (f) Shape of the free mucosal graft in the dimensions of the graft bed. (g) Fixation of the graft with interrupted sutures in the coronal portion and crossover external mattress sutures. (h) Situation after graft harvesting, with clearly visible subepithelial connective tissue. (i) Situation after application of tissue glue (Histoacryl, B. Braun). In addition, a palatal protector is fabricated from transparent plastic and given to the patient (to be inserted in the event of bleeding and/or while eating).

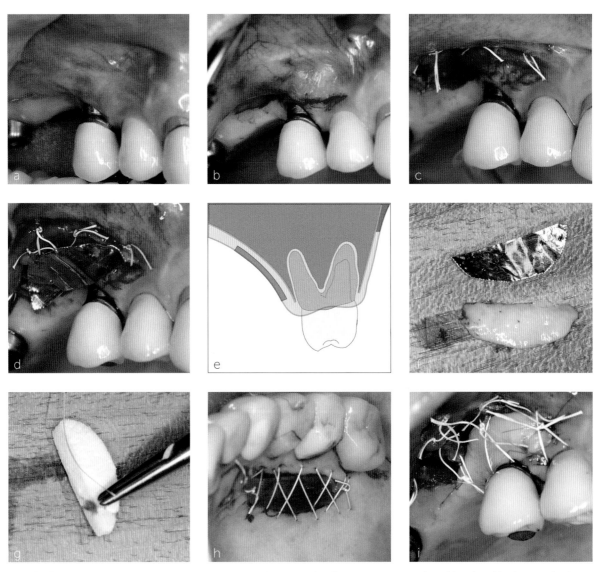

Fig 15-4   Free mucosal graft to widen the keratinized gingiva for the purpose of peri-implantitis therapy in the maxillary right second premolar region. (a) Preoperative situation shows alveolar mucosa adjacent to the implant and soft tissue dehiscence on the vestibular aspect. (b) Incision prior to mucosal flap elevation. (c) Periosteal fixation of the dissected alveolar mucosa (apical). (d) Measuring the graft dimensions with the aid of sterile foil. (e) Schematic diagram of the graft dimensions and surgical depth. (f) Graft in relation to the template. (g) Congruent dimensioning of a xenogeneic collagen matrix as a wound dressing in the donor region. (h) Situation after adaptation and fixation of the collagen matrix (Mucograft, Geistlich) with interrupted sutures and continuous external mattress sutures. (i) Fixation of the graft with interrupted sutures in the coronal portion and with crossover external mattress sutures. In addition, a palatal protector is fabricated from transparent plastic and given to the patient (to be inserted in the event of bleeding and/or while eating).

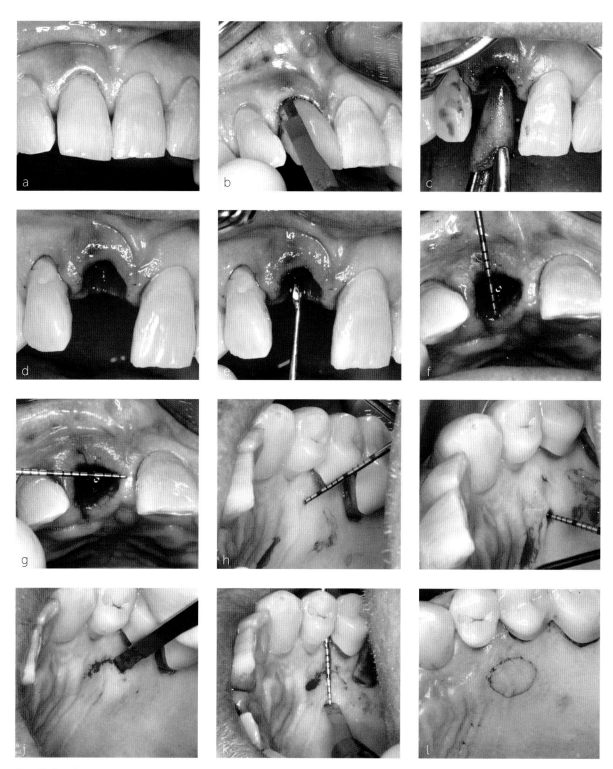

Fig 15-5 Grafting of a mucosal patch from the palate as part of a minimally invasive extraction (diagnosis: external cervical resorption of the maxillary right central incisor). (a) Preoperative situation. (b) Intrasulcular incision to detach the periodontal ligament fibers. (c) Extraction by the Ögram system. (d) Extraction socket. (e) Curettage of the socket to remove granulation tissue. (f and g) Measuring the socket. (h and i) Measuring and marking the donor site on the palate in the maxillary right first and second premolar region. (j to l) Incision.

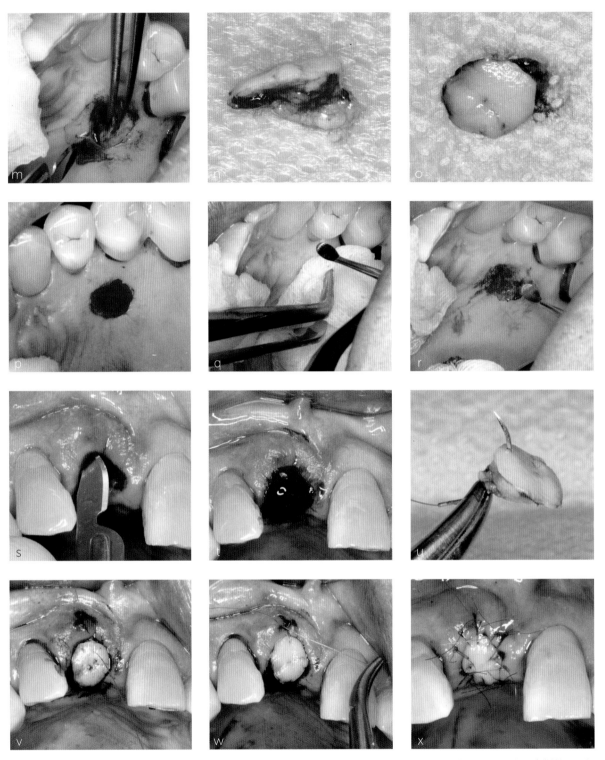

Fig 15-5 (continued)   (m) Full-thickness patch harvesting. (n and o) View of the patch after harvesting. (p) Wound in the palate immediately after graft harvesting. (q and r) Application of Histoacryl glue. (s) De-epitheliailization in the area of the sulcus epithelium. (t) Socket with coagulum. (u) Ligation of the patch. (v to x) Fixation of the patch with 7-0 monofilament suture material.

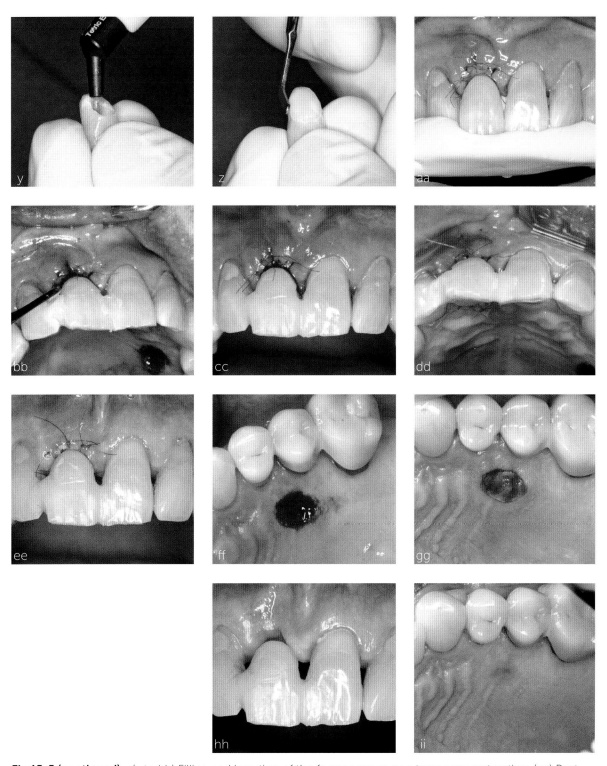

Fig 15-5 (continued) (y to bb) Filling and insertion of the former crown as a temporary restoration. (cc) Postoperative frontal view. (dd) Postoperative occlusal view. (ee) Frontal view 1 day postoperatively. (ff) Palatal wound. (gg) Palatal wound 5 days postoperatively. (hh and ii) Frontal view and palatal wound 2 weeks postoperatively.

continuously with diamond-coated surgical forceps, but not compressed.)

■ Wound closure is carried out with 6-0 monofilament suture material (continuous horizontal suture with a crossover external mattress suture as a support suture).

Trap-door technique

■ In addition to the incision 2 mm apical to the marginal gingiva (see single-incision technique, first cut), two vertical releasing incisions are made, each overlapping at the ends of the first cut[25].

■ The rest of the procedure for harvesting connective tissue is the same as for the single-incision technique (second to fifth cut).

■ Wound closure is carried out with 6-0 monofilament suture material (continuous horizontal suture, interrupted sutures in the area of the releasing incisions, and a crossover external mattress suture as a support suture).

Full-thickness graft

Secondary extraoral de-epithelialization[29,33]:

■ Harvesting of a full-thickness graft (epithelium and connective tissue) is identical to the procedure for obtaining a free mucosal graft.

■ The aim should be to achieve a graft thickness (equal to the cutting depth) of 2 to 2.5 mm[34].

■ Harvesting of a full-thickness graft is followed by secondary wound healing.

■ Wound care involves the use of Histoacryl glue or fixation of xenogeneic collagen fleece with 6-0 monofilament suture material.

■ Note: The single-incision technique and trap-door technique allow connective tissue to be harvested from the deep (basal) mucosal layer (in the direction of the periosteum), whereas harvesting of

full-thickness grafts that are de-epithelialized extraorally represents the connective tissue of the upper (apical) mucosal layer. Compared with apical grafts, the basal grafts contain more fatty and glandular tissue, which has to be removed from the graft extraorally. In addition, the connective tissue of apical grafts is firmer and more stable than that of basal grafts.

■ After harvesting the connective tissue, extraoral storage should be on a sterile board, covered with a sterile swab soaked in sterile 0.9% NaCl solution.

4. Integration of the graft into the recipient bed and wound closure
Integration of the free mucosal graft (Figs 15-2 to 15-4)

■ The free mucosal graft can be fixed with the aid of interrupted sutures (preferably 7-0 monofilament suture material) along the coronal edge of the graft to the coronal wound margin of the recipient bed and with crossover external mattress sutures (6-0 monofilament suture material).

■ There is the alternative option of fixing the graft using Histoacryl glue on the periosteal surface of the recipient bed.

■ For both types of fixation, a minimum distance of 2 mm should be maintained between the underside of the graft and the apical wound margin. (Note: Care should be taken to ensure that the alveolar mucosa of the apical wound margin does not extend beyond the graft or form a fold.)

Integration of the connective tissue graft (Figs 15-7, 15-11, 15-13, and 15-14)

■ Optional: During the course of soft tissue augmentation around the teeth (e.g. for recession coverage), there is the option of using enamel matrix derivatives to improve wound healing and possibly formation/ repair of the cementum layer for a connective tissue attachment between the tooth surface and the newly inserted connective tissue. (Note: See the relevant literature for the use of enamel matrix derivatives[1,2,20].)

■ When the **tunnel technique** is used, the connective tissue is pulled into the graft bed through one of the lateral transsulcular accesses with the aid of a vertical mattress suture and is ultimately fixed laterally with transepithelial interrupted sutures (6-0 monofilament suture material).

■ For **combined flap elevation** and **mucosal flap elevation** (see Fig 15-11m), the connective tissue is fixed directly to the periosteum and/or with a sling suture (around the tooth or implant) using resorbable suture material (size 6-0).

■ For all techniques of graft bed dissection, the mucosal flap is advanced coronally with the aid of internal vertical mattress sutures (it is also possible to use a Laurell suture) and suspension sutures at the interproximal tooth contact points (in the interproximal spaces).

5. Follow-up phase

■ Irrigate the surgical site with sterile 0.9% NaCl solution.

■ Careful digital adaptation of the graft on the graft bed using a gauze patch soaked in sterile 0.9% NaCl solution for a few minutes.

■ Insert the palatal protector and explain wearing time and care to the patient.

■ Postoperative information, medication, and oral hygiene instructions.

■ Document the procedure (including photographs).

■ Arrange appointments for postoperative follow-up and suture removal.

Wound care and closure

The procedure for wound care of the recipient and donor regions was described above under Step-by-step clinical procedure. Therefore, only the specific characteristics related to wound care in the donor region are addressed below.

A basic distinction must be made as to whether primary or secondary wound healing ensues in the area of the donor region. When a **free mucosal graft** is harvested, there is some disintegration of the palatal mucosa because the epithelium is grafted at the same time. Therefore, secondary wound healing processes always follow, which can involve a number of complications such as postoperative pain, bleeding, and wound healing complications. Wearing the palate-spanning protector can prevent injuries, and, in the event of postoperative bleeding, can help to control the bleeding as a kind of pressure dressing. Histoacryl glue or a xenogeneic collagen fleece can be used to dress the palatal wound. The advantages of Histoacryl glue are that it stems bleeding rapidly and is very easy and quick to use. One disadvantage of the glue is that a rough surface can arise as it sets, which can lead to irritation. Dressing the palatal wound with a xenogeneic collagen fleece is relatively more elaborate because it is fixed to the palatal mucosa with a continuous crossover horizontal mattress suture. Advantages of the collagen fleece are that the wound is fully covered, bleeding is rapidly stemmed, and secondary healing (keratinization) follows an uncomplicated course.

When a **connective tissue graft** is harvested by either the single-incision technique or the trap-door technique, wound closure can be carried out with continuous external horizontal mattress sutures, interrupted sutures, and crossover external mattress sutures (support suture). The advantage of these two harvesting techniques lies in primary wound healing. If epithelial tissue thickness is sufficient (minimum:

1 mm) and uniform, necrosis of the mucosa is less common and primary healing follows a rapid and uneventful course[5]. Wound care for full-thickness connective tissue grafts is identical to that following the harvest of a free mucosal graft. A palatal protector should also be inserted after the harvest of a connective tissue graft.

Postoperative controls and course

Immediately after the surgical procedure, a recall appointment should be arranged. For outpatient surgical interventions, it might be appropriate to arrange a telephone appointment for the evening immediately after the procedure. This enables the clinician to inquire about the patient's well-being, provide any needed instructions, and address any unanswered questions. An appropriate emergency regimen should be discussed as a matter of routine. This might include, for example, attendance at the dental emergency service in the event of bleeding. Patients should already have been given a cooling pack to take home with them. Cooling of the surgical site can curtail reactive hyperemia and hence control the severity of postoperative swelling and pain. Patients should continue to cool the site at home the next day. However, intermittent cooling is recommended instead of continual cooling. A cold washcloth is enough to provide the necessary cooling. During the night following the procedure, patients should sleep in a cool environment with the head slightly elevated.

The first pain medication (e.g. ibuprofen 600 mg) can be taken in the immediate postoperative period while the local anesthetic is still effective. It is essential to check the patient's history when prescribing pain medication (taking into account the anticoagulant effect of certain analgesics).

The first follow-up appointment should be on the day after the procedure or the following day. Irrespective of general medical parameters (e.g. swelling, hematoma, infection), patients should be thoroughly instructed on oral hygiene, in particular. Rinsing the oral cavity with alcohol-free 0.1% chlorhexidine mouthwash for a period of about 2 weeks should be planned postoperatively[23]. In the wound region, mechanical oral hygiene with a toothbrush (regardless of type) should definitely be avoided in order to promote uncomplicated wound healing. However, so that the teeth are cleaned daily, it is advisable to clean the teeth in the surgical field with cotton swabs soaked in 0.1% chlorhexidine.

Mechanical oral hygiene with a toothbrush can be resumed in the donor region after about 1 week. In the recipient region, patients should only use the toothbrush again after about 4 weeks.

After about a week to 10 days, another check-up should take place. Sutures are removed from the palate (if there are any) and professional wound cleansing is carried out (0.1% chlorhexidine solution). After a total of 12 to 14 days, sutures are removed in the recipient region, another professional wound cleansing is carried out, and the patient is reinstructed and remotivated with regard to oral hygiene. Professional mechanical cleaning of all teeth (including removal of possible discoloration caused by chlorhexidine) should take place another 2 weeks later. In the following 2 weeks, patients should resume mechanical oral hygiene in the recipient region using a soft toothbrush. They can resume regular oral hygiene and use of all hygiene aids after a total of 6 weeks.

Healing progress should continue to be monitored clinically according to the individual appointment schedule and, after a period of about 6 months postoperatively, the result can be assessed with relative certainty. The key healing and remodeling processes are completed after this period of time. (Note: This applies especially when assessing the result after recession coverage.)

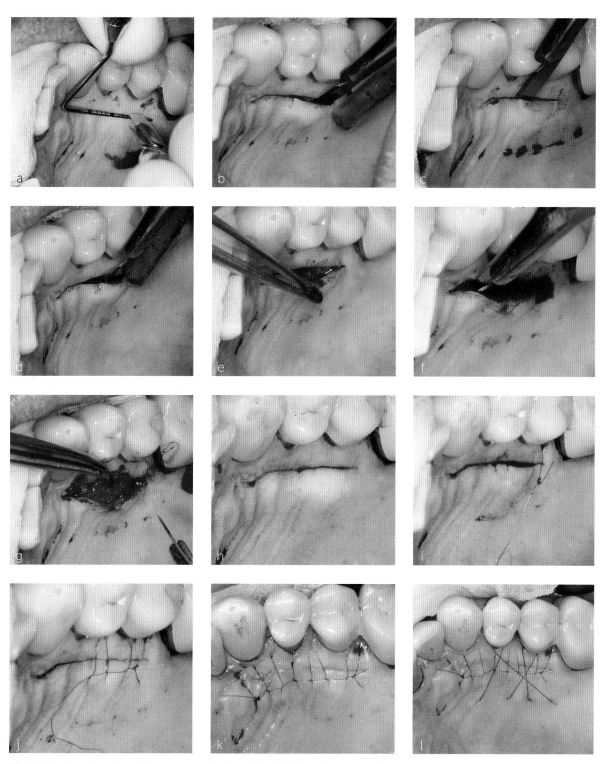

Fig 15-6 Continuation of the case study from Fig 15-5 after 6 months. Connective tissue graft for the preprosthetic augmentation of the alveolar ridge in the maxillary right central incisor region. (a) Incision path with the aid of a periodontal probe to assess the correct graft dimension. (b to d) Incision parallel to the epithelial surface approximately 1 mm subepithelial. (e) Visualization of the epithelium with uniform layer thickness of 1.5 mm. (f) Third cut parallel to the second cut, approximately 2.5 mm more basal. (g) Removal of the connective tissue. (h) Situation after graft harvesting. (i) Start of wound care at the posterior end of the incision (bleeding stops). (j to l) Wound care with a continuous horizontal external mattress suture and external crossover mattress sutures (support sutures).

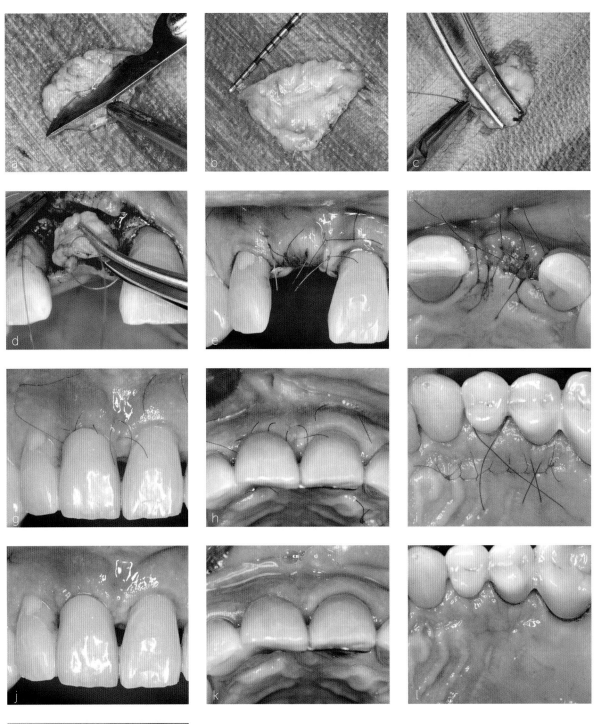

Fig 15-7   Continuation of the case study from Fig 15-6. Application of the connective tissue graft in the recipient region. (a) Removal of glands and fatty tissue. (b) Processed connective tissue. (c) Ligation of the connective tissue with 6-0 resorbable suture material. (d) Placement and suturing of the connective tissue in the mucosal flap pocket in the region of the maxillary right central incisor using 6-0 resorbable suture material (crossover external mattress suture). (e and f) Wound closure with 6-0 monofilament suture material. (g to i) Twelve days postoperatively. (j to l) Six weeks postoperatively. (m) Situation after prosthetic restoration 1 year postoperatively.

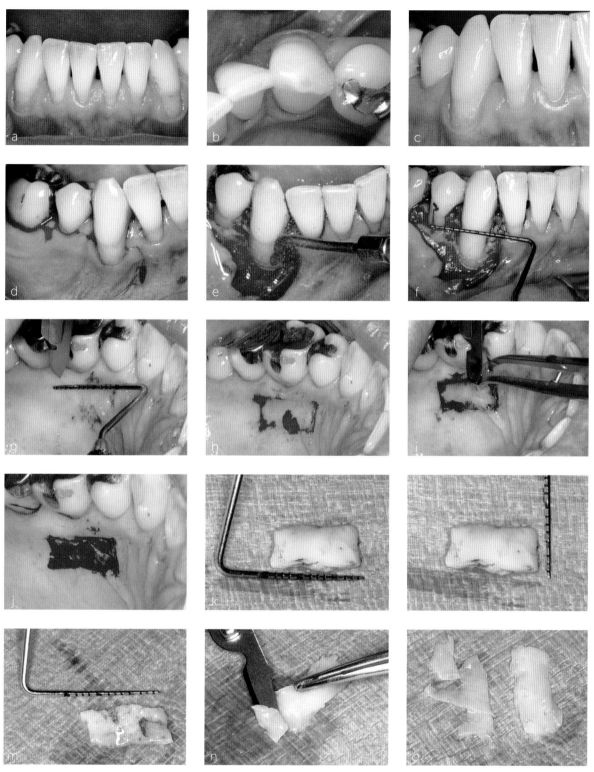

Fig 15-8 Recession coverage of the mandibular canines with the aid of full-thickness connective tissue grafts. (a to c) Preoperative situation. (d) Incision path for a mucosal-mucoperiosteal-mucosal flap. (e) Decontamination and planing of the root surface. (f) Measuring the recipient bed. (g) Measuring the donor region. (h and i) Incision and dissection of the full-thickness graft. (j) After graft harvesting. (k to m) Measuring the graft. (n and o) De-epithelialization of the connective tissue.

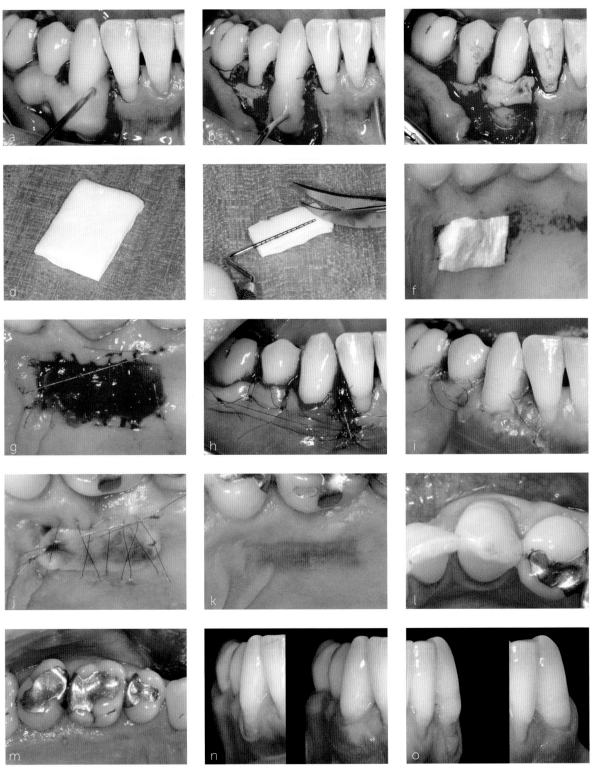

Fig 15-9   Continuation of the case study from Fig 15-8. (a) Application of EDTA for conditioning. (b) Application of enamel matrix proteins to the root surface. (c) Adaptation of the connective tissue graft with 6-0 resorbable suture material. (d and e) Preparation of the xenogeneic collagen fleece. (f and g) Wound care on the palate: Application and fixation of the collagen fleece with 6-0 monofilament suture material. (h) Coronal advancement of the flap. (i and j) One week postoperatively. (k and l) Four weeks postoperatively. (m) Six months postoperatively. (n) Preoperative and final situation after 6 months, right canine. (o) Preoperative and final situation after 6 months, left canine.

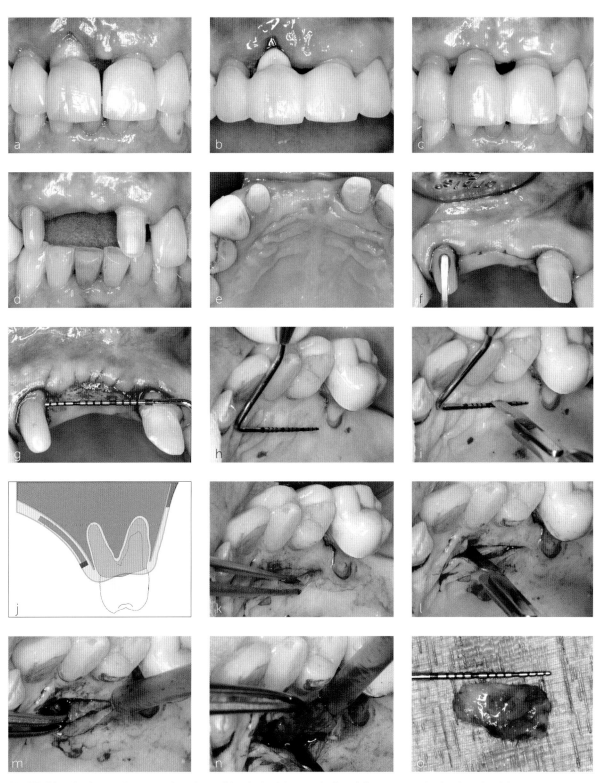

Fig 15-10 Grafting of connective tissue (single-incision technique) for preprosthetic alveolar ridge augmentation in a patient with stage IV, grade B periodontitis. (a) Preoperative situation. (b) Situation after extraction of the maxillary right central incisor and provisional splinting. (c) Situation 6 months after nonsurgical periodontitis treatment (completion of steps 1 and 2). (d and e) Provisional preparation. (f) Incision with mucosal flap elevation. (g) Measuring the recipient bed. (h and i) Measuring and incision in the donor region. (j) Diagram of the planned graft harvesting. (k to n) Individual steps of graft harvesting. (o) Connective tissue graft.

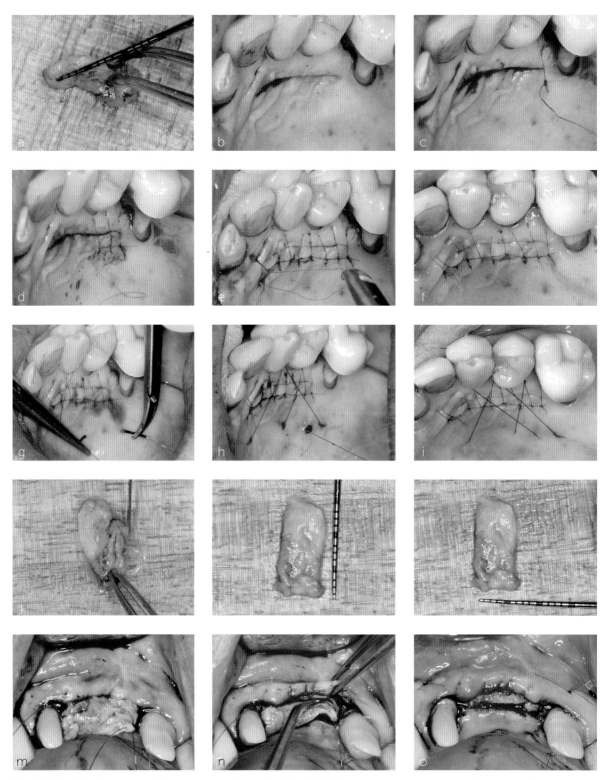

Fig 15-11 Continuation of the case study from Fig 15-10. (a) Removal of glandular and fatty tissue from the graft. (b to i) Stepwise wound care with a continuous horizontal external mattress suture and external crossover mattress sutures. (j to l) Measuring the graft. (m to o) Insertion of the graft underneath the mucosal flap on the periosteum and adaptation with 6-0 monofilament suture material in the lateral recipient bed areas using interrupted suturing.

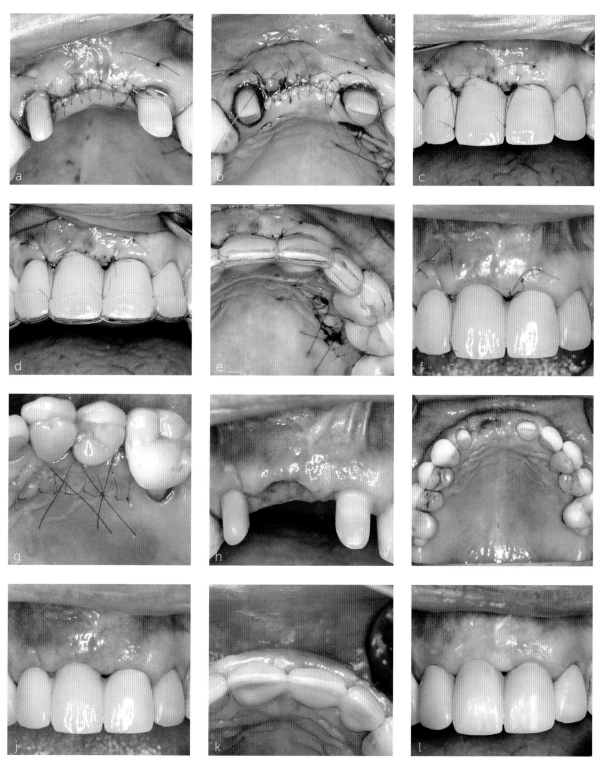

Fig 15-12 Continuation of the case study from Fig 15-11. (a and b) Wound closure with 7-0 monofilament suture material for the interrupted sutures and 6-0 monofilament suture material for the vertical internal mattress sutures. (c) Situation after placement of the provisional prosthesis. (d and e) Insertion of the palatal protector. (f and g) Two weeks postoperatively. (h and i) Four weeks postoperatively. (j) Frontal view 4 weeks postoperatively. (k and l) Two years postoperatively (Prosthodontics: Prof Dr Beuer, Department of Prosthodontics, Charité—Universitätsmedizin Berlin).

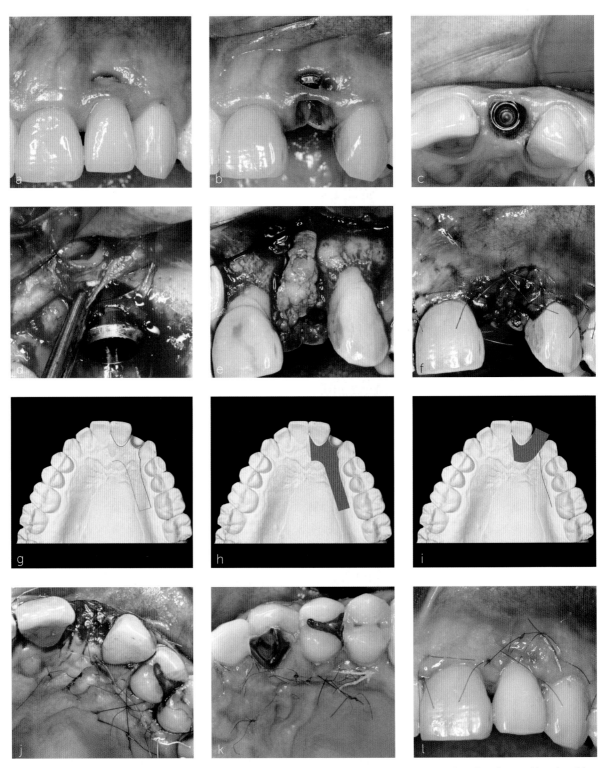

Fig 15-13 Variation of the single-incision technique: Connective tissue pedicle rotation flap for peri-implantitis and peri-implant soft tissue defect vestibular to the maxillary left lateral incisor implant. (a) Preoperative situation. (b and c) Preoperative situation after removal of the implant crown and visualization of the peri-implant soft tissue defect. (d) Removal of the encapsulated cementum remnant. (e) Vestibular fixation of the rotation flap with 6-0 resorbable suture material. (f) Coronally repositioned flap and fixation with 6-0 monofilament suture material (interrupted sutures, interproximal internal vertical mattress sutures). (g to i) Schematic diagrams for planning the connective tissue pedicle rotation flap. (j) Situation after wound closure. (k and l) Two weeks postoperatively.

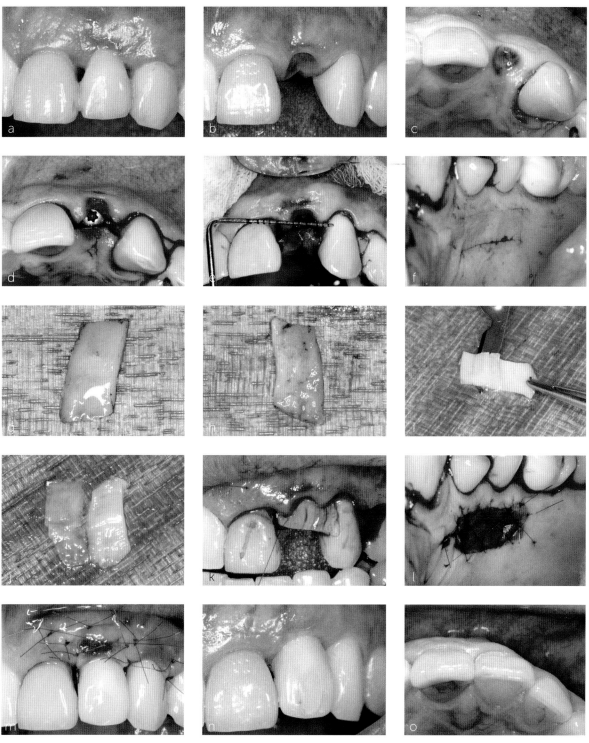

Fig 15-14 Continuation of the case study from Fig 15-13. Exposure and renewed restoration of the implant in the maxillary left lateral incisor region. (a) One year after first surgery (see Fig 15-13). (b and c) After removal of the provisional retainer partial denture. (d) Incision for raising the mucoperiosteal-mucosal flap. (e) Measuring the recipient bed. (f) Incision in the donor region. (g) Epithelial view of the graft. (h) Basal view of the graft. (i and j) De-epithelialization of the graft. (k) Insertion of the graft underneath the mucosal flap on the periosteum and adaptation with 6-0 monofilament suture material in the lateral recipient bed areas by means of an interrupted suture. (l) Adaptation and suturing of the xenogeneic collagen fleece. (m) Situation after wound closure. (n and o) One year postoperatively (Prosthodontics: Prof Dr Beuer, Department of Prosthodontics, Charité—Universitätsmedizin Berlin).

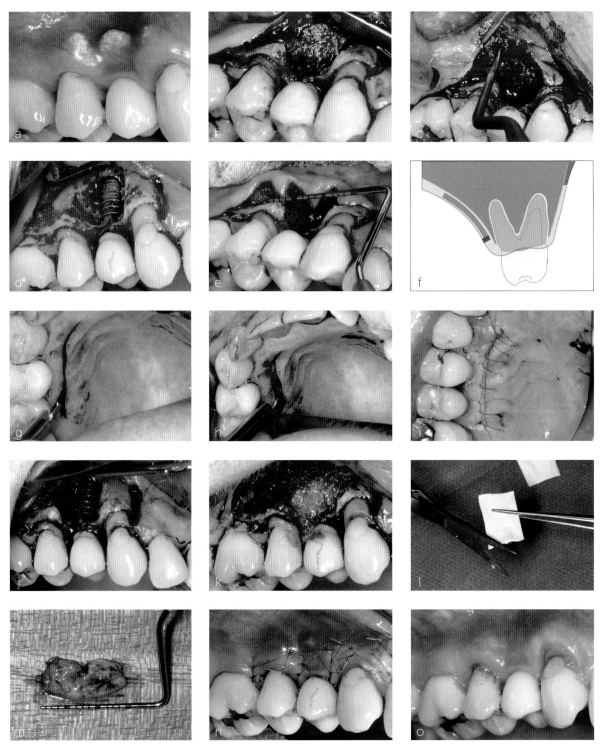

Fig 15-15   Peri-implantitis treatment following augmentation performed at another dental practice and encapsulation of the grafted bone substitute in the maxillary right first premolar region. (a) Preoperative situation. (b) Exposure of the site. (c) Careful removal of the encapsulated material. (d) Situation after decontamination of the implant threads. (e) Measuring the recipient bed. (f) Schematic diagram of the planned graft harvesting. (g and h) Incision to harvest the connective tissue graft (single-incision technique). (i) Wound closure of the donor region. (j) Situation after cleaning the bone defect. (k) Application of a bovine bone substitute. (l) Contouring a xenogeneic resorbable membrane. (m) Measuring the graft. (n) Wound closure after graft insertion to correct the soft tissue defect in the maxillary right first premolar region. (o) Six months postoperatively.

References

1. Aydinyurt HS, Tekin Y, Ertugrul AS: The effect of enamel matrix derivatives on root coverage: A 12-month follow-up of a randomized clinical trial. Braz Oral Res 2019;33:e006.

2. Barootchi S, Tavelli L, Ravida A, Wang CW, Wang HL: Effect of EDTA root conditioning on the outcome of coronally advanced flap with connective tissue graft: A systematic review and meta-analysis. Clin Oral Investig 2018;22: 2727–2741.

3. Basegmez C, Karabuda ZC, Demirel K, Yalcin S: The comparison of acellular dermal matrix allografts with free gingival grafts in the augmentation of peri-implant attached mucosa: A randomised controlled trial. Eur J Oral Implantol 2013;6:145–152.

4. Bertl K, Melchard M, Pandis N, Muller-Kern M, Stavropoulos A: Soft tissue substitutes in non-root coverage procedures: A systematic review and meta-analysis. Clin Oral Investig 2017;21:505–518.

5. Bhatavadekar NB, Gharpure AS: Controlled palatal harvest technique for harvesting a palatal subepithelial connective tissue graft. Compend Contin Educ Dent 2018;39:e9–e12.

6. Burkhardt R, Hämmerle CH, Lang NP, Research Group on Oral Soft Tissue Biology and Wound Healing: Self-reported pain perception of patients after mucosal graft harvesting in the palatal area. J Clin Periodontol 2015;42:281–287.

7. Cairo F, Barbato L, Selvaggi F, Baielli MG, Piattelli A, Chambrone L: Surgical procedures for soft tissue augmentation at implant sites. A systematic review and meta-analysis of randomized controlled trials. Clin Implant Dent Relat Res 2019;21:1262–1270.

8. Cairo F, Barootchi S, Tavelli L, Barbato L, Wang HL, Rasperini G, Graziani F, Tonetti M: Aesthetic-and patient-related outcomes following root coverage procedures: A systematic review and network meta-analysis. J Clin Periodontol 2020;47:1403–1415.

9. Cevallos CAR, de Resende DRB, Damante CA, Sant'Ana ACP, de Rezende MLR, Greghi SLA, Zangrando MSR: Free gingival graft and acellular dermal matrix for gingival augmentation: A 15-year clinical study. Clin Oral Investig 2020;24:1197–1203.

10. Chambrone L, de Castro Pinto RCN, Chambrone LA: The concepts of evidence-based periodontal plastic surgery: Application of the principles of evidence-based dentistry for the treatment of recession-type defects. Periodontol 2000 2019;79:81–106.

11. Dragan IF, Hotlzman LP, Karimbux NY, Morin RA, Bassir SH: Clinical outcomes of comparing soft tissue alternatives to free gingival graft: A systematic review and meta-analysis. J Evid Based Dent Pract 2017;17:370–380.

12. Giannobile WV, Jung RE, Schwarz F, Groups of the 2nd Osteology Foundation Consensus Meeting: Evidence-based knowledge on the aesthetics and maintenance of peri-implant soft tissues: Osteology Foundation Consensus Report Part 1 – effects of soft tissue augmentation procedures on the maintenance of peri-implant soft tissue health. Clin Oral Implants Res 2018;29(Suppl 15):7–10.

13. Jepsen S, Caton JG, Albandar JM, Bissada NF, Bouchard P, Cortellini P, Demirel K, de Sanctis M, Ercoli C, Fan J et al.: Periodontal manifestations of systemic diseases and developmental and acquired conditions: Consensus report of workgroup 3 of the 2017 World Workshop on the Classification of Periodontal and Peri-Implant Diseases and Conditions. J Clin Periodontol 2018;45(Suppl 20):S219–S229.

14. Jung RE, Siegenthaler DW, Hammerle CH: Postextraction tissue management: A soft tissue punch technique. Int J Periodontics Restorative Dent 2004;24:545–553.

15. Karring T, Lang NP, Loe H: The role of gingival connective tissue in determining epithelial differentiation. J Periodontal Res 1975;10:1–11.

16. Kumar A, Sood V, Masamatti SS, Triveni MG, Mehta DS, Khatri M, Agarwal V: Modified single incision technique to harvest subepithelial connective tissue graft. J Indian Soc Periodontol 2013;17:676–680.

17. Langer B, Calagna LJ: The subepithelial connective tissue graft. A new approach to the enhancement of anterior cosmetics. Int J Periodontics Restorative Dent 1982;2:22–33.

18. Lorenzana ER, Allen EP: The single-incision palatal harvest technique: A strategy for esthetics and patient comfort. Int J Periodontics Restorative Dent 2000;20:297–305.

19. McGuire MK, Scheyer ET: Randomized, controlled clinical trial to evaluate a xenogeneic collagen matrix as an alternative to free gingival grafting for oral soft tissue augmentation. J Periodontol 2014;85:1333–1341.

20. Mercado F, Hamlet S, Ivanovski S: Subepithelial connective tissue graft with or without enamel matrix derivative for the treatment of multiple class III–IV recessions in lower anterior teeth: A 3-year randomized clinical trial. J Periodontol 2020;91:473–483.

21. Pelekos G, Lu JZ, Ho DKL, Graziani F, Cairo F, Cortellini P, Tonetti MS: Aesthetic assessment after root coverage of multiple adjacent recessions with coronally advanced flap with adjunctive collagen matrix or connective tissue graft: Randomized clinical trial. J Clin Periodontol 2019;46:564–571.

22. Ramesh KSV, Swetha P, Krishnan V, Mythili R, Rama Krishna Alla, Manikandan D: Assessment of thickness of palatal masticatory mucosa and maximum graft dimensions at palatal vault associated with age and gender – a clinical study. J Clin Diagn Res 2014;8:ZC09–ZC133.

23. Sanz M, Herrera D, Kebschull M, Chapple I, Jepsen S, Beglundh T, Sculean A, Tonetti MS; EFP Workshop Participants and Methodological Consultants. Treatment of stage I–III periodontitis – the EFP S_3 level clinical practice guideline. J Clin Periodontol 2020;47(Suppl 22):4–60.

24. Sanz M, Simion M; Working Group 3 of the European Workshop on Periodontology. Surgical techniques on periodontal plastic surgery and soft tissue regeneration: Consensus report of Group 3 of the 10th European Workshop on Periodontology. J Clin Periodontol 2014;41(Suppl 15):S92–S97.

25. Scharf DR, Tarnow DP: Modified roll technique for localized alveolar ridge augmentation. Int J Periodontics Restorative Dent 1992;12:415–425.

26. Sullivan HC, Atkins JH: Free autogenous gingival grafts. 3. Utilization of grafts in the treatment of gingival recession. Periodontics 1968;6:152–160.

27. Sullivan HC, Atkins JH: Free autogenous gingival grafts. I. Principles of successful grafting. Periodontics 1968;6:121–129.

28. Tavelli L, Barootchi S, Ravida A, Oh TJ, Wang HL: What is the safety zone for palatal soft tissue graft harvesting based on the locations of the greater palatine artery and foramen? A systematic review. J Oral Maxillofac Surg 2019;77: e271–e279.

29. Tavelli L, Ravida A, Lin GH, Del Amo FS, Tattan M, Wang HL: Comparison between subepithelial connective tissue graft and de-epithelialized gingival graft: A systematic review and a meta-analysis. J Int Acad Periodontol 2019;21:82–96.

30. Tavelli L, Ravida A, Saleh MHA, Maska B, Del Amo FS, Rasperini G, Wang HL: Pain perception following epithelialized gingival graft harvesting: A randomized clinical trial. Clin Oral Investig 2019;23:459-468.

31. Thoma DS, Benic GI, Zwahlen M, Hammerle CH, Jung RE: A systematic review assessing soft tissue augmentation techniques. Clin Oral Implants Res 2009;20(Suppl 4):146–165.

32. Thoma DS, Naenni N, Figuero E, Hammerle CHF, Schwarz F, Jung RE, Sanz-Sanchez I: Effects of soft tissue augmentation procedures on peri-implant health or disease: A systematic review and meta-analysis. Clin Oral Implants Res 2018;29(Suppl 15):32–49.

33. Zucchelli G, Mele M, Stefanini M, Mazzotti C, Marzadori M, Montebugnoli L, de Sanctis M: Patient morbidity and root coverage outcome after subepithelial connective tissue and de-epithelialized grafts: A comparative randomized-controlled clinical trial. J Clin Periodontol 2010;37:728–738.

34. Zucchelli G, Mounssif I, Mazzotti C, Montebugnoli L, Sangiorgi M, Mele M, Stefanini M: Does the dimension of the graft influence patient morbidity and root coverage outcomes? A randomized controlled clinical trial. J Clin Periodontol 2014;41:708–716.

Recession coverage

16

Adrian Kasaj

Indications

By definition, recession means the marginal gingiva lies apical to the cementoenamel junction (CEJ), and hence the root surface is exposed. This clinical condition is widespread and affects patients with both good and poor oral hygiene. Although recessions are associated with loss of attachment and may concern the patient, they only rarely result in tooth loss and do not require treatment in every case. The main indications for surgical recession coverage are the esthetic correction of exposed root surfaces and the treatment of dentinal hypersensitivity[11]. However, when patients with dentinal hypersensitivity do not want to undergo esthetic gingival correction, less invasive treatment methods (desensitizing products) should first be used to reduce the pain. In addition, if root caries and/or non-carious cervical lesions (NCCLs) are present, surgical root coverage combined with restorative procedures can be utilized. Recession coverage is also indicated if unfavorable forms of recession or a lack of keratinized tissue compromise mechanical plaque control.

Contraindications

There are only a few specific contraindications for surgical recession coverage. The absolute contraindications relate to patients with serious systemic diseases and/or conditions (e.g. acute-phase myocardial infarction, acute leukemia, deficient immune system) that generally preclude oral surgery interventions. The relative contraindications include an increased bleeding tendency (hemorrhagic diathesis), wound healing complications, acute inflammation in the oral cavity, untreated periodontitis, nicotine use, poor compliance, and unrealistic patient expectations. The decision to perform recession coverage should generally be based on an individual risk analysis and a careful risk–benefit assessment, while taking the patient's preferences into account.

Specific risks

In the hands of an experienced surgeon, surgical recession coverage is a low-risk procedure. However, complications can still occur in isolated cases, and the maxim "there is no surgery without risk" is always true.

Apart from the general risks associated with surgery (swelling, wound infection, bleeding, pain), the main risk related to surgical recession coverage lies in necrosis of the advanced flap and/or the grafted tissue. The consequences may be the formation of visible scar tissue as well as inadequate root coverage and a poor soft tissue condition. Therefore, during flap elevation, attention should always be paid to underlying biologic aspects such as satisfactory flap vascularization and primary tension-free wound closure. In addition, when autologous subepithelial connective tissue grafts are used, care should be taken to ensure that these are perfectly adapted to the recipient site and that coverage is as complete as possible in order to avoid graft exposure and subsequent necrosis. Another specific risk relates to the harvesting of connective tissue grafts from the palate. A bleeding event can occur during harvesting, both intraoperatively and in the early healing phase. However, observing the anatomical limits and ensuring sufficient wound closure can minimize the risk of bleeding. In rare cases, paresthesia (e.g. numbness) can occur at the palatal donor site, but this is only temporary and does not result in permanent functional impairments affecting the palate.

Step-by-step clinical procedure

During the course of recession coverage, an adequate anesthetic effect in both the maxilla and mandible can usually be achieved by vestibular and oral infiltration anesthesia. To avoid bleeding that will compromise visibility during flap elevation and possibly graft adaptation, the author prefers to use a local anesthetic containing 4% articaine and a vasoconstrictor (adrenaline/epinephrine 1:100,000).

Palatal infiltration anesthesia as well as a nerve block in the area of the greater palatine foramen and incisive foramen are suitable when harvesting soft tissue grafts from the palate. Any direct injection of anesthetic into the soft tissue graft should be avoided, if possible, so that blood flow in the graft is not impaired.

If enough depth of anesthesia is not achieved by buccal/lingual infiltration anesthesia during recession coverage in the mandible, a nerve block of the inferior alveolar nerve or the mental nerve can be carried out. However, this is usually not necessary.

Nowadays, surgeons performing coverage of gingival recessions have a wide choice of surgical techniques and combinations of those techniques with different soft tissue grafts. The principle of most surgical techniques involves mobilizing the surrounding keratinized tissue in the form of pedicle flaps and thereby covering the exposed root surface[2]. The pedicle flap techniques can be divided into rotational flaps (laterally positioned or lateral sliding flap, double-papilla flap) and advanced flaps (coronally advanced flap, semilunar flap, tunnel technique). In the case of soft tissue grafts (see Section 15), a distinction is made between the free gingival graft, subepithelial connective tissue graft, and soft tissue substitutes (xenogeneic and allogeneic collagen matrices). The choice of surgical technique is guided by the morphology of the recession, the amount of keratinized tissue around the recession, and the periodontal phenotype. The interproximal height of bone and soft tissue is a crucial factor in the prognosis of recession coverage. Thus, complete root coverage is possible with type 1 (no interproximal attachment loss) and type 2 (interproximal attachment loss equal to or less than buccal attachment loss) recessions[1]. Generally, an inflammation-free soft tissue condition as well as effective biofilm control should be established before any surgical recession coverage. Carious lesions, cervical fillings, and overextended crown margins must be removed before recession coverage, and the exposed root surfaces must be mechanically treated.

The coronally advanced flap is currently the most popular surgical technique for recession coverage and is the first choice in the treatment of single gingival recessions[4]. The presence of at least 2 mm of keratinized tissue apical to the recession is therefore advocated. Preparation of the coronally advanced flap starts with two horizontal incisions, which are placed mesial and distal to the marginal gingiva. These incision lines correspond to the coronal border of the surgical papillae. The height at which the horizontal incision lines are made is determined by the recession depth + 1 mm and is measured from the tip of the anatomical papilla. As a result, the flap can be positioned 1 mm coronal to the CEJ in order to compensate for possible tissue contraction. Starting from the horizontal incisions, two slightly divergent and bevelled oblique incisions are made, which are extended beyond the mucogingival junction into the area of the alveolar mucosa. This is followed by split-thickness elevation of the surgical papillae. The soft tissue apical to the recession is then elevated full-thickness with a periosteal elevator approximately 3 to 4 mm beyond the buccal bone dehiscence. To allow tension-free, coronal mobilization of the flap, the apical portion of the flap is elevated split-thickness, and the muscle insertions are additionally removed from the inside of the flap. Finally, the anatomical papillae are de-epithelialized, the flap is mobilized coronally, and the surgical papillae are secured onto the de-epithelialized anatomical papillae.

The procedure described above for a coronally advanced flap to treat single recessions can also be applied to multiple recessions (Fig 16-1). In a modified form of the coronally advanced flap, oblique incisions are made in the area of the interdental papillae without vertical releasing incisions[10] (Fig 16-2, Video 16-1). The advantages of this technique are that it ensures a good blood supply to the flap and avoids the formation of scar tissue.

If sufficiently wide and thick keratinized tissue is available apical to the recession, the coronally advanced flap can be performed alone or in combination with enamel matrix proteins. In thin soft tissue conditions, however, the coronally advanced flap should be used in combination with a connective tissue graft in order to achieve marginal soft tissue thickening. Harvesting of the connective tissue graft from the palate can either be subepithelial or performed as a free gingival graft with subsequent de-epithelialization. The connective tissue graft should cover the bone dehiscence at the recipient site and be fixed slightly apical to the CEJ. Combination therapy consisting of a coronally advanced flap with a connective tissue graft is currently regarded as the gold standard for surgical coverage of gingival recessions[2]. Xenogeneic collagen matrices can be used as a tissue substitute when patients do not have enough donor tissue or feel uncomfortable with palatal tissue harvesting.

Like the coronally advanced flap, the modified tunnel technique is widely used in the treatment of multiple recessions (Fig 16-3). The characteristic features of this technique are that vertical releasing incisions are not used and the papillae are fully preserved. Starting from

intrasulcular incisions, undermining dissection of the buccal soft tissue is performed with tunneling instruments. The dissection can be performed as a mucosal or mucoperiosteal flap, depending on tissue thickness, and extends apically beyond the mucogingival junction. In addition, the papillae are undermined and mobilized to allow better coronal advancement of the tunneled flap. After flap mobilization, a connective tissue graft is inserted into the tunnel and secured. Finally, tension-free coronal advancement and fixation of the tunneled flap are performed. This technique is particularly suitable for the treatment of shallow and moderate recessions with a sufficiently deep vestibule in the mandibular anterior region.

The majority of recession defects can be successfully treated by the above-mentioned coronally advanced flap techniques alone or in combination with a connective tissue graft. For particularly deep recessions in which there is not enough keratinized tissue apically for coronal advancement, a laterally positioned flap[6] (Fig 16-4) can be used instead. This involves mobilization of the tissue lateral to the recession and subsequent flap rotation to cover the exposed root surface. Other surgical techniques, for example, the double-papilla flap[3], semilunar flap[9], or free gingival graft[8] (Fig 16-5) are only rarely used nowadays.

Wound care and closure

Wound closure for the coronally advanced flap is performed with a sling suture and interrupted sutures in the area of the vertical releasing incisions. For the modified coronally advanced flap without releasing incisions, the flap is accordingly fixed only with sling sutures. A sling suture can also be used for flap fixation in the modified tunnel technique. Alternatively, suspended sutures can be used; these are placed over the

Fig 16-1 Recession coverage with coronally advanced flap in combination with a connective tissue graft:

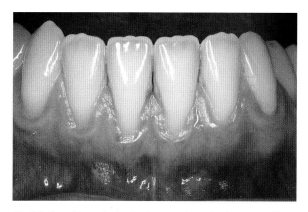

Fig 16-1a   Type 1 gingival recessions in the mandibular central incisor region.

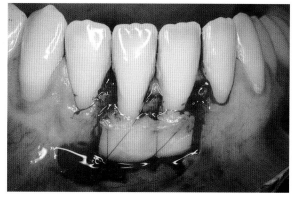

Fig 16-1b   Situation after elevation of a coronally advanced flap and fixation of a de-epithelialized free gingival graft. The anatomical papillae are de-epithelialized and serve as a base for the surgically created papillae.

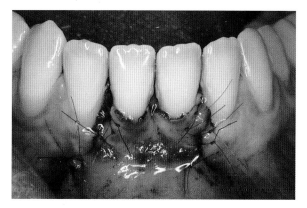

Fig 16-1c   Tension-free coronal flap positioning with sling sutures and interrupted sutures in the area of the vertical releasing incisions.

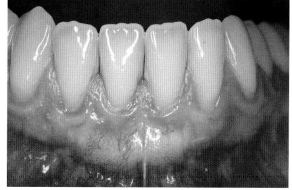

Fig 16-1d   Clinical situation 22 months postoperatively.

interproximal contact points previously blocked out with composite, or they are fixed on the buccal tooth surface.

Wound care in the donor region following connective tissue harvesting from the palate is dictated by the harvesting technique. Interrupted sutures, cross sutures, or continuous sutures can be used for wound closure following subepithelial connective tissue harvesting using the trap-door technique[5] or the single-incision technique[7]. When a free gingival graft is being harvested, the wound surface should be covered with a collagen fleece secured with cross sutures. The donor site can additionally be covered with a cyanoacrylate-based tissue adhesive. It is usually not necessary to use a palatal stent.

Fig 16-2 Recession coverage with a modified coronally advanced flap in combination with a connective tissue graft:

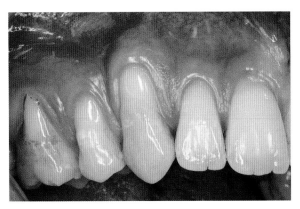

Fig 16-2a   Multiple type 1 gingival recessions in the right maxilla, from central incisor to first molar.

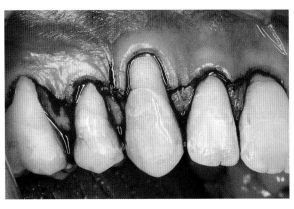

Fig 16-2b   Oblique interdental incisions based on the technique of Zucchelli and De Sanctis[10].

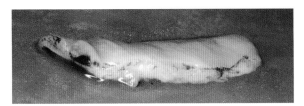

Fig 16-2c   Approximately 2-mm–thick free gingival graft harvested from the palate.

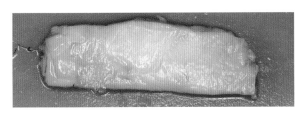

Fig 16-2d   Graft after removal of the epithelial layer.

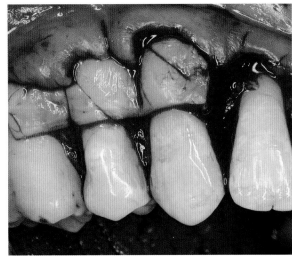

Fig 16-2e   Fixation of the graft with cross sutures.

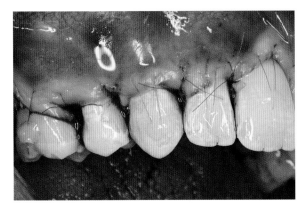

Fig 16-2f   Wound closure with sling sutures and additional suspended sutures, which are fixed buccally with flowable composite.

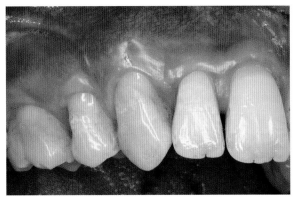

Fig 16-2g   Clinical situation 6 months postoperatively.

Fig 16-3 Recession coverage by the modified tunnel technique in combination with a connective tissue graft:

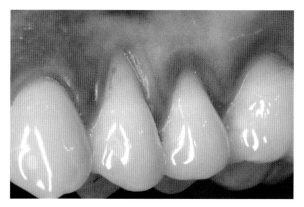

Fig 16-3a Type 1 gingival recessions in the maxillary left first and second premolar region.

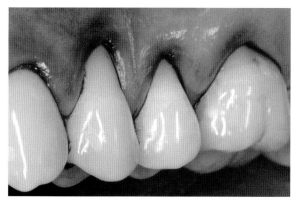

Fig 16-3b Situation after intrasulcular incision from the canine to the first molar, preserving the interdental papillae, and buccal tunnel preparation.

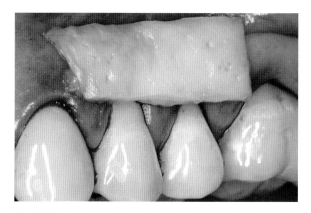

Fig 16-3c Preparation of a de-epithelialized free gingival graft.

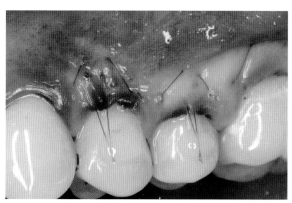

Fig 16-3d Situation after insertion of the graft and coronal fixation of the tunnel flap with modified sling sutures. Buccally suspended sutures are additionally secured with flowable composite.

Video 16-1 Modified coronally advanced flap without vertical releasing incisions in combination with a subepithelial connective tissue graft.

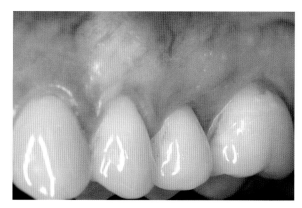

Fig 16-3e Clinical situation 24 months postoperatively.

Fig 16-4 Recession coverage with a laterally positioned flap in combination with a connective tissue graft:

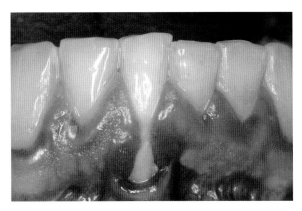

Fig 16-4a   Type 1 gingival recession in the mandibular right central incisor region with < 1 mm of keratinized tissue apical to the recession.

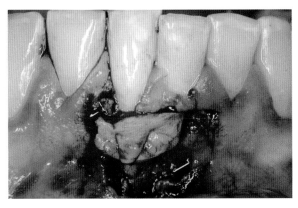

Fig 16-4b   Fixation of a subepithelial connective tissue graft with a cross suture after flap elevation. A recipient bed is first created by de-epithelialization of the gingiva distal and apical to the recession. In the area of the donor site mesially, a horizontal paramarginal incision and an oblique vertical incision are made, and then a mucosal flap is raised.

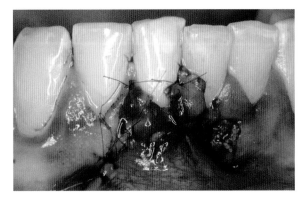

Fig 16-4c   Wound closure of the laterally and coronally positioned flap using a sling suture and interrupted sutures along the vertical incision.

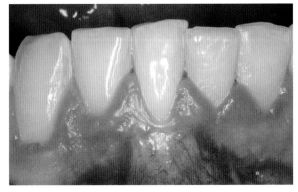

Fig 16-4d   Clinical situation 6 months postoperatively.

Postoperative controls and course

Patients are instructed not to carry out any mechanical oral hygiene at the surgical site postoperatively and to rinse daily with 0.12% chlorhexidine solution for a period of 14 days. Patients are also instructed to avoid tensing the lip and cheek areas as much as possible during this period. An initial wound check can take place 1 week postoperatively, which includes removal of the sutures on the palate and in the area of the vertical releasing incisions. The remaining sutures should be taken out 1 week later, after a total of 14 days postoperatively. The surgical site should then be cleaned carefully with an extra-soft toothbrush for a period of 4 weeks.

Fig 16-5 Recession coverage with a free gingival graft:

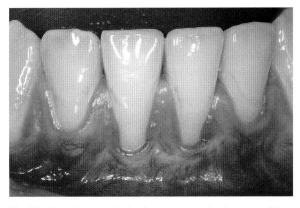

Fig 16-5a Type 1 gingival recessions in the mandibular central incisor region with thin tissue conditions and a shallow vestibule.

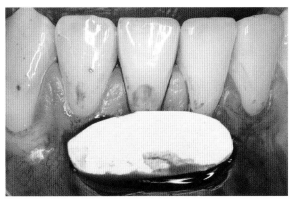

Fig 16-5b Situation after preparation of a recipient bed and adaptation of a template for graft harvesting.

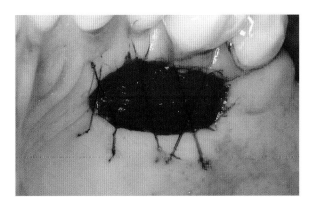

Fig 16-5c Coverage of donor area with collagen fleece and suturing with cross sutures.

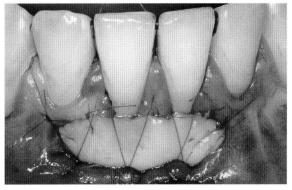

Fig 16-5d Fixation of the free gingival graft on the prepared recipient bed with interrupted and cross sutures.

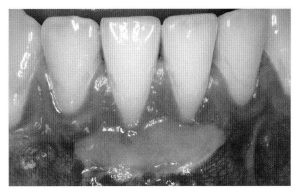

Fig 16-5e Clinical situation 6 months postoperatively.

References

1. Cairo F, Nieri M, Cincinelli S, Mervelt J, Pagliaro U: The interproximal clinical attachment level to classify gingival recessions and predict root coverage outcomes: an explorative and reliability study. J Clin Periodontol 2011;38:661–666.

2. Cairo F: Periodontal plastic surgery of gingival recessions at single and multiple teeth. Periodontol 2000 2017;75:296–316.

3. Cohen DW, Ross SE: The double papillae repositioned flap. J Periodontol 1968;39:65–70.

4. De Sanctis M, Zucchelli G: Coronally advanced flap: a modified surgical approach for isolated recession-type defects: three-year results. J Clin Periodontol 2007;34:262–268.

5. Edel A: Clinical evaluation of free connective tissue grafts used to increase the width of keratinised gingiva. J Clin Periodontol 1974;1:185–196.

6. Grupe HE, Warren RF: Repair of gingival defects by a sliding flap operation. J Periodontol 1956;27:92–95.

7. Hürzeler MB, Weng D: A single-incision technique to harvest subepithelial connective tissue grafts from the palate. Int J Periodontics Restorative Dent 1999;19:279–287.

8. Sullivan HC, Atkins JH: Free autogenous gingival grafts. I. Principles of successful grafting. Periodontics 1968;6:121–129.

9. Tarnow DP: Semilunar coronally repositioned flap. J Clin Periodontol 1986;13:182–185.

10. Zucchelli G, De Sanctis M: Treatment of multiple recession-type defects in patients with esthetic demands. J Periodontol 2000;71:1506–1514.

11. Zucchelli G, Mounssif I: Periodontal plastic surgery. Periodontol 2000 2015;68:333–368.

Salivary stone removal

17

Fabio Saccardin, Sebastian Kühl

A salivary stone (sialolith or ptyalolith) is a calcified concretion of inorganic and organic matter (calcium phosphate, glycoproteins, mucopolysaccharides, lipids, cell debris, etc) that is located within the salivary gland or an excretory duct. A sialolith can measure a few millimeters to several centimeters, and multiple sialoliths can occur. A manifestation or symptoms of a sialolith is referred to as sialolithiasis.

The estimated prevalence of sialoliths in the population is around 1.2%[3]. They predominantly affect middle-aged males.

Indications

Sialoliths are mostly asymptomatic and are discovered by chance during a dental examination (Fig 17-1). However, painful swellings can occur in rare cases, especially before and during meals, because of a buildup of saliva (salivary stone colic). These swellings may additionally be accompanied by a bacterial infection (obstructive sialadenitis). To date, the etiology and pathogenesis of sialoliths have not been fully resolved. The following are probable contributory factors:

- Dehydration,
- Elevated salivary calcium concentration,
- Change in salivary pH,
- Increased salivary viscosity,
- Salivary flow rate and flow direction in conjunction with the morphology of the system of salivary ducts (angled areas of the parotid duct and submandibular duct),
- Sialadenitis (microorganisms and food remnants in the salivary gland excretory ducts),
- Medication (e.g. diuretics, anticholinergics),
- Nicotine use,
- Primary hyperparathyroidism.

Sialoliths are predominantly formed in the major salivary ducts: The submandibular gland is affected in around 85% of cases, the parotid gland in approximately 10% of cases, and the sublingual gland in about 5% of cases. Sialoliths only rarely develop in the minor salivary glands of the mucosa as well. From a topographic viewpoint, sialoliths can be localized in the ductal area (in the distal duct system), hilar area (the transition of the glandular parenchyma to the excretory duct), and the intraglandular area (in the glandular parenchyma) (Fig 17-2). However, a sialolith should ideally be located in the ductal region for it to be surgically removable by a dentist or oral surgeon (sialodochotomy).

Diagnosis involves general history taking but also a thorough clinical examination. This comprises the inspection and also bimanual palpation of the major salivary glands, including their excretory ducts (Figs 17-3 and 17-4). In most cases, this will enable the clinician to distinguish a ductal stone location from a hilar or even intraglandular site with certainty. Furthermore, the affected salivary gland should be swabbed, and the saliva assessed in terms of quantity expelled (salivary congestion), viscosity, and appearance (clear, cloudy, putrid/purulent) (Fig 17-5). It can be helpful to compare the affected side with the contralateral salivary gland. In individual cases, the excretory duct can be probed with a periodontal probe (0.5-mm diameter), a Bowman probe (#00 = 0.7-mm diameter) or a catheter (Fig 17-11). If a surgical procedure is imminent, the intactness of the lingual neve and the facial nerve should always be checked.

In radiologic terms, if sialoliths are located in the ductal area of the submandibular duct or sublingual duct, they can be visualized on a mandibular occlusal radiograph (Fig 17-6). The exposure time is reduced by 50% for better radiographic visualization of the sialoliths. It should be noted that ultrasound is considered the gold standard imaging technique in human medicine. In some cases, however, more

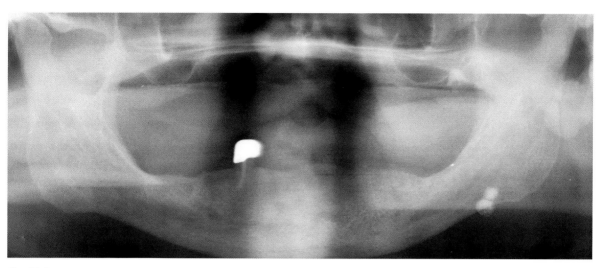

Fig 17-1 With the aid of a panoramic radiograph, two sialoliths are discovered by chance in the area of the left submandibular gland of a 76-year-old patient. The patient had not had any discomfort at any time.

Fig 17-2 In the major salivary ducts, sialoliths can occur in a ductal (a), hilar (b) or intraglandular (c) location. With regard to the submandibular duct (Wharton's duct), sialoliths are found in the ductal system in 34% of cases, in the hilar in 57% of cases, and in the intraparenchymal duct system in 9% of cases. In the parotid duct (Stensen's duct), by comparison, sialoliths have a ductal location in 64% of cases, a hilar location in 13% of cases, and an intraparenchymal location in 23% of cases[4].

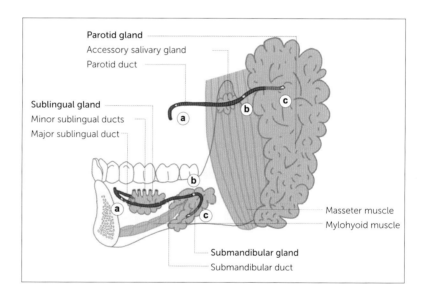

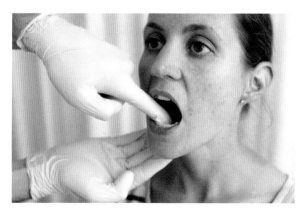

Fig 17-3 Bimanual palpation of the submandibular and sublingual glands.

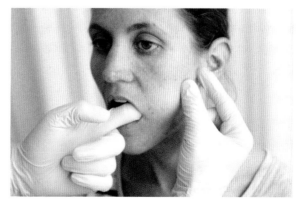

Fig 17-4 Bimanual palpation of the parotid gland.

detailed diagnostic assessment is necessary, for example with the aid of sialendoscopy, magnetic resonance sialography (heavily T2-weighted sequence) or other (functional) radiologic methods (panoramic tomography, cone beam computed tomography, computed tomography or sialography).

Before surgical removal of a sialolith, an attempt should first be made to bring about spontaneous expulsion of the sialolith through conservative therapy. It is possible for sialoliths of < 3 mm in diameter to pass spontaneously through the opening of a salivary gland excretory duct. Saliva-stimulating measures such as hydration (drinking water), mouthwashes, salivary gland massage, drug treatment with sialogogues (e.g. pilocarpine), vitamin C powder, and the use of chewing gum or the sucking of acidic sweets can aid the spontaneous passage of a sialolith. If a patient additionally has sialadenitis, cold should be applied (cool compress) and an anti-inflammatory medication and/or a broad-spectrum antibiotic (e.g. amoxicillin or clindamycin) should be prescribed. If conservative therapy is not successful, other treatment options should be considered:

- Interventional sialendoscopy,
- Sialodochotomy (duct slitting),
- Extracorporeal shock wave lithotripsy (ESWL),
- Combined endoscopic and surgical sialolith retrieval,
- Sialoadenectomy (as a last resort, in cases of recurrent symptomatic sialolithiasis).

The choice of therapeutic approach is guided by the salivary gland affected, which means the location of the obstruction within the gland or excretory duct as well as the cause. The individually listed treatment options can be utilized on their own or in combination[1]. However, this section will only examine in detail the procedure for sialodochotomy. Sialodochotomy is particularly well suited to a salivary stone location in the submandibular or sublingual ducts because these ducts immediately follow a submucous course over a lengthy distance and are hence readily accessible.

Contraindications

Properly performed diagnosis and treatment of salivary stones in a hilar or even intraglandular location fall outside the scope of treatments provided by dental practitioners. In these cases, patients should be referred to an oral and maxillofacial surgeon or an ear, nose, and throat specialist for further diagnosis and treatment.

The following are the most common complications associated with sialodochotomy mentioned in the literature: dry mouth, wound infections, damage to the lingual nerve, and recurrence of sialoliths. Complications are significantly more frequent with a hilar or intraglandular stone location than with a ductal location[2].

In addition, it is more difficult to perform a sialodochotomy on the parotid duct than the submandibular duct because the parotid duct runs deeply through the buccinator muscle immediately after the parotid papilla. Sialodochotomy on the parotid duct is no longer performed due to the extremely high risk of scarring (Figs 17-7 to 17-10).

Other contraindications are general medical impairments that preclude surgery.

Step-by-step clinical procedure

For sialoliths in the submandibular duct and sublingual duct, a nerve block applied to the lingual nerve is not absolutely essential; it is usually enough to perform infiltration anesthesia several times into the floor of the mouth. Especially

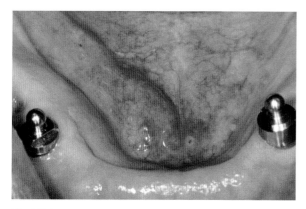

Fig 17-5 A sialolith is located directly in front of the ostium of the submandibular duct on the right. The affected area is slightly reddened and swollen. In this case, bimanual palpation readily reveals a ductal stone location.

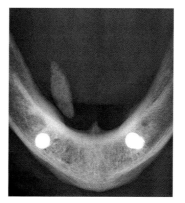

Fig 17-6 Mandibular occlusal radiograph corresponding to Fig 17-5. The exposure time should be reduced by 50% for better radiographic visualization of a sialolith. However, only one-third of all sialoliths can be adequately visualized by radiographic methods.

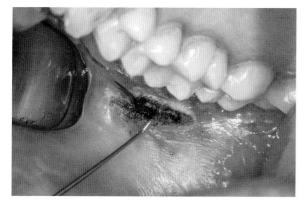

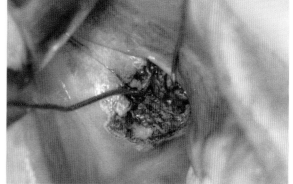

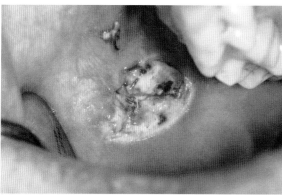

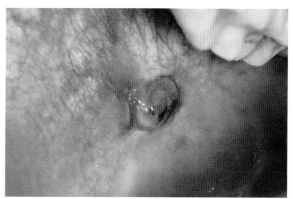

Figs 17-7 to 17-10 Sialodochotomy is often difficult in the area of the parotid duct because, directly after the parotid papilla, this duct runs deeply through the buccinator muscle. Sialodochotomy on the parotid duct is no longer performed due to the extremely high risk of scarring.

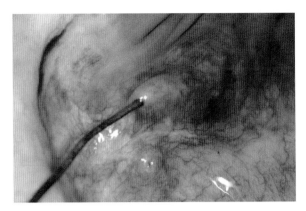

Fig 17-11 Locating the submandibular duct with a thin Bowman probe. In this case, the probe could be advanced as far as the sialolith.

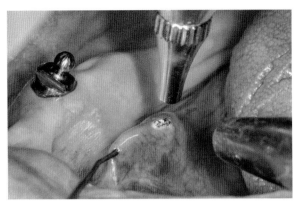

Fig 17-12 With the aid of CO_2 laser, the mucosa is opened along the Bowman probe in the vicinity of the sialolith. The probe can be slightly elevated to do this.

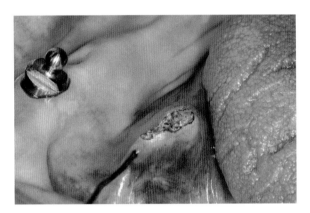

Fig 17-13 After incision with CO_2 laser. The incision does not necessarily have to extend as far as the sublingual caruncle.

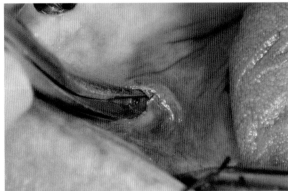

Fig 17-14 Using dissecting scissors for blunt, minimal widening of the opened site.

for younger patients, the application of a surface anesthetic and the use of small needles for administering local anesthetic may be appropriate. The local anesthetic should ideally include an adrenaline/epinephrine additive in order to create bloodless conditions and hence maintain better visibility.

The submandibular duct or sublingual duct can then be visualized using a thin Bowman probe, which is carefully advanced into the particular duct (Fig 17-11, Videos 17-1 and 17-2). With the aid of CO_2 laser (tapered attachment, char-free mode, frequency 140 to 180 Hz, pulse duration 450 µs; see Section 3), the mucosa is then incised above the probe or along the probe, so that the former smaller opening in the area of the excretory duct is enlarged enough to make the sialolith clearly visible (Figs 17-12 and 17-13). Dissecting scissors are used next for blunt, minimal widening of this newly created opening until

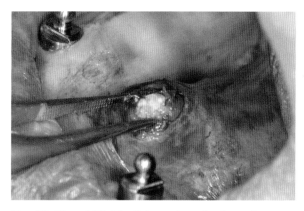
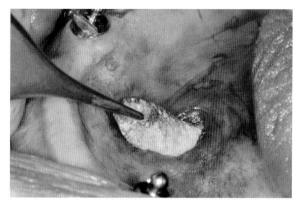

Figs 17-15 and 17-16 Extraoral application of pressure (with the finger from the submandibular direction) and raising the floor of the mouth will squeeze the sialolith outwards. The now clearly visible sialolith can be grasped and removed with surgical tweezers.

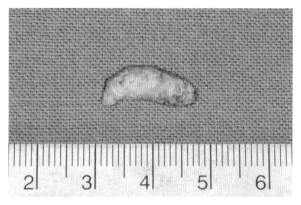
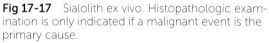

Fig 17-17 Sialolith ex vivo. Histopathologic examination is only indicated if a malignant event is the primary cause.

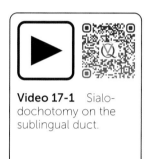

Video 17-1 Sialodochotomy on the sublingual duct.

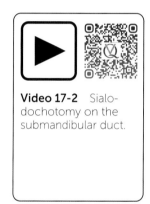

Video 17-2 Sialodochotomy on the submandibular duct.

the sialolith is able to slide through (Fig 17-14). Extraoral application of pressure (with the finger from the submandibular direction) and raising the floor of the mouth will squeeze the sialolith outwards. As a result, the stone can be grasped and removed more easily with surgical tweezers (Figs 17-15 to 17-17). If sialodochotomy is performed with CO_2 laser, no further care of the wound site is required (Figs 17-18 and 17-19). However, if a scalpel is used for the incision, it is advisable to evert the wound margins and suture them to the surrounding mucosa (marsupialization). This prevents adhesion of the wound margins or scarring (with the risk of duct obliteration), and a neo-ostium is able to form.

Antiseptic and analgesic (paracetamol or a nonsteroidal anti-inflammatory drug, preferably ibuprofen) are dispensed postoperatively. Dose and dosage need to be adjusted to the patient's body weight and age.

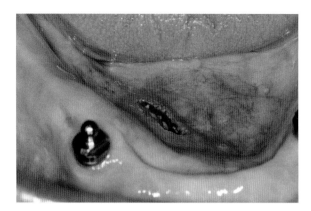

Fig 17-18   Clinical situation of the wound after the sialodochotomy. If the incision is made with CO_2 laser, no further wound care is required.

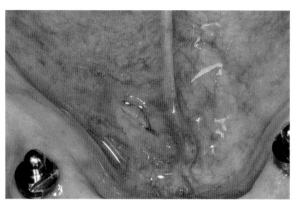

Fig 17-19   Wound conditions 2 weeks after surgery show no irritation.

Postoperative controls and course

The first wound check-up is carried out on the second day postoperatively. During this check-up, the wound site is disinfected with an antiseptic. Follow-up can then take place after 1 week and 1 month.

References

1.   Al-Nawas B, Beutner D, Geisthoff U, Guntinas-Lichius O, Günzel T, Iro H, Koch M, Lell M, Lüers JC, Schröder U, Sproll C, Teymoortash A, Ußmüller J, Vogl T, Wittekindt C, Zengel P, Zenk J: S2k-Leitlinie (Langfassung): Obstruktive Sialadenitis. DGHNO-KHC 2020;4:1–26.

2.   Dong SH, Kim SH, Doo JG, Jung AR, Lee YC, Eun YG: Risk factors for complications of intra-oral removal of submandibular sialoliths. J Oral Maxillofac Surg 2018;76:793–798.

3.   Harrison JD: Causes, natural history, and incidence of salivary stones and obstructions. Otolaryngol Clin North Am 2009;42:927–947.

4.   Sproll C, Naujoks C: Entzündungen und obstruktive Speicheldrüsenerkrankungen. MKG-Chirurg 2015;8:128–141.

Recommended literature

Lommen J, Sproll C: Speichelsteine und deren Behandlung. In: Filippi A, Waltimo T (Hrsg.): Speichel. Berlin: Quintessenz, 2020.

Zenk J, Constantinidis J, Al-Kadah B, Iro H: Transoral removal of submandibular stones. Arch Otolaryngol Head Neck Surg 2001;127:432–436.

Cystostomy and cystectomy

18

Sebastian Kühl, Khaled Mukaddam, Daniel Baumhoer

Indications

Cysts are empty or fluid-filled cavities lined by epithelium that can develop in all tissues, including bone. In the jaws, cysts should generally be removed since leaving them untreated can result in secondary complications, including superinfection, loosening of teeth, fractures, and very rarely also malignant transformation (Fig 18-1). A cystectomy (or enucleation) is always indicated if the cyst can be removed in its entirety without injuring vital neighboring structures. A cystostomy (or marsupialization) is always indicated if injury to vital neighboring structures (nerves, blood vessels, adjacent roots, maxillary sinus, floor of the nose) cannot be safely excluded by curettage during a cystectomy (Figs 18-2 and 18-3). This involves simply opening the cyst or creating a stoma to reduce pressure within the cyst (decompression), enabling bone apposition toward the lumen to take place.

Contraindications

Absolute contraindications mainly arise from the general medical history when patients are inoperable because of their general state of health

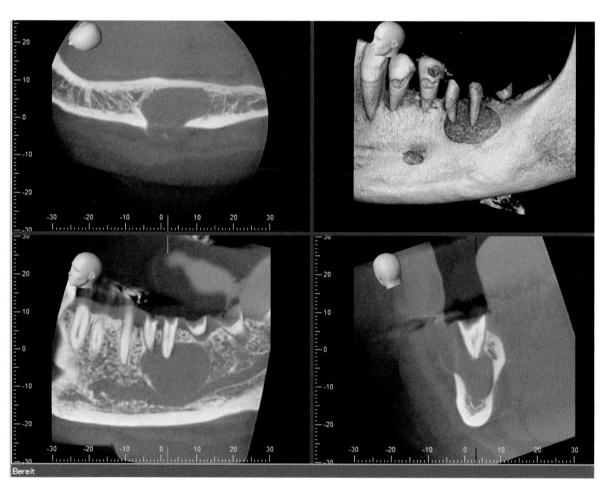

Fig 18-1   Sizeable radicular cyst that led to mild paresthesia in the innervation region of the mental nerve because of pressure on the roof of the canal.

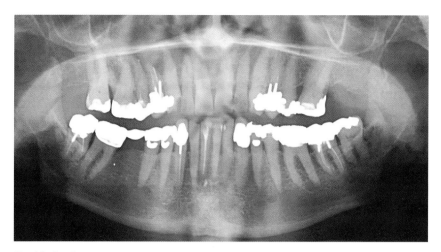

Fig 18-2 Sizeable radicular cyst in the right maxilla. A three-dimensional radiograph is required to correctly assess the dimensions and hence decide on the most appropriate treatment.

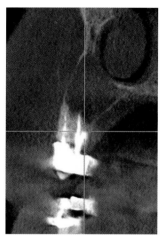

Fig 18-3 Detail from the CBCT in Fig 18-2: maxillary right first premolar region. There is no bony border to the sinus membrane, which is why a cystostomy was planned first in this case.

(e.g. undergoing chemotherapy or diagnosed with terminal-stage cancer). Provisional triple anticoagulation that will be switched to bi- or monotherapy in the foreseeable future is one example of a temporary contraindication. An acute local infection may also be regarded as a temporary contraindication because sufficient depth of anesthesia during the surgical procedure might not be achievable, and the risk of a postoperative wound infection is also increased. A distinction between a cystectomy and cystostomy must also be made with regard to contraindications. The size of a cyst can be a temporary contraindication for a cystectomy if it borders vital structures such as the inferior alveolar nerve, maxillary sinus or tooth roots, and is no longer separated from these vital structures by bone. In these circumstances, a clean cystectomy without injury to these vital structures can no longer be guaranteed, and a cystostomy should be performed as an initial step to reduce the size of the cyst (Figs 18-4 and 18-5).

Specific risks

The specific risks arise from the nature of the surgical procedure (cystectomy versus cystostomy) and the patient's specific anatomy. A cystectomy in the mandible can result in injury to the inferior alveolar nerve or the mental nerve, given the proximity of vital structures. Likewise, in the maxilla, perforation of the maxillary sinus or the floor of the nose can occur if there is no longer a bony separation between the cyst and the sinus membrane or the nasal mucosa. Given the proximity of tooth roots, during curettage of the cyst sac there is a risk of causing direct mechanical damage to the root surface, which can lead to resorptions and hence tooth loss.

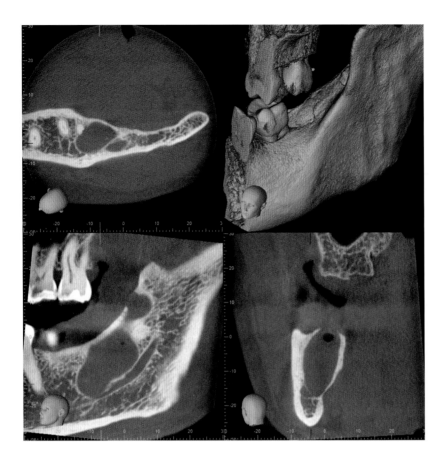

Fig 18-4 In the anterior region, there is no longer a bony border between the odontogenic keratocyst and the mandibular canal. Clean curettage is not possible without injury to the neurovascular bundle; therefore, a cystostomy was initially performed.

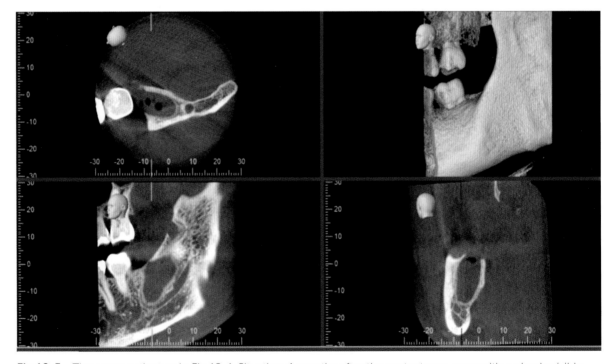

Fig 18-5 The same patient as in Fig 18-4. Situation 4 months after the cystostomy, now with a clearly visible bony border that allows clean curettage to be performed without any damage to the neurovascular bundle.

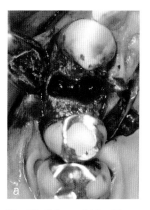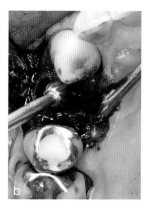

Fig 18-6 (a and b) The same case as in Figs 18-2 and 18-3. Tooth extraction followed by widening of the socket with round burs to gain access to the cyst.

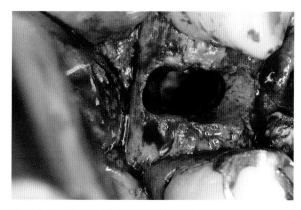

Fig 18-7 The sufficiently widened socket now serves as the access for a tamponade of the cyst.

Especially when large cysts are removed, there is the additional risk of postoperative infection and destabilization of the blood clot.

As with any surgical procedure, the general risks in the form of pain, swelling, wound infection, and bleeding have to be accepted.

Step-by-step clinical procedure

Local anesthesia is guided by the location of the cyst being removed and/or the localization of the access. If a cyst is being removed from a buccal location in the maxilla, infiltration anesthesia mesially and distally of the cyst is advisable. As cysts can extend a long way palatally, local anesthesia should be additionally administered in the palate in the area of the greater palatine foramen or the incisive foramen.

In the mandible, a nerve block of the inferior alveolar nerve should be carried out, together with buccal infiltration mesially and distally of the cyst. Infiltration should be avoided in the area where the cyst is largest because, in many cases, there is no bony border to the cyst here, and inadvertent perforation of the cyst with the

tip of a needle can make an eventual cystectomy more difficult. Local anesthetics with vasoconstrictors should be used to achieve bloodless conditions.

The clinical procedure is dependent on the localization and size of the cyst. For a cystostomy, an access to the cyst is created, through which a tamponade can be placed for several weeks or months. It is therefore advantageous, if at all possible, to place the access in the area of the attached and hence keratinized gingiva. In this respect, large radicular cysts are very amenable to a transalveolar tamponade following tooth extraction and socket widening (Figs 18-6 to 18-11). This is the most comfortable form of access for patients after a cystostomy. After tooth extraction, a round bur is used to widen access to the cyst, while preserving the buccal alveolar wall (i.e. the bur is used on the mesial, distal, and palatal/lingual aspects), sufficiently to allow adequate visibility and good access (see Figs 18-6 and 18-7). In this context, a tissue sample should ideally be obtained to confirm the diagnosis histologically. Cysts can also present as cavities filled with a gelatinous and sometimes yellowish material. However, pseudocysts (not lined by epithelium) and cystic tumors can show

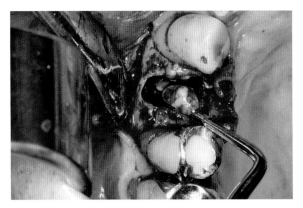

Fig 18-8 Detection of the gelatinous material may indicate the diagnosis of a cyst but is no substitute for taking a tissue sample from the cyst sac.

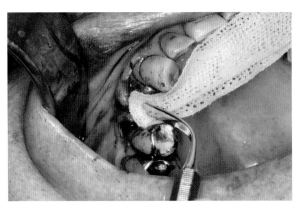

Fig 18-9 An iodine–petroleum jelly tamponade being applied to the cyst to keep the access open.

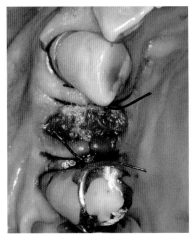

Fig 18-10 Cyst with a tamponade and interrupted sutures. The tamponade should be changed every week.

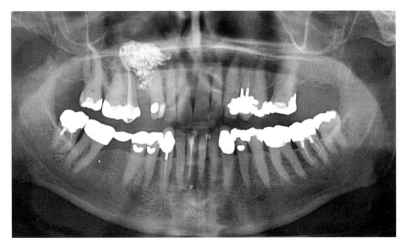

Fig 18-11 Panoramic tomograph showing the size of the cyst that has been treated by a tamponade.

similar findings, which is why tissue should always be sent for histologic examination in those cases to confirm the diagnosis (see Fig 18-8). However, this can also occur with pseudocysts or cyst-like tumors and hence is not a definite indication of a cyst, which is why a histologic examination should always be carried out. Before a tamponade of the cyst lumen is placed, it is advisable to irrigate the lumen first with an iodine solution. If a patient is allergic to iodine, sterile isotonic saline can also be used to remove all the gelatinous material from the cyst lumen. Then, the lumen should be packed, loosely at first so that drainage can still take place (see Figs 18-9 to 18-11). After the initial tamponade has been placed, the switch to an obturator prosthesis can be made (Figs 18-12 to 18-14). This is far more pleasant for the patient to taste, although it is essential to ensure that daily irrigation of the cyst lumen takes place at home. A control radiograph

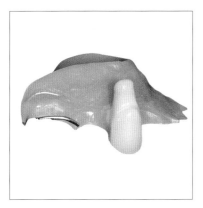

Fig 18-12 Obturator prosthesis for a cystostomy.

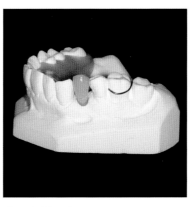

Fig 18-13 Obturator prosthesis.

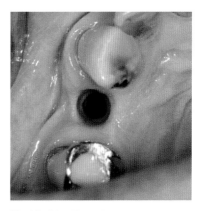

Fig 18-14 The obturator prosthesis keeps the socket open and thereby allows the cyst lumen to decrease in size.

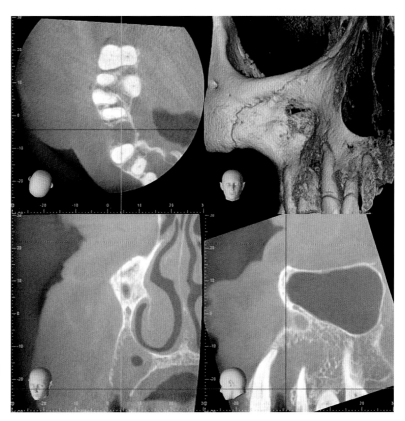

Fig 18-15 In comparison with the preoperative situation (Fig 18-3), there is now a bony border between the sinus membrane and the cyst lumen so that a cystectomy can take place.

is taken about 3 months after the cystostomy. The focus is to check whether the vital structure that justified the cystostomy now has a complete bony border to the cyst lumen (Fig 18-15) and permits clean curettage of the cyst on the

bony foundation without jeopardizing that vital structure.

In the case of a cystectomy, access should also be chosen with care in order to ensure that the cyst lumen can be fully opened for complete

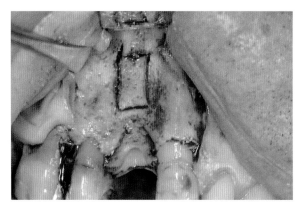

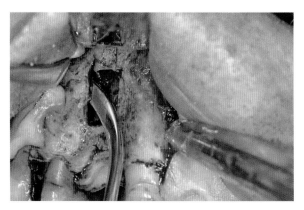

Fig 18-16   After a crestal incision and vertical releasing incisions (trapezoidal flap) are made, a bone window is dissected in the buccal area by piezosurgery. The window must permit access to the entire cyst lumen.

Fig 18-17   Blunt curettage of the cyst with special cyst elevators.

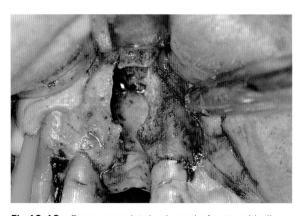

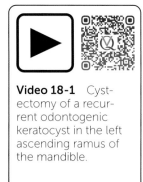

Video 18-1   Cystectomy of a recurrent odontogenic keratocyst in the left ascending ramus of the mandible.

Fig 18-18   Bone completely cleared of cyst epithelium.

curettage. Transalveolar access is usually insufficient for this purpose (Fig 18-16). Piezosurgery enables the bone cover to be shaped in order to allow good access to the cyst lumen (Fig 18-17). The cyst sac is ideally detached bluntly from the underlying bone with special elevators, then undergoes histopathologic examination (Fig 18-23). The more carefully the cystectomy is carried out, the lower the risk of recurrence (Fig 18-18). Freshening the bone can be useful, especially in the case of odontogenic keratocysts with a tendency to recur (Video 18-1). Furthermore, when dealing with an odontogenic keratocyst, the stoma and the surrounding mucosa, which has meanwhile fused with the cyst, also need to be removed since evaginations presenting as microcysts or satellites might be present and increase the risk of recurrence[1]. This involves microscopically small, self-contained outgrowths and separate lesions, which definitely have to be removed at the same time. To seal the access again, fresh osteotomies can be made in the alveolar process and the bone cover by piezosurgery, which then help when repositioning and fixing the bone cover with resorbable sutures (Figs 18-19 and 18-20). In the

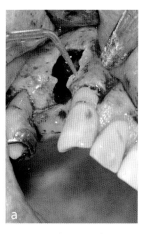 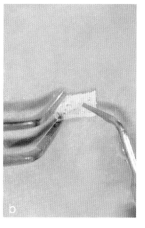

Fig 18-19 (a and b) Osteotomies are created by piezosurgery so that the bone cover can be repositioned again after the cystectomy.

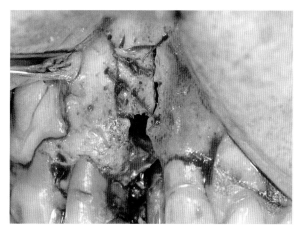

Fig 18-20 Bone cover repositioned and fixed with resorbable sutures.

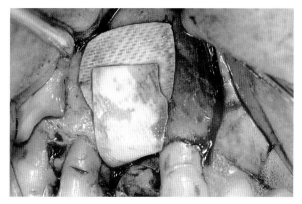

Fig 18-21 Additional coverage with a resorbable membrane, as in the guided bone regeneration technique.

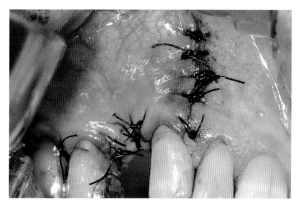

Fig 18-22 Suturing.

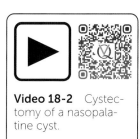

Video 18-2 Cystectomy of a nasopalatine cyst.

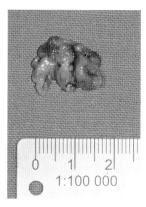

Fig 18-23 Cyst sac after removal and before histopathologic examination.

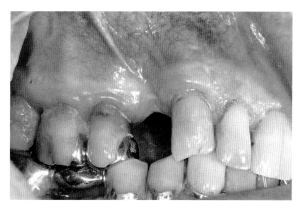

Fig 18-24 Clinically unremarkable situation 3 weeks after suture removal.

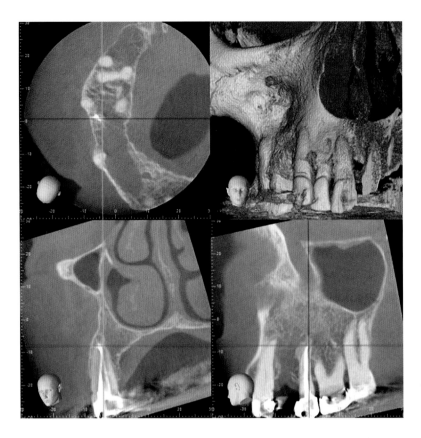

Fig 18-25   Radiographic follow-up 1 year after the cystectomy. There is almost complete bony consolidation of the former cyst lumen.

same way as for the guided bone regeneration technique, the next step is to carry out coverage with a resorbable collagen membrane and tight wound closure with sutures (Figs 18-21 and 18-22). Provided there is no tunneling defect, the former cyst lumen does not necessarily have to be filled with filling materials such as bone substitute or collagen fleece (Video 18-2). Monitoring of treatment outcome is then documented clinically and radiographically (Figs 18-24 and 18-25). If the treatment has been successful, a definitive prosthetic restoration can be provided (Fig 18-26).

Pseudocysts, including solitary and aneurysmal bone cysts, are distinct from odontogenic cysts, both histologically and genetically. They lack an epithelial lining and are considered true neoplasms with recurrent genetic alterations. Pseudocysts have a predilection for the body and the posterior aspects of the mandible and

can reach a considerable size (Fig 18-27). In the anterior mandible, a two-layer procedure may be recommended as an alternative to marginal incision (Figs 18-28 to 18-30). After the initial surface incision in the vestibule (see Fig 18-28), a second, horizontal cut is made more caudally on the bone. The subsequent dissection of the periosteum caudally gives rise to a two-layer flap (Figs 18-31 to 18-35).

Wound closure is adaptive, with interrupted sutures for both the palatal and vestibular access. A tight seal is not essential. If a marginal access had been chosen, either interrupted sutures or vertical mattress sutures can be used for the papillae. It is advisable to fill the former cyst lumen if a tunneling defect is present[2]. This situation mainly occurs with radicular cysts, which are treated in conjunction with an apicectomy (see Section 10) or with nasopalatine cysts (see Video 18-2).

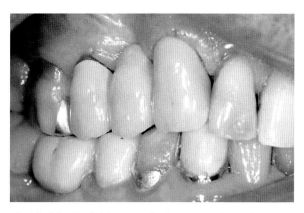

Fig 18-26 Definitive prosthetic restoration using a bridge (reconstruction by Dr Inga Mollen).

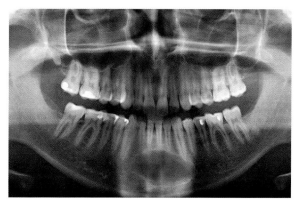

Fig 18-27 Panoramic radiograph with sizeable radiolucent area in the anterior mandible. All the teeth are vital.

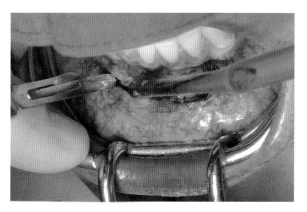

Fig 18-28 Initial incision in the area of the mucosa.

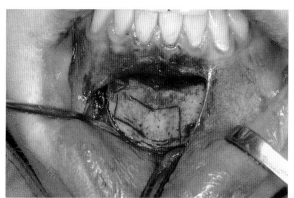

Fig 18-29 Second incision much further caudally, creating a two-layer flap.

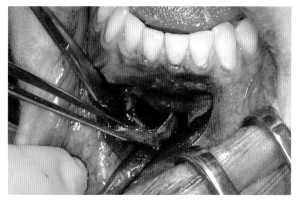

Fig 18-30 Placement of bone cover.

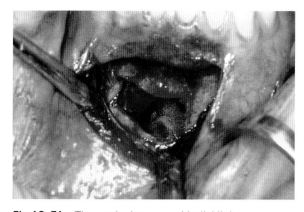

Fig 18-31 The cavity has no epithelial lining.

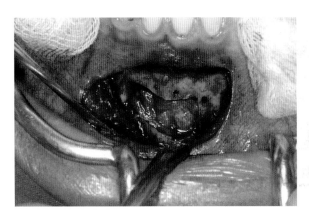

Fig 18-32   After cleansing, collagen fleece is packed into the wound.

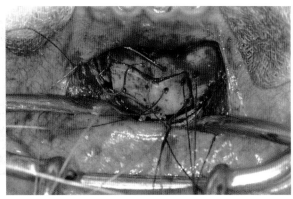

Fig 18-33   Perforations in the bone cover and locally for adaptation of the bone cover with resorbable suture material.

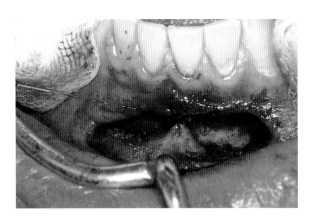

Fig 18-34   Deep two-layer wound closure with resorbable suture material.

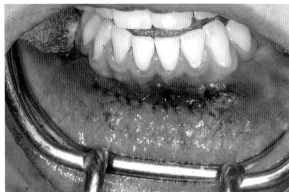

Fig 18-35   Surface view of the two-layer wound closure.

Postoperative controls and course

The first clinical check-up after a cystectomy usually takes place on the second day after surgery. During the appointment, wound disinfection can be performed with 1% hydrogen peroxide or with povidone iodine. It is important to encourage patients to resume their habitual oral hygiene measures and clean the wounds with a soft toothbrush. Pain medication, depending on the individual case history, either takes the form of ibuprofen or paracetamol. Administration of antibiotics is not generally required after a cystostomy. In the case of cystectomies, the indication is determined by the size of the cyst lumen:

The larger the lumen, the more advisable it is to prescribe an antibiotic. An aminopenicillin with clavulanic acid is usually recommended; clindamycin at a dose dependent on body weight is used for patients who are allergic to penicillin.

References

1.   Stoelinga PJ: Long-term follow-up on keratocysts treated according to a defined protocol. Int J Oral Maxillofac Surg 2001;30:14–25.

2.   von Arx T, AlSaeed M: The use of regenerative techniques in apical surgery: A literature review. Saudi Dent J 2011;23:113–127.

3.   Weiss P, Baumhoer D, Lambrecht JT, Filippi A: Pseudozysten im Kieferbereich. Quintessenz 2011;62:931–939.

Removal of exostoses

19

Silvio Valdec, Bernd Stadlinger

Indications

Absolute indications for the removal of exostoses are discomfort or pain, dehiscence or exposure, and a mucosa-supported complete denture worn by an edentulous patient.

Relative indications comprise impairment of tongue movement, corresponding speech difficulties, interference with oral hygiene, and periodontal problems such as pseudopockets.

In addition, the possibility of Gardner syndrome (autosomal dominant inherited, familial adenomatous polyposis coli) must be considered and investigated, if appropriate.

Contraindications

Absolute and temporary contraindications relate to notable issues in a patient's medical history. Patients receiving ongoing treatment with anti-resorptive medication should be referred to a specialist.

Specific risks

The specific risks consist of bleeding, wound healing complications, dehiscence, infections, and nerve lesions (mandible: lingual nerve; also, inferior alveolar nerve in the retromolar region).

Step-by-step clinical procedure

The surgical field is numbed by infiltration anesthesia (if appropriate, a nerve block) using articaine 4% with 1:200,000 adrenaline/epinephrine.

The following treatment steps then take place (Video 19-1):

Incision:

■ Midline open-door (double "Y") incision in the maxilla for palatal tori (Figs 19-1 and 19-2); intrasulcular or mucosal incision for exostoses with a vestibular location (Figs 19-11 and 19-12), depending on the size and localization.

■ Lingual intrasulcular incision in the mandible (Figs 19-15, 19-16, and 19-36 to 19-39); crestal incision in the edentulous jaw segment (Figs 19-24, 19-25, 19-45, 19-46, and 19-52), depending on the size and localization.

After a mucoperiosteal flap has been raised, the exostosis is fully exposed (Figs 19-2, 19-12, 19-16, 19-26, 19-29, 19-39, 19-46, and 19-52).

Using piezoelectric surgery, risk-free segmentation or particulation can be performed, followed by smoothing of sharp bone edges with diamond-coated piezoelectric surgery attachments or with a rose bur or diamond round bur. (Caution: complete excision of the exostosis with a rose bur or diamond bur makes it impossible to perform a histopathologic examination) (Figs 19-3 to 19-7, 19-13, 19-17 to 19-19, 19-21, 19-27, 19-28, 19-30, 19-31, 19-33, 19-40 to 19-42, 19-47 to 19-50, 19-53, and 19-55).

Then, the bone chips should be irrigated with sterile isotonic saline. After irrigation, the mucoperiosteal flap is repositioned (sizeable exostoses may additionally require adaptation of excess tissue, provided that any risk to nerves or blood vessels is unlikely), and primary wound closure takes place (Figs 19-8, 19-14, 19-20, 19-22, 19-32, 19-51, and 19-54).

Primary wound closure involves the use of interrupted sutures or vertical mattress sutures for an intrasulcular incision (usually with nonresorbable suture material in order to avoid accumulation of plaque; resorbable suture material can be used in children and patients with poor compliance).

Postoperative controls and course

A recall to check the wound normally takes place after 2 to 3 days, and suture removal is performed after 7 to 10 days (Figs 19-9, 19-10, 19-23, 19-34, 19-35, 19-43, 19-44, and 19-56).

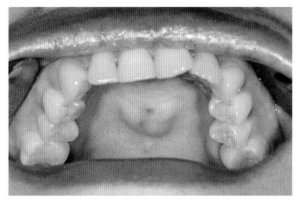

Fig 19-1 Case 1: Clinical image of a sizeable palatal torus in the typical midline position in the area of the hard palate.

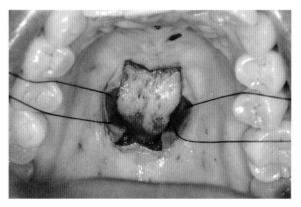

Fig 19-2 Case 1: Midline incision on the exostosis with two anterolateral and posterolateral releasing incisions. The elevated flap is then retracted with stay sutures on both sides.

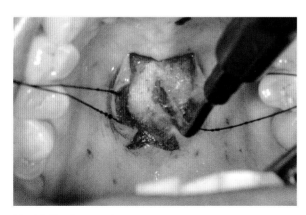

Fig 19-3 Case 1: Segmentation by piezoelectric surgery.

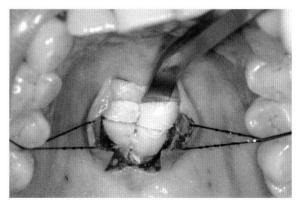

Fig 19-4 Case 1: The exostosis segments are excised with a chisel.

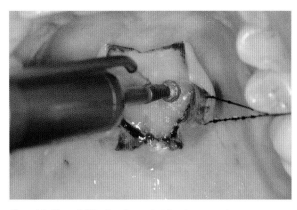
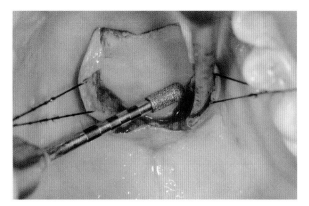

Figs 19-5 and 19-6   Case 1: The bone edges are smoothed with a rotary diamond round bur and/or by piezo-electric surgery with a diamond-coated attachment.

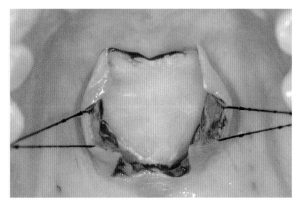
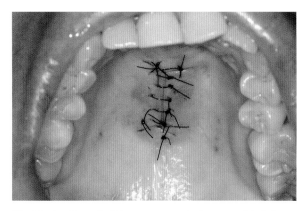

Fig 19-7   Case 1: The surgical field is irrigated with saline.

Fig 19-8   Case 1: Primary wound closure with 5-0 interrupted sutures.

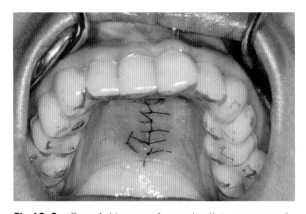
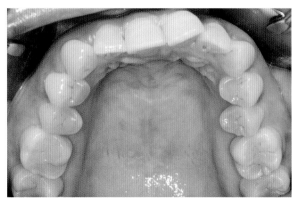

Fig 19-9   Case 1: Vacuum-formed splint as a wound protector; clinical situation 8 days postoperatively.

Fig 19-10   Case 1: Clinical situation 3 months postoperatively.

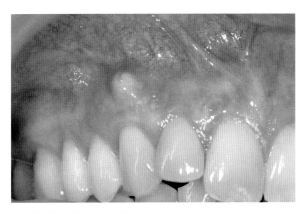

Fig 19-11 Case 2: Clinical image of a buccal exostosis in the maxillary right canine region.

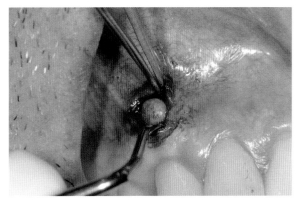

Fig 19-12 Case 2: Vestibular incision at the margin of the exostosis.

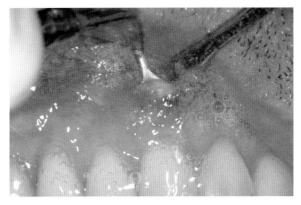

Fig 19-13 Case 2: The exostosis is excised by piezoelectric surgery.

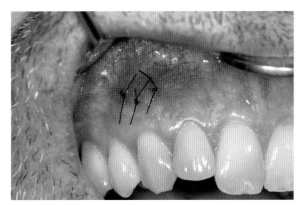

Fig 19-14 Case 2: Clinical situation 7 days postoperatively, immediately before suture removal.

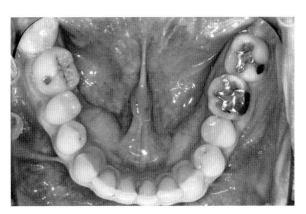

Fig 19-15 Case 3: Bilateral lingual exostoses in the mandible; typical localization of mandibular tori.

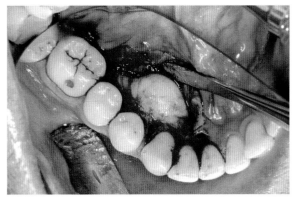

Fig 19-16 Case 3: Intrasulcular incision from the central incisor to the first molar in the right mandible and exposure of the exostosis.

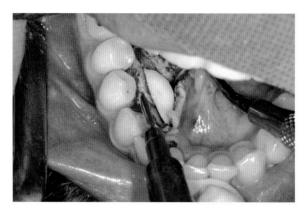

Fig 19-17   Case 3: Osteotomy by means of piezo-electric surgery without penetrating the soft tissue.

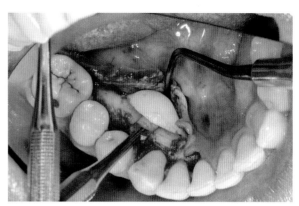

Fig 19-18   Case 3: Resection with a chisel.

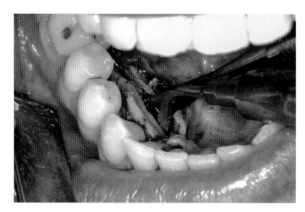

Fig 19-19   Case 3: The excess and sharp edges are smoothed by piezoelectric surgery with a diamond-coated attachment.

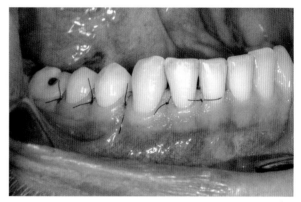

Fig 19-20   Case 3: Primary wound closure with vertical mattress sutures (5-0) in the area of the papillae (vestibular view).

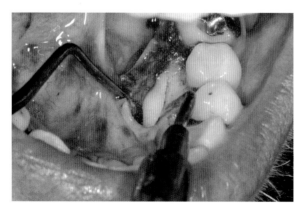

Fig 19-21   Case 3: Marginal incision from the mandibular left lateral incisor to the first molar for exposure of the opposite exostosis and resection by piezoelectric surgery in the same way as on the contralateral side.

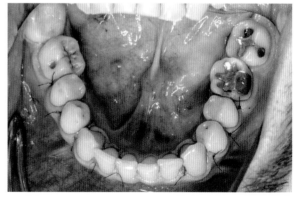

Fig 19-22   Case 3: Primary wound closure with vertical mattress sutures (5-0) in the area of the papillae (occlusal view).

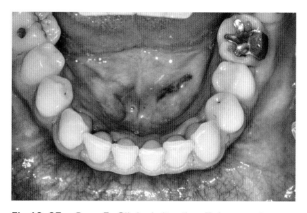

Fig 19-23 Case 3: Clinical situation 7 days postoperatively, immediately after suture removal.

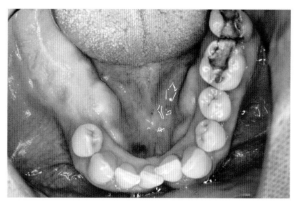

Fig 19-24 Case 4: Bilateral lingual exostoses in the mandible; typical localization of a mandibular tori. In this case, the fabrication of a removable prosthetic restoration was impeded by the exostosis.

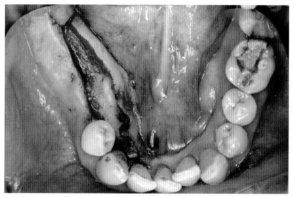

Fig 19-25 Case 4: Intrasulcular incision made lingually of the mandibular right central incisor over the crest to the mandibular right first and second molars with an unobtrusive distal releasing incision in the lingual direction. (Caution: Only place a lingual releasing incision crestally in an edentulous jaw and never too far distally in order to avoid harming the lingual nerve.)

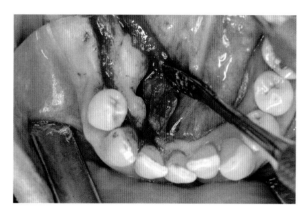

Fig 19-26 Case 4: Exposure of the exostosis in the mandibular right canine to first molar region.

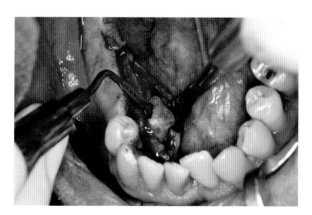

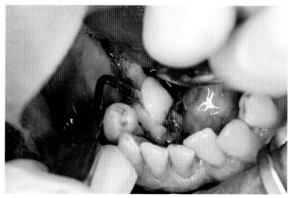

Figs 19-27 and 19-28 Case 4: Osteotomy by means of piezoelectric surgery without penetrating the soft tissue.

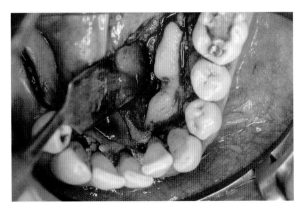

Fig 19-29   Case 4: Exposure of the contralateral exostosis in the mandibular left lateral incisor to first molar region.

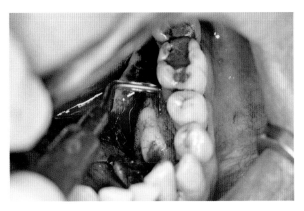

Fig 19-30   Case 4: Osteotomy by means of piezo-electric surgery without penetrating the soft tissue; in this case, with a double-angled attachment.

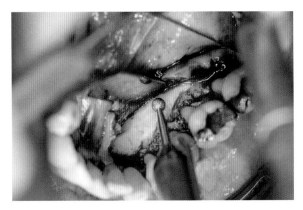

Fig 19-31   Case 4: The excess and sharp edges are smoothed with a diamond round bur.

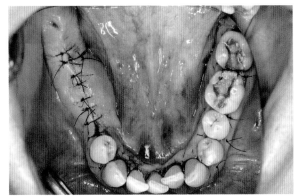

Fig 19-32   Case 4: Primary wound closure with vertical mattress sutures in the area of the papillae and interrupted sutures (5-0) (occlusal view).

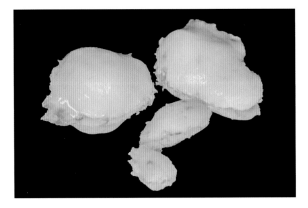

Fig 19-33   Case 4: Parts of the osteotomized exostoses before fixation in formalin and histopathologic examination.

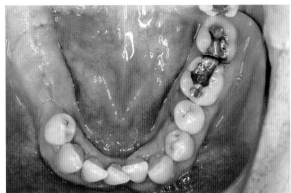

Fig 19-34   Case 4: Clinical situation 7 days postoperatively, immediately after suture removal.

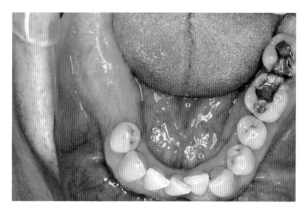

Fig 19-35 Case 4: Clinical situation 6 months post-operatively.

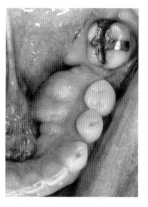

Fig 19-36 Case 5: Prominent lingual exostosis in the mandibular left quadrant.

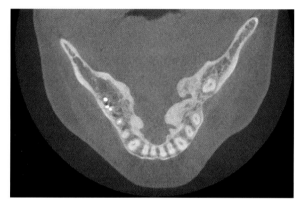

Fig 19-37 Case 5: Axial CBCT view of the exostosis.

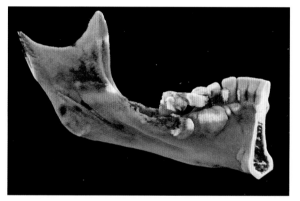

Fig 19-38 Case 5: Cinematic rendering of the CBCT data set: Sagittal view with slight cranial angulation.

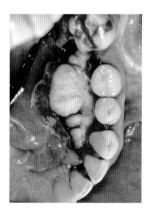

Fig 19-39 Case 5: Intra-sulcular incision from the mandibular left central incisor to the second molar: Exposure of the significant exostosis.

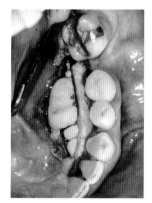

Fig 19-40 Case 5: Osteotomy by means of piezoelectric surgery without penetrating the soft tissue.

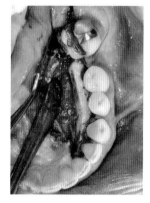

Fig 19-41 Case 5: The excess and sharp edges are smoothed.

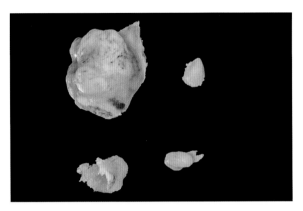

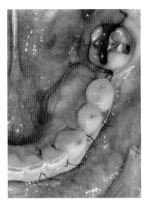

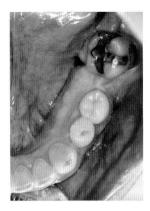

Fig 19-42 Case 5: Parts of the removed exostoses before fixation in formalin and histopathologic examination.

Fig 19-43 Case 5: Clinical situation 7 days postoperatively, immediately before suture removal. It is advisable to monitor progress in this case because of the significant soft tissue excess.

Fig 19-44 Case 5: Clinical situation 4 months postoperatively. Soft tissue adaptation can be seen.

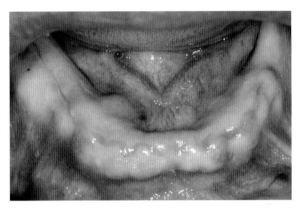

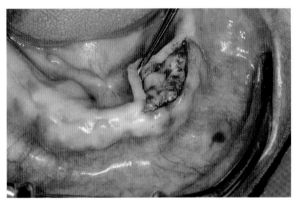

Fig 19-45 Case 6: Bilateral lingual exostoses in the edentulous mandible; referral for removal of exostoses prior to restoration with a complete denture.

Fig 19-46 Case 6: Crestal incision in the mandibular left quadrant; in this case, without releasing incisions because of the minimal size and proximity to the alveolar ridge.

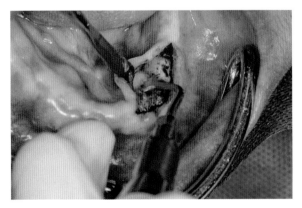

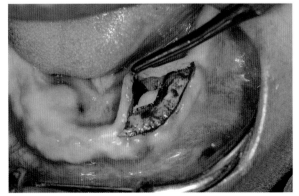

Figs 19-47 and 19-48 Case 6: Osteotomy by means of piezoelectric surgery without penetrating the soft tissue.

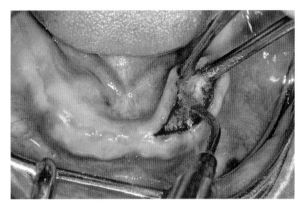

Fig 19-49 Case 6: The excess and sharp edges are smoothed by piezoelectric surgery with a diamond-coated attachment.

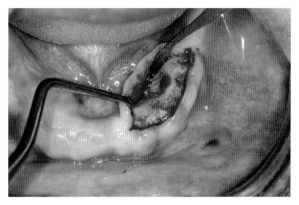

Fig 19-50 Case 6: Clinical situation after irrigation with saline.

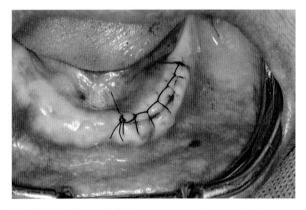

Fig 19-51 Case 6: Primary wound closure in the mandibular left quadrant with continuous sutures (4-0) in the area of the alveolar ridge.

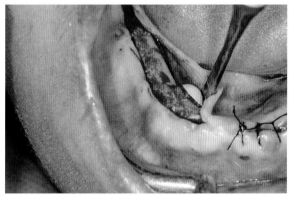

Fig 19-52 Case 6: Crestal incision in the mandibular right quadrant without releasing incisions; an osteotomy by piezoelectric surgery.

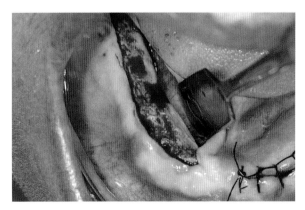

Fig 19-53 Case 6: The excess and sharp edges are smoothed by piezoelectric surgery with a diamond-coated attachment.

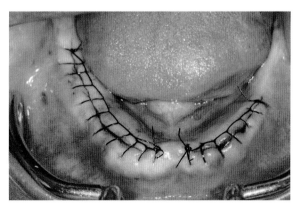

Fig 19-54 Case 6: Primary wound closure in the mandibular right quadrant with continuous sutures (4-0) in the area of the alveolar ridge.

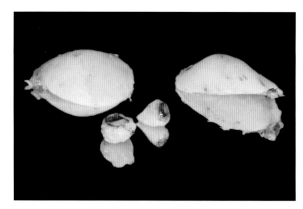

Fig 19-55   Case 6: Parts of the removed exostoses before fixation in formalin and histopathologic examination.

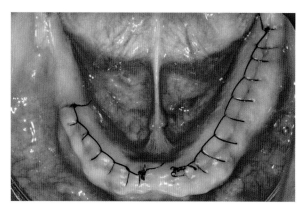

Fig 19-56   Case 6: Clinical situation 7 days postoperatively, immediately before suture removal.

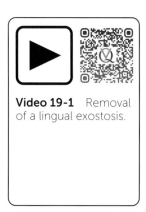

Video 19-1   Removal of a lingual exostosis.

Recommended literature

García-García AS, Martínez-González JM, Gómez-Font R, Soto-Rivadeneira A, Oviedo-Roldán L: Current status of the torus palatinus and torus mandibularis. Med Oral Patol Oral Cir Bucal 2010;15:e353–e360.

Lambrecht JT (Hrsg.): Zahnärztliche Operationen. Berlin: Quintessenz, 2008.

Loukas M, Hulsberg P, Tubbs RS, Kapos T, Wartmann CT, Shaffer K, Moxham BJ: The tori of the mouth and ear: a review. Clin Anat 2013;26:953–960.

Surgical revisions of the alveolar process

20

Stephan Acham, Michael Schwaiger, Norbert Jakse,
Jürgen Wallner, Wolfgang Zemann

Revisions of the alveolar ridge may become necessary if surgical procedures, foremost tooth extractions, or traumata, such as pressure points of dentures, are followed by impaired wound healing processes. The consequences may be pain, swelling, fistulas, and/or bone exposure. In rare cases they occur spontaneously. The particular indications are painful and/or inflammatory processes affecting the jawbone that:

■ Cannot be controlled by purely conservative measures,
■ Cannot be expected to remain sustainably symptom-free in the long term after suspension of conservative treatment,
■ Are following a progressive course,
■ Are suspected to be (latently) progressing.

Such changes should be thoroughly investigated and the indication for surgical revision should be considered.

In addition to the clear indication for the removal of symptomatic bone splinters and sharp bone edges, retained mobile root remnants, and (infected) foreign bodies, the following three diagnoses usually require a surgically assisted intervention:

■ Alveolitis or alveolar osteitis (AO),
■ Osteonecrosis of the jaw (ONJ) (medication-related osteonecrosis of the jaw [MRONJ], osteoradionecrosis [ORN]),
■ Osteomyelitis (OM).

Alveolitis or alveolar osteitis

Blum reports 18 different definitions of alveolar osteitis (AO)[4]. The most appropriate description is "postoperative pain increasing in severity as time progresses, which occurs between the first and third day post-extraction, accompanied by (partial) loss of the blood clot from the dental socket with or without halitosis."

Gowda et al discuss 12 etiologically relevant factors that can favor the development of alveolitis[8] (Figs 20-1 and 20-2). They can be subdivided into:

■ **Patient-specific factors** (e.g. age, hormonal factors, systemic diseases, smoking, local infections, mechanical removal of the blood clot),
■ **Factors intrinsic to the treatment** (e.g. region and level of difficulty of the procedure, experience of the surgeon, nature and administration of local anesthesia).

The incidence correlates with the level of difficulty and duration of tooth extraction. While the prevalence ranges between 0.5% and 5% for routine tooth extractions, it varies between 1% and 37.5% for third molar extractions[10]. The course of the disease is self-limiting in the majority of cases. Conservative local measures and appropriate pain therapy mainly serve to reduce the symptoms.

Surgical revision with primary wound closure is indicated if there is no subjective or objective improvement in the clinical situation within 3 to 5 days despite adequate conservative **local treatment and medication**.

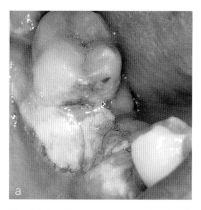 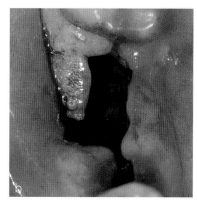 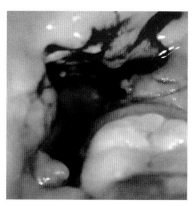

Fig 20-1   Poor postoperative hygiene in the area of the extraction sockets favors the development of primarily infectious alveolar osteitis (AO), usually with a smeary coating of mixed, mycobacterial colonization (a). After removal of the coating, an empty socket (dry socket) can be visualized (b).

Fig 20-2   Typical image of a dry socket after wisdom tooth extraction. Radiographic evaluation to visualize root remnants, bone splinters, exclusion of a fracture, and the course of the mandibular canal in relation to the tooth socket is essential (see Figs 20-6 to 20-8).

Osteonecrosis of the jaw

Medication-related osteonecrosis of the jaw (MRONJ)

The term osteonecrosis of the jaw (ONJ) covers a rare but serious complication of drug treatments, which was first described in 2003 in connection with bisphosphonates. Nowadays, anti-bone resorption therapies are mainly used in the treatment of various hemato-oncologic diseases, but also for reducing bone resorption in osteoporosis.

Definition

The following common features are attributed to MRONJ[1,14]:

■ Currently ongoing or previous treatment with antiresorptive or antiangiogenic drugs,

■ Exposed bone over a period of 8 weeks (from the time the diagnosis is made),

■ No history of radiotherapy and definite exclusion of metastases in the oral and maxillofacial region.

Etiology

As well as reducing bone turnover by irreversibly impairing osteoclast activity, bisphosphonates are toxic to many different cell lines (e.g. mucosa, vessel wall). Long-term binding to bone is a key aspect of this group of active substances. Different bisphosphonate drugs with variable potency and a correlating risk of ONJ are available[7,9].

Denosumab (brand names: Xgeva, Prolia) is a monoclonal immunoglobulin G_2 (IgG_2) antibody, which reduces overall osteoclast activity by selectively binding to the cellular surface protein RANKL (receptor activator of nuclear factor kappa B ligand) and preventing the transformation of pre-osteoclasts into fully functioning osteoclasts; as a result, bone resorption is inhibited[7].

Risk stratification

The risk of developing MRONJ while on antiresorptive therapy largely depends on external variables and individual risk factors (Fig 20-3).

The following treatment-related factors are decisive in terms of the individual risk:

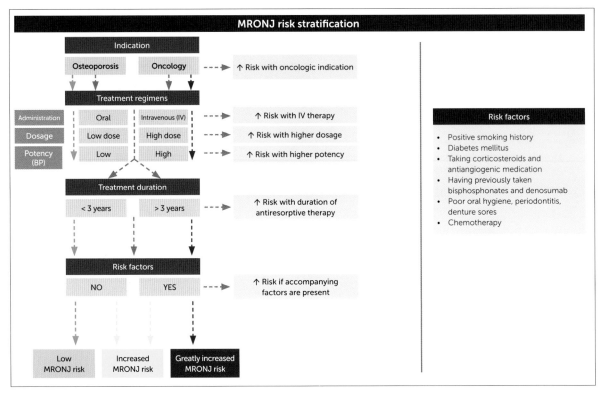

Fig 20-3   Risk stratification of MRONJ.

- Dose and dosage interval,
- Duration of treatment,
- For bisphosphonates, the active substance and route of administration (oral or intravenous).

Patient-specific risk factors such as the presence of systemic diseases like diabetes mellitus and cortisone therapy as well as a history of smoking, genetic predisposition, anatomical factors, and individual hygiene capability have an additional influence.

The dosage of antiresorptive drugs to treat osteoporosis is usually significantly lower than for oncologic indications. Consequently, the risk of patients with osteoporosis developing the side effects of MRONJ is hugely reduced compared with the risk in oncology patients[11].

Clinical and radiologic features

The **clinical symptoms** of MRONJ range from nonspecific jaw pain and nonhealing extraction sockets to large areas of exposed bone, the formation of bone sequestra, the formation of intraoral and extraoral fistulas, and pathologic jaw fractures. Infections of exposed, necrotic bone are typical and, in most cases, aggravate the clinical picture. MRONJ affects the mandible far more frequently (65%) than the maxilla (28.4%). Both jaws are affected in 6.5% of cases. In rare cases (0.1%), extraoral localizations are additionally observed. Local bony prominences such as the area of the mylohyoid line, bony exostoses, and tori are particularly susceptible to developing MRONJ[9].

Radiologic changes comprise areas of bony sclerosis, a thickened lamina dura, and

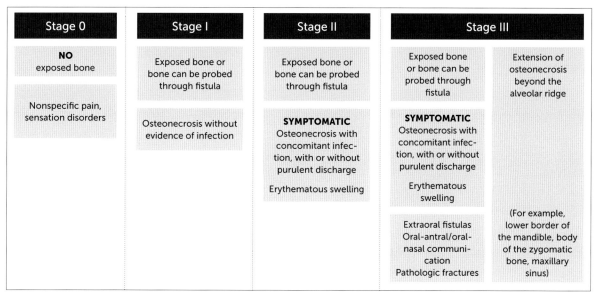

Stage 0	Stage I	Stage II	Stage III	
NO exposed bone	Exposed bone or bone can be probed through fistula	Exposed bone or bone can be probed through fistula	Exposed bone or bone can be probed through fistula	Extension of osteonecrosis beyond the alveolar ridge
Nonspecific pain, sensation disorders	Osteonecrosis without evidence of infection	**SYMPTOMATIC** Osteonecrosis with concomitant infection, with or without purulent discharge	**SYMPTOMATIC** Osteonecrosis with concomitant infection, with or without purulent discharge	
		Erythematous swelling	Erythematous swelling	
		Extraoral fistulas Oral-antral/oral-nasal communication Pathologic fractures		(For example, lower border of the mandible, body of the zygomatic bone, maxillary sinus)

Fig 20-4 The staging of MRONJ (according to the AAOMS 2014 classification[1]).

persistent extraction sockets. This can often be observed even in the very early stages of the disease. However, a diagnosis of MRONJ always requires a clinical and morphologic correlation. Osteolytic areas of bone are likely in advanced cases, so that it is particularly important to look out for pathologic fractures and disruptions of bone continuity.

Staging

The severity of existing MRONJ is graded into stages according to the AAOMS 2014 classification[14] (Fig 20-4).

The staging of osteonecrosis is crucial to the therapeutic approach adopted and hence of major clinical relevance[13].

When determining whether surgical revision is indicated in oncologic disease, particular attention should be paid to the course and prognosis of the underlying disease as well as the possibility of managing the consequences of MRONJ by conservative measures. The curative approach should be

chosen when a patient is in good general health and has a correspondingly good life prognosis, in the same way as for the complication of MRONJ in osteoporosis patients. The best possible local and systemic infection control is a crucial prerequisite for any successful surgical intervention. It thus determines the choice of timing and increases the success of the intervention.

Osteoradionecrosis of the jaw

The term osteoradionecrosis of the jaw (ORN) refers to a rare but serious side effect of radiotherapy for the purpose of treating head and neck tumors. Prevalence rates of 0% to 25% are mentioned in the literature. The mandible is far more commonly affected than the maxilla at a ratio of 24:1[6]. The average time until ORN clinically manifests after completion of radiotherapy varies: a mean of 13 months has been reported, although cases with a significantly delayed onset are not uncommon (up to 40 years after radiotherapy).

Definition[6]
- Condition post-radiotherapy of the head and neck region,
- Exposed, irradiated bone for a period of 3 months,
- Tumor activity in the oral and maxillofacial region excluded.

Etiology
The pathomechanism of ORN is thought to be vascular inflammation of the irradiated region (radiation arteritis), which results in changes to the bone being supplied and the surrounding mucosa. Ultimately, these changes can result in ischemic necrosis of the bone and poor mucosal barrier function, which clinically manifests as ORN.

Apart from the spontaneous development of ORN, there is generally a direct correlation between the formation of ORN and mucosal and bone trauma of the irradiated jawbone, as in the case of oral surgery procedures or denture sores.

Risk stratification
The following are influencing factors associated with the risk of ORN[2]:
- Type of radiotherapy technique,
- Level of the cumulative radiation dose (doses around 70 Gy are associated with a greatly increased ORN risk; at doses below 50 Gy ["cumulative limit dose"], the ORN risk can be classified as low),
- Procedures performed on the alveolar process (pre- and post-radiation),
- Health risk factors and comorbidities (e.g. cigarette smoking, alcohol consumption, marginal periodontitis, and/or diabetes mellitus).

Symptoms
The symptoms of ORN range from nonspecific pain, accompanying neurologic symptoms, and trismus to serious clinical situations with suppurating intraoral and extraoral fistulas and pathologic fractures, which hugely impair the quality of life and general health of patients and sometimes require drastic therapeutic measures.

Tables 20-1 and 20-2 list the most common clinical and radiologic symptoms (Video 20-1).

Many treatment-resistant cases of ORN actually conceal a recurrence or a newly developed tumor. Therefore, differential diagnosis must also consider the possibility of cancerous activity. Confirmation of the diagnosis by biopsy and histopathology is absolutely essential.

Staging
In view of the fact that ORN affects the mandible several times more frequently than the maxilla, systems for classifying ORN relate specifically to this anatomical region.

The classification proposed by Notani et al[12] is simple to apply in everyday clinical practice. According to this classification, ORN is classified into three degrees of severity, where the degree of severity relates to the clinical extent of the ORN (Fig 20-5).

Indications for surgical revision of ORN in a dental or oral surgery setting are confined to:
- Small, localized processes that are amenable to primary tension-free coverage (Caution: inelastic irradiated soft tissue with reduced blood supply), and
- The removal of bone sequestra in the surface layer.

Patients with more extensive ORN should immediately be referred to a maxillofacial specialist.

Table 20-1 Clinical symptoms of ORN[6].

Clinical symptoms of ORN	
Nonspecific symptoms	**Morphologic symptoms**
• Pain	• Ulceration of the mucosa
• Sensory disorders	• Exposed, necrotic bone (bone sequestra)
• Trismus	• Local irritation of surrounding tissue
• Halitosis	• Suppuration and secondary infection
• Difficulty eating	• Fistula formation (intraoral and extraoral)
	• Pathologic fractures
	• Loss of continuity

Table 20-2 Radiologic signs of ORN[6].

Radiologic signs of ORN
• Osteosclerotic changes
• Osteolysis
• Bone sequestra
• Persistent extraction sockets
• Pathologic fractures
• Loss of continuity in the jawbone

Video 20-1 CBCT of ORN: The bone pattern of the depicted slices reflects the clinical situation in Figs 20-32 to 20-37. As well as reactive osteosclerotic areas, extensive osteolytic bone areas with loss of continuity of the cortical structures and embedded bone sequestra are visualized. As a result of the chronic nature of the condition, the borders of the former extraction sockets (usually persisting for a long time) already appear significantly fused.

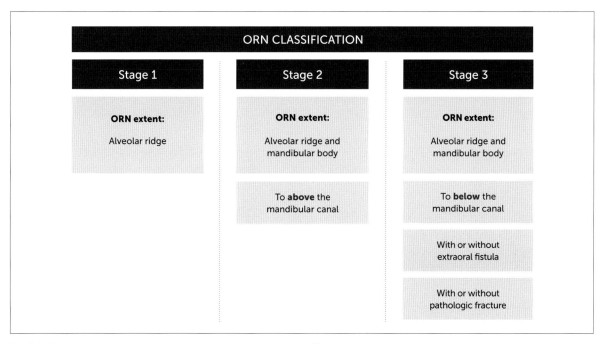

Fig 20-5 Classification of ORN according to Notani et al[12].

Osteomyelitis

The term osteomyelitis (OM) describes an inflammatory process of the cancellous bone and surrounding bony structures typically caused by microorganisms. The inflammatory process affecting the bone and the associated intraosseous reactions (including edema and purulent discharge) will compromise the regional blood supply[16]. The development of necrotic areas of bone and the formation of bone sequestra are generally further consequences of the process (Video 20-2). Rapid and sometimes extensive therapeutic action is required to halt the ongoing inflammatory process and to restore balance in bone metabolism.

Whereas hematogenic forms of the spread of OM are mainly described in the rest of the skeletal system, in the jaw area it is predominantly local causes (e.g. trauma, odontogenic causes) that can lead to the development of OM of the jaw. Regardless of the causal factors in OM of the jaw, there are known to be various forms of the disease.

Definition

A distinction is made between three principal forms of OM[3]:

■   Acute OM,
■   Secondary chronic OM,
■   Primary chronic OM.

Video 20-2   CBCT of osteomyelitis (OM): The CBCT slicing is confined to the core of the region in the left mandible affected in the course of chronic OM. In keeping with the relatively short history, osteosclerotic areas are identifiable as discontinuities; a central rarefication of the bone pattern suggestive of edema is noticeable in the anterior marginal region. The full picture (bone sequestra embedded centrally in osteolytic areas) cannot be visualized, as might be expected from the acute nature of the condition.

The acute and secondary chronic forms are the same form of the inflammatory process but refer to different phases. Both are classified as infections with pathogenic, purulent microorganisms leading to the development of typical symptoms. The acute phase of OM is, by definition, limited to a duration of 4 weeks. If symptoms persist beyond that time, the OM is considered to have become chronic.

Primary chronic OM describes a rare bony inflammatory process of uncertain origin and will not be addressed further here.

Symptoms

The symptoms of acute and secondary chronic OM are similar, but the two forms differ mainly in the manifestation and timing of onset of clinical symptoms (Table 20-3).

Risk stratification[3]

The risk of developing acute and secondary chronic OM increases in the case of:

■   Impaired microcirculation (e.g. denture pressure),
■   Reduced immunocompetence (e.g. immunosuppression, diabetes mellitus),
■   Local risk factors (e.g. marginal periodontitis),
■   Poor oral and denture hygiene,
■   Smoking and alcohol abuse.

In OM, there is a clear indication for surgical intervention:
■ If the surgical release of local abscesses is necessary,
■ In the presence of foreign bodies,
■ In the presence of odontogenic inflammatory foci.

Minimally invasive debridement can usually be performed on an outpatient basis, but an inpatient setting is advisable for decortication and all major resective procedures.

Table 20-3 Symptoms of acute and secondary chronic OM.

Acute OM	Secondary chronic OM
Common	**Common**
• Pain • Swelling • Hypoesthesia of the inferior alveolar nerve (Vincent's symptom) • Abscess formation or purulent discharge • Limited mouth opening • Intraoral fistulas • Loose teeth	• Pain • Swelling • Hypoesthesia of the inferior alveolar nerve (Vincent's symptom) • Abscess formation or purulent discharge • Limited mouth opening • Intraoral fistulas • Extraoral fistulas • Bone sequestra • Pathologic fractures • Exposed bone
Rare	
• Extraoral fistulas • Bone sequestra • Exposed bone • Pathologic fractures	

Contraindications (absolute and temporary)

Where pathologic processes do not respond to appropriate conservative therapeutic measures within a maximum of 2 weeks, a delay in focused diagnostic assessment can cause a loss of treatment time that cannot be recovered.

Therefore, cases where a local or systemic malignant process cannot be definitively excluded in the differential diagnosis will require immediate, focused diagnostic investigation.

Alveolitis

Surgical revision is generally contraindicated in the case of alveolitis as long as adequate infection and pain control and a tendency to complete healing are feasible with purely conservative methods in a patient with an unremarkable history.

Osteonecrosis of the jaw (MRONJ and ORN) and osteomyelitis

Contraindications for conservative therapeutic measures

Absolute contraindications for conservative therapeutic measures are an intolerance of or allergy to individual substances applied.

Contraindications for surgical revision

Surgical measures generally have to be considered in terms of the chosen timing but also against the background of the underlying disease and the patient's general health. A strict risk–benefit assessment dependent on the patient's medical history and life prognosis therefore plays a key role, especially in ONJ in the context of oncologic diseases.

Absolute contraindications for surgical revision exist if:

■ The general state of health is substantially compromised,

■ There is a systemic spread of the underlying malignant disease, and a (secondary or metastatic) neoplastic lesion underlies the condition affecting the jawbone,

- A curative treatment places an inappropriate burden on palliative care patients.

Temporary or relative contraindications exist if:

- An essential oncologic treatment (e.g. polychemotherapy, neoangiogenesis inhibitors, tyrosine kinase inhibitors) must not be interrupted,
- Long-term disease control can be guaranteed by conservative measures,
- Within the first 6 months after locoregional radiotherapy in the craniofacial region in the case of radiotherapy.

Specific risks

> The specific risks of the required procedure arise from the localization, nature, and extent of the procedure and the change (destruction, induration) underlying the particular condition. A surgical intervention performed during the phase of acute inflammation may spread the infection more deeply. Surgical interventions that are extended too far can cause a significantly larger bone defect, which in turn can necessitate follow-up operations.

Alveolitis or alveolar osteitis

- Aggressive therapy (curettage, decortication) can lead to stimulation of the inflammatory condition and can increase discomfort,
- Delayed or nonexistent therapy may encourage progression and may even lead to chronic OM.

Osteonecrosis of the jaw (MRONJ and ORN)

- Fundamentally high risk of recurrence, depending on the stage,
- Purely conservative therapy; possibility of the necrosis progressing to higher stages of the disease,
- Extensive resective procedure, potentially unnecessarily large defect; reconstruction necessary with outcome often uncertain,
- Risk of subtotal necrosis removal with a restrictive or resective procedure,
- In the case of ORN:
  - Tension-free soft tissue coverage made difficult by radiation-induced induration of the tissue,
  - Increased risk of dehiscence due to the tendency of delayed soft tissue healing.

Osteomyelitis

- Chronification, pathologic fractures, extension into organs.

Local anesthesia and general anesthesia or intubation anesthesia

> The choice of the correct type of anesthesia is guided by:
> - Localization and extent of the disease process,
> - Invasiveness and extent of resection of the planned procedure,
> - Involvement of relevant anatomical structures,
> - Current degree of inflammation in the affected region of the jaw,
> - Patient's psychomotor condition.

Alveolitis or alveolar osteitis

Local anesthesia (infiltration anesthesia or a nerve block) is indicated as an option for conservative treatment. Local anesthesia is also the method of choice for the rarely indicated surgical revision.

Osteonecrosis of the jaw (MRONJ and ORN)

Small-dimension osteonecrosis of the jaw (MRONJ and ORN) can be safely resected under local anesthesia, and the alveolar ridge can then be shaped by an alveoloplasty. Advanced stages, which necessitate an extensive resective and/or reconstructive approach in topographic relationship to anatomically relevant structures, must be rehabilitated under general anesthesia.

Osteomyelitis

As with ONJ, the choice of the type of anesthesia offered to the patient is basically guided by the scale of the surgery:

- Local curettage of infected bone and limited debridement of local foci of infection can be performed safely under local anesthesia,
- Indications for the planning of the intervention under general anesthesia on an in-patient basis are:
    - Extensive decortications with or without neurolysis,
    - Extended periosteal resections and (partial) resections of affected jaw segments,
    - Cases with progressive, chronic OM due to poor anesthetic effect in the inflamed area,
    - Pathologic fractures, extension into organs.

Step-by-step clinical procedure

The cornerstones of the clinical procedure are:
- General and specific history taking,
- Targeted clinical examination (intraoral and extraoral, including swabbing),
- Appropriate radiologic exploration.

These steps are also essential for individual surgical planning.

Two-dimensional visualization of the affected region by means of a panoramic radiograph is a basic diagnostic tool for all situations described in this section. For extended diagnostics, the three-dimensional techniques of CBCT or CT are primarily used for hard tissue imaging (root remnants [Fig 20-6]; bone sequestra and fractures [Fig 20-7]), demarcating the affected areas, topographic assessment of the path of the mandibular canal (Fig 20-8), and searching for foreign bodies.

Nuclear medicine imaging (bone scintigraphy) and hybrid techniques (positron emission tomography [PET] or CT) will fine-tune the information gained in the search, differential diagnosis, and differentiation of inflammatory or (secondary) neoplastic tissue areas, especially in MRONJ and ORN.

In OM, reactive changes in the medullary bone and adjacent soft tissue can also be clearly visualized by MRI.

In every case, the purpose of the intervention is to restore bone and mucosal integrity so that the symptoms subside, and, ideally, complete resolution can be achieved.

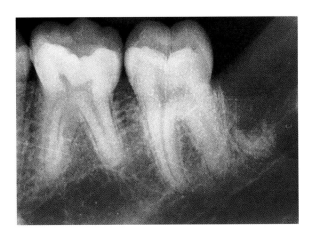

Fig 20-6   A root remnant in the mandibular left third molar region can be identified as the cause of alveolitis.

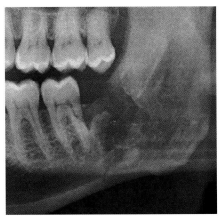

Fig 20-7   Fractures must be radiographically excluded as a cause of postextraction inflammation and require appropriate treatment (conservative, surgical stabilization).

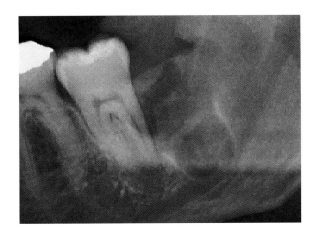

Fig 20-8   Before any manipulation of the affected alveoli, the anatomical relationship to the mandibular canal in the region of the mandibular third molar should be radiologically verified (panoramic radiograph and possibly CBCT or CT). Accordingly, the use of neurotoxic substances must be avoided, and special attention should be paid to the topography of the inferior alveolar nerve if excochleation is carried out.

Alveolitis or alveolar osteitis

Medication management

The primary aim is to control the pain, reduce the local microbial load, and prevent any progression of the condition, e.g. into OM. Pain treatment should be systemic and at a sufficient dosage. The basic medication is a nonsteroidal anti-inflammatory drug (diclofenac, ibuprofen, dexibuprofen, metamizole; various coxibs; alternatively, paracetamol), to which an opioid (tramadol, dihydrocodeine) can be added, especially at night for severe pain conditions (Step 2 of the WHO analgesic ladder for pain management). This group of medications has a slight sedative side effect, which can help the patient to sleep at night. Systemic antibiotic treatment should only be introduced if there are complications or signs of progression with use of topical treatment. Topical analgesics can also be used.

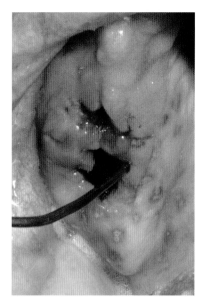

Fig 20-9 Sounding probe to exclude a maxillary sinus perforation prior to alveolar irrigation.

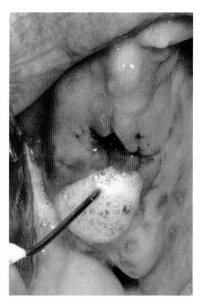

Fig 20-10 Thorough irrigation of the tooth socket before cleansing and antiseptic treatment with 3% H_2O_2 solution.

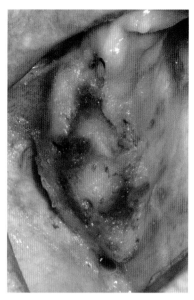

Fig 20-11 The thoroughly irrigated socket (especially after photodynamic therapy) is covered with adhesive ointment to prevent saliva and food debris from entering the socket and to promote local mucosal healing.

Interventional procedure

Especially in the acute phase, any manipulation in the affected region of the jaw is associated with severe additional pain, which is why local anesthesia is also advisable with a conservative approach.

In particular, sounding of the maxillary sinus should be performed in the maxillary posterior dentition before any intervention takes place (Fig 20-9); in the mandible, the path of the nerve should be tracked (see Fig 20-8).

In most cases, conservative local measures are adequate to treat AO. These consist of local antimicrobial mouthwashes (Fig 20-10), optional photodynamic therapy (low-level laser therapy with a soft laser at an appropriate wavelength and with a photosensitizer in the form of methylene blue or toluidine blue), and, if necessary, analgesic dressings (containing lignocaine or eugenol, e.g. Alveogyl, Septodont) or covering the socket with adhesive ointments (Fig 20-11).

Careful surface debridement (with tweezers or a bone curette) of loose, granulated, mobile, infected hard tissue and remaining food debris can assist irrigation measures. In the majority of cases, excochleation is not a suitable measure for achieving rapid healing of AO. Any aggressive manipulation in terms of curettage or even decortication should be avoided because this can cause the inflammation to spread more deeply, prolong the inflammatory process, and hence enlarge the bone defect (see above under Contraindications).

Postoperative controls and course (Figs 20-12 and 20-13)

The patient or an authorized person should be instructed in the use of irrigation and dressing application because they need to perform these measures properly as a matter of routine three to four times a day (at least after eating). Wound closure occurs spontaneously after the inflammation has resolved.

Regular follow-up appointments at intervals dictated by the patient's progress should be carried out to monitor and professionally assist such progress. If there is no appreciable improvement in the symptoms and the local clinical situation after 1 week, a reevaluation regarding the indication for surgical revision with facultive tension-free soft tissue coverage or possible differential diagnoses is required.

Osteonecrosis of the jaw – MRONJ

Medication management

Concomitant antibiotic treatment

Planned oral surgery interventions must be accompanied by antibiotic prophylaxis. For this purpose, the oral or intravenous administration of a bone-penetrating broad-spectrum antibiotic (e.g. amoxicillin with clavulanic acid if the patient has no penicillin allergy) or adjustment of the antibiotic spectrum (depending on the result of an optional swab test) is recommended. Antibiotic administration should start 1 to 2 days before the procedure and should last for at least 7 days (until suture removal).

> Note that mixed infections with yeasts (e.g. *Candida albicans*, *Candida glabrata*) that require treatment can often be found.

Drug holiday

Even though there is no consensus among experts, the authors recommend temporary suspension of antiresorptive therapy, a so-called drug holiday, until the wound region has healed. However, the break from antiresorptive medication must be agreed upon with the prescriber in an interdisciplinary manner and should be kept to as short a duration as possible. The regimen set out in Table 20-4 can be used as a guide.

Interventional procedure

In the pretreatment preceding surgical intervention (Video 20-3), the main focus is on reducing the infection and minimizing the mucosal defect, e.g. by removing sharp bone edges (Figs 20-14 to 20-17).

Local anesthetic should be administered as far away as possible from the site of inflammation and safely cover the affected region. The size of the soft tissue flap already defined by the **incision** (Fig 20-18) must be decided upon on the basis of clinical and radiologic findings. In the process, the periosteal supply to the alveolar bone should only be interrupted when raising the mucoperiosteum as much as is necessary to gain a proper overview of the entire affected bone.

Teeth involved in the necrotic zone must be extracted (Fig 20-19). Strategically troublesome or unnecessary neighboring teeth should also be extracted during the course of rehabilitation.

The affected alveolar bone must be removed sparingly but sufficiently (Fig 20-20) to ensure that definitively vital and hence properly perfused bone is identifiable (decortication). Bone edges must be excised by an alveoloplasty (Fig 20-21), and, using a piezotome or rotary instruments, ablatively shaped to be as round as possible so that they do not penetrate the overlying mucosa at a later stage.

Tension-free **soft tissue coverage** (Figs 20-22 and 20-23) is crucial to the long-term success of the revision. Layer-by-layer wound closure is therefore recommended for the closure of sizeable flaps (Figs 20-24 and 20-25).

Fig 20-12 Alveolar osteitis after tooth extractions in the maxilla (4 days postextraction).

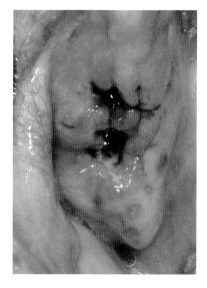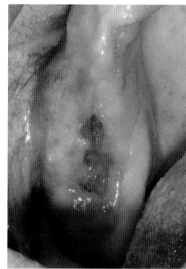

Fig 20-13 Clinical findings after 1 week of conservative local treatment.

Table 20-4 Recommendations for perioperative medication management (modified from Campisi et al[5]).

Drug suspension protocol		
Active substance	**Minimum interval between the last dose and the intervention**	**Minimum interval between the intervention and the next dose**
Perioperative management for oncologic indications		
Bisphosphonates	1 week	4–6 weeks
Denosumab (Xgeva)	3 weeks	
Bevacizumab	5–8 weeks	
Sunitinib	1 week	
Perioperative management for osteometabolic indications		
Bisphosphonates (> 3 years of therapy)	1 week	4–6 weeks
Denosumab (Prolia)	5 months	

Video 20-3 Removal of MRONJ: Video recording of a planned decortication in the mandible for ONJ in the mandibular left first molar to right canine region with retrospectively inadequate planning. After detection of a pathologic fracture of the mandibular body, partial resection of the mandible and insertion of a reconstruction plate take place (described step by step in the video).

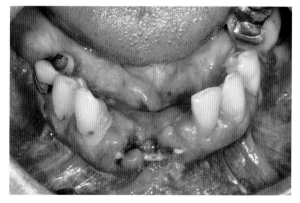

Fig 20-14 Sharp bone edges are often the cause of MRONJ. As long as they are present, however, they will interfere with spontaneous healing or prevent the existing mucosal dehiscence from shrinking.

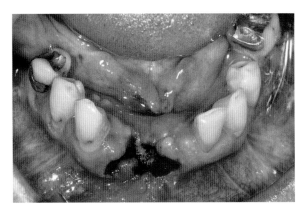

Fig 20-15   After decontaminating irrigation, under antibiotic prophylaxis, sharp bone edges that are preventing a positive healing process are trimmed.

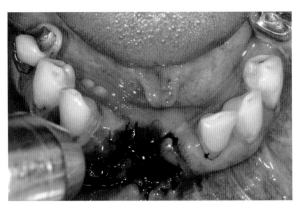

Fig 20-16   After decontamination and photodynamic therapy, the mucosal defect is covered in order to guarantee that the bone condition is as clean as possible and thereby promote a spontaneous healing process.

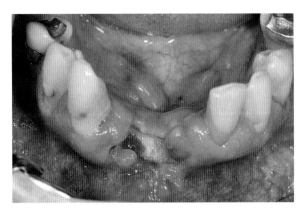

Fig 20-17   The mucosal defect has shrunk, and the patient is now in symptom-free Stage I preoperatively. The conditions for revision with antibiotic administration are thus ideal.

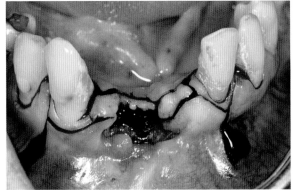

Fig 20-18   After local infiltration anesthesia, cutting around the mucosal defect to freshen the future wound margins. The incision is extended far enough laterally to ensure mobilization of the flap, the margins of which will come to lie over intact bone in the course of wound closure.

Step-by-step MRONJ surgical technique

- Planning of the procedure and marking of the incision path,
- A nerve block and/or regional anesthesia, depending on osteonecrosis localization,
- Incision: freshening wound margins on all sides and cutting around fistula tracts; this can already be fully integrated into the incision stage,

- Gentle mobilization of the mucoperiosteal flap and exposure of the osteonecrosis,
- Bone resection and/or removal of bone sequestra:
  - Using a piezoelectric method or rose burs (alternatively Er:YAG laser),
  - Note: The extent of resection must be sufficient to allow identification of well-perfused, entirely vital bone,

- Smoothing the bone edges (alveoloplasty),
- Releasing the periosteum and performing layer-by-layer, tension-free wound closure:
    - Deep periosteal stay sutures, resorbable suture material (e.g. Vicryl 3-0),
    - Mucosal wound closure: nonresorbable suture material (e.g. Ethilon 4-0).

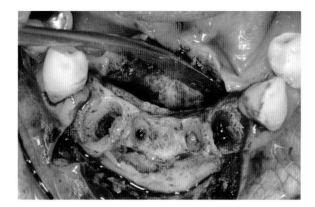

Fig 20-19   After mobilization of the mucoperiosteal flap, the extent of the osteonecrosis becomes visible. Here, the partly involved adjacent teeth have been extracted.

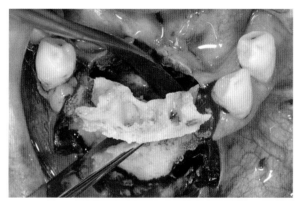

Fig 20-20   Sparing osteotomy, preferably by a piezotome, and lifting out of the necrotic bone in toto.

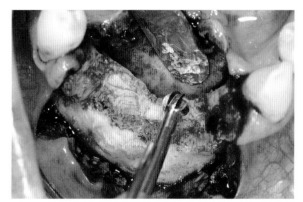

Fig 20-21   Alveoloplastic contouring of the bone under efficient cooling.

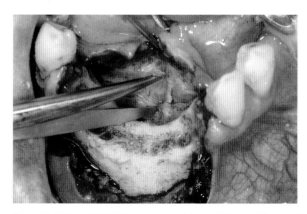

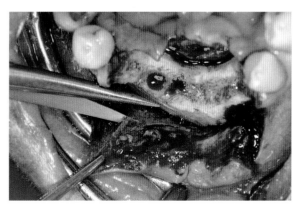

Figs 20-22 and 20-23   Appropriate splitting of the periosteum is crucial for tension-free wound closure, which in turn is an essential condition for stable soft tissue healing.

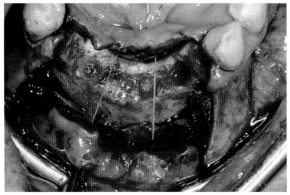

Fig 20-24   Placing stay sutures. These later ensure secure multilayer wound closure. Resorbable sutures do not require removal.

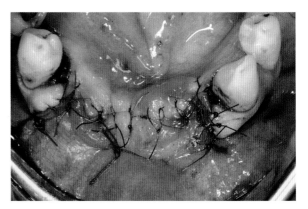

Fig 20-25   Performing tension-free wound closure with interrupted sutures.

Postoperative controls and course

Systemic measures involve continuing antibiotic administration at least until suture removal, hence a minimum of 7 to 14 days. Adequate analgesia must be guaranteed, merely to enable the patient to carry out essential **local accompanying measures**. This mainly relates to mechanical wound cleansing and rinsing with 0.2% chlorhexidine or 3% H_2O_2 solution three times a day.

Food should be cut into small pieces to protect the surgical site. Use of mucosa-supported dentures should be strictly avoided for at least 4 weeks. Dentures and gingival stents are only permissible if they are periodontally or implant-supported.

Suture removal should take place at least 7 days after wound closure. Functionally important (resorbable) periosteal stay sutures should remain in place for at least 2 weeks[9].

Postoperative progress in the first 3 months needs to be closely monitored, depending on the situation, so that the clinician can react promptly to any dehiscence that may appear and can reassign the patient to a conservative treatment regimen. Prosthetic restoration should only be performed with the approval of the surgeon (Figs 20-26 and 20-27).

Osteonecrosis of the jaw – ORN

Medication management
Concomitant antibiotic treatment is along the same broad lines as for MRONJ. However, in view of the reduced local blood flow and delayed wound healing, the antibiotic treatment should generally be continued for longer.

- Initially, bone-penetrating broad-spectrum antibiotic (e.g. amoxicillin with clavulanic acid),
- Subsequently, antibiotic treatment should be adjusted depending on microbiologic findings (a swab test is strongly recommended for targeted antibiotic administration),
- Planned oral surgery procedures for ORN revision absolutely require antibiotic prophylaxis:
  - Start the antibiotic at least 1 day prior to surgery,
  - Continue antibiotic administration to at least beyond suture removal (10 to 14 days postoperatively).

Interventional procedure
The interventional procedure for ORN (Fig 20-28) is strongly guided by the localization and extent of the ORN (see Fig 20-5, Video 20-1). Generally,

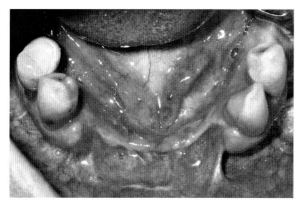

Fig 20-26 Recall after 12 weeks and approval for renewed prosthetic restoration. In the interim, the patient was fitted with a purely cosmetic partial denture not supported by the mucosa.

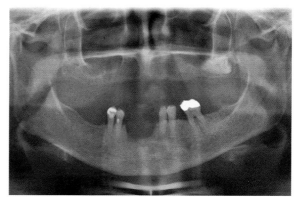

Fig 20-27 Radiographic outcome 12 weeks after surgical rehabilitation.

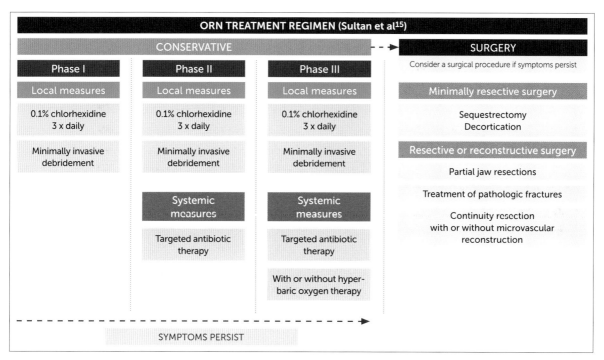

ORN TREATMENT REGIMEN (Sultan et al[15])			
CONSERVATIVE			SURGERY
Phase I	**Phase II**	**Phase III**	Consider a surgical procedure if symptoms persist
Local measures	Local measures	Local measures	Minimally resective surgery
0.1% chlorhexidine 3 x daily	0.1% chlorhexidine 3 x daily	0.1% chlorhexidine 3 x daily	Sequestrectomy Decortication
Minimally invasive debridement	Minimally invasive debridement	Minimally invasive debridement	Resective or reconstructive surgery
	Systemic measures	Systemic measures	Partial jaw resections
	Targeted antibiotic therapy	Targeted antibiotic therapy	Treatment of pathologic fractures
		With or without hyperbaric oxygen therapy	Continuity resection with or without microvascular reconstruction
SYMPTOMS PERSIST			

Fig 20-28 Step-by-step regimen for ORN treatment (Sultan et al[15]).

surgical revision of necrotically altered bone should be considered quickly if the symptoms are severe. If there are extensive findings, rehabilitation should take place in an in-patient setting (Figs 20-29 to 20-31). Before the procedure is performed, the diagnosis should be confirmed by histopathology, if possible, so that tumor recurrence can be reliably excluded. Preparatory and concurrent conservative measures resemble those applied to MRONJ (local washes and chlorhexidine gel, antibiotic treatment with or without hyperbaric oxygen therapy).

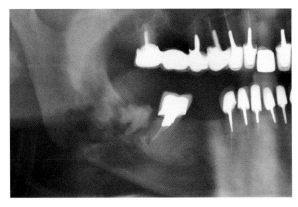

Fig 20-29 Radiologic preoperative situation with ORN in the right mandible. The 67-year-old patient was in a compromised general condition following tonsillar carcinoma and primary radiotherapy 7 years earlier. Clinically, the patient exhibits putrid exudation intraorally and extraorally. In addition, pathologic fracture of the mandible is present.

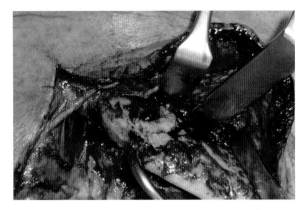

Fig 20-30 Extraoral view: Dramatic findings of a pathologic mandibular fracture. The procedure performed is a partial mandibular resection and reconstruction with an osteosynthesis plate and pectoral muscle flap.

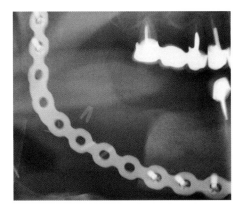

Fig 20-31 Postoperative radiograph after partial mandibular resection and plate reconstruction.

Oral surgery procedures for ORN revision basically follow the same principles as for MRONJ. However, soft tissue management is considered more important due to postradiogenic reduced microcirculation and local fibrosis in ORN.

All the necrotic bone should be resected, and demonstrably vital bone structures should be present throughout the surgical bed (Figs 20-32 to 20-37). This is particularly important in order to ensure that sufficient soft tissue coverage of the bony defect can be achieved subsequently. Postradiogenic and inflammatory soft tissue indurations and associated reduced elasticity of the tissue must be taken into account and incorporated into surgical planning beforehand. The incision path and design of the mucoperiosteal flap should ensure that absolutely tension-free closure of the wound region becomes possible.

Step-by-step ORN surgical technique
The surgical procedure for ORN (Video 20-4) follows the same approach as for MRONJ.

Note: The reduced soft tissue elasticity and decreased microcirculation require special expertise in the flap closure technique, and stay sutures have to remain in place longer.

Postoperative controls and course
Systemic measures involve continuing antibiotic administration at least until the sutures are removed, hence a minimum of 10 to 14 days.

Local measures:
- **Mechanical wound cleansing** and rinsing with 0.2% chlorhexidine or 3% H_2O_2 solution three times a day,
- **Food intake:** Liquid diet for 2 to 4 weeks, possibly nasogastric tube for 5 to 7 days,
- **No denture wearing** until wound healing is completed (2 to 4 weeks) if the denture covers the wound region,

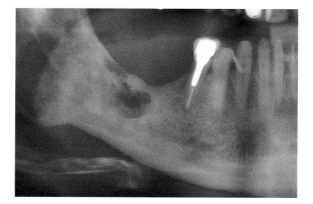

Fig 20-32 A 60-year-old patient with a history of primary radiotherapy of an oropharyngeal carcinoma 13 years earlier. Preoperative radiographic findings are highly suggestive of osteoradionecrosis (ORN) in the right mandible. The extent of the ORN in the right mandible appears to be radiologically clear and confined to the crestal portion of the jawbone (Stage II ORN). No pathologic fracture is present.

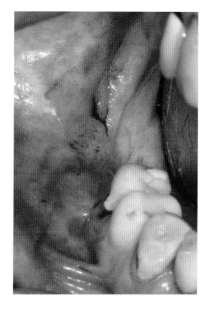
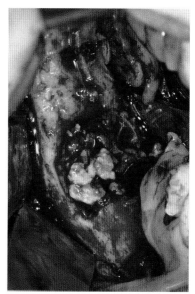

Fig 20-33 Intraoral clinical photograph of the same patient: Unremarkable local clinical findings accompanying severe pain symptoms and radiologic changes.

Fig 20-34 The procedure performed is decortication in the right mandible under intubation anesthesia. After reflection of the surgical site, the mandibular bone appears locally destroyed and necrotically altered. Regions of cancellous bone have been replaced by granulation tissue.

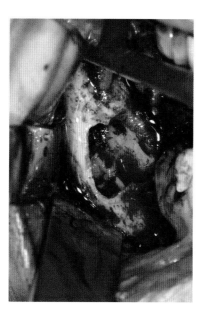
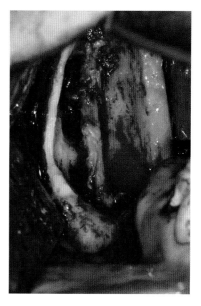

Fig 20-35 After removal of the granulation tissue, the extent of the cancellous bone defect is apparent. Caudally, the inferior alveolar nerve becomes visible. Devitalized bone is resected and sharp bone edges are removed.

Fig 20-36 Pronounced tub-shaped bone defect after removal of the necrotically altered bone. Next, tension-free wound closure is carried out with interrupted and mattress sutures. First, two deep stay sutures are placed with Vicryl 3-0, which are intended to reduce the tension. Nonresorbable suture material (e.g. Ethilon 4-0) is used for definitive wound closure.

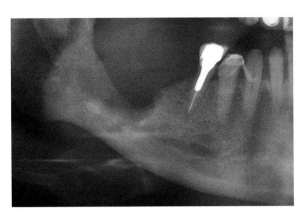

Video 20-4 ORN procedure: Video recording of the decortication of radiogenic osteonecrosis in the mandibular left first molar to right lateral incisor region after extraction of the residual mandibular dentition that was largely involved (described step by step in the video).

Fig 20-37 Postoperative panoramic radiograph after decortication of radiogenic osteonecrosis in the mandibular right first to third molar region.

- **Mucosal suture removal** at least 10 to 14 days after wound closure,
- Routine clinical check-ups with respect to the underlying disease as part of oncology aftercare by the relevant department treating the disease.

Osteomyelitis

Treatment of the acute and secondary chronic forms of OM consists of a combination of conservative and surgical measures.

The three cornerstones of treatment are:
- Antibiotic therapy,
- Surgical intervention,
- Hyperbaric oxygen therapy.

It is the first two of these cornerstones that play a decisive role. Hyperbaric oxygen therapy is recommended as a supportive measure.

Medication management
Antibiotic therapy
Antibiotic therapy should be as targeted as possible. A broad-spectrum antibiotic is indicated until an antibiogram has been assessed.

Antibiotics are usually administered in conjunction with surgical interventions. Antibiotic treatment as a standalone measure only has a reliable effect if it is started promptly after the onset of symptoms (within the first 3 days).

Hyperbaric oxygen therapy
Hyperbaric oxygen therapy is recommended as a supportive measure. The available studies describe an improvement in local perfusion and a reduction of anaerobic microorganisms, while the effectiveness in the acute and secondary chronic forms is not entirely clear.

Interventional procedure
The primary aim of the surgical intervention is to relieve the medullary bone in the acute phase and excise infected and necrotic bone (Video 20-2, Figs 20-38 to 20-40). This will improve the local microcirculation and the immune response so that resolution of the disease can be achieved.

Step-by-step OM surgical technique
The surgical procedure follows the same approach as for MRONJ and ORN.

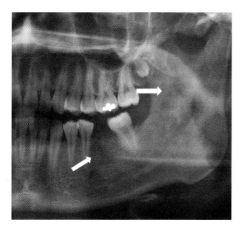

Fig 20-38 Panoramic radiograph of a 23-year-old patient with symptoms in the left ascending ramus (top arrow). According to the case history, the mandibular left first molar had been extracted 6 months earlier (bottom arrow). Secondary chronic OM is suspected on the basis of case history, clinical findings, and primary radiologic diagnostics.

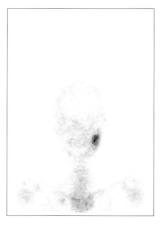

Fig 20-39 Further nuclear medicine diagnostics by means of skeletal scintigraphy; there is a distinctly increased uptake noticeable in the left mandible.

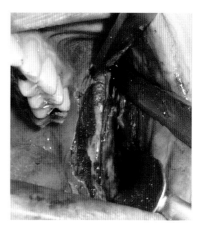

Fig 20-40 Intraoperative condition of the ascending ramus of the left mandible. Ample resection of bone altered by inflammation.

The extent of the alveolar ridge revision varies widely depending on indication, localization, and progression of the condition. Depending on these factors, it comprises:

- Curettage of granulation and scar tissue (excochleation),
- Relieving abscess formations,
- Removing loose foreign bodies and teeth,
- Removing avascular bone sequestra (sequestrectomy),
- Relieving the cancellous bone by removing the oral cortical bone of the jawbone and minimally invasive surgical debridement (saucerization),
- Ample removal of bone areas altered by osteonecrosis and OM (decortication),
- Continuity resection of the jaw with or without surgical reconstruction.

Postoperative controls and course

Systemic measures involve continuing the antibiotic therapy at least until suture removal, hence a minimum of 10 to 14 days. It is advisable to consult an infectiologist before the antibiotic therapy is stopped.

Local measures:

- **Mechanical wound cleansing** and rinsing with 0.2% chlorhexidine or 3% H_2O_2 solution three times a day,
- **Food intake:** Liquid diet for 2 to 4 weeks, possibly nasogastric tube for 5 to 7 days,
- **No denture wearing** until wound healing is completed (2 to 4 weeks) if the denture covers the wound region,
- **Mucosal suture removal** should take place at least 10 to 14 days after wound closure.

References

1. Ruggiero SL, Dodson TB, Aghaloo T, Carlson ER, Ward BB, Kademani D. American Association of Oral and Maxillofacial Surgeons' Position Paper on Medication-Related Osteonecrosis of the Jaws–2022 Update. J Oral Maxillofac Surg 2022;80:920–943. doi:10.1016/j.joms.2022.02.008. Epub 2022 Feb 21. PMID:35300956.

2. Aarup-Kristensen S, Hansen CR, Forner L, Brink C, Eriksen JG, Johansen J: Osteoradionecrosis of the mandible after radiotherapy for head and neck cancer: risk factors and dose-volume correlations. Acta Oncol 2019;58:1373–1377.

3. Baltensperger M, Eyrich G: Osteomyelitis Therapy – General Considerations and Surgical Therapy. In: Baltensperger M, Eyrich G (eds): Osteomyelitis of the Jaws. Berlin, Heidelberg: Springer, 2009.

4. Blum IR: Contemporary views on dry socket (alveolar osteitis): a clinical appraisal of standardization, aetiopathogenesis and management: a critical review. Int J Oral Maxillofac Surg 2002;31:309–317.

5. Campisi G, Mauceri R, Bertoldo F, Bettini G, Biasotto M, Colella G, et al.: Medication-Related Osteonecrosis of Jaws (MRONJ) Prevention and Diagnosis: Italian Consensus Update 2020. Int J Environ Res Public Health 2020;17:5998.

6. Chronopoulos A, Zarra T, Ehrenfeld M, Otto S: Osteoradionecrosis of the jaws: definition, epidemiology, staging and clinical and radiological findings. A concise review. Int Dent J 2018;68:22–30.

7. Eguia A, Bagan-Debon L, Cardona F: Review and update on drugs related to the development of osteonecrosis of the jaw. Med Oral Patol Oral Cir Bucal 2020;25:e71–e83.

8. Gowda GG, Viswanath D, Kumar M, Umashankar DN: Dry socket (alveolar osteitis): incidence, pathogenesis, prevention and management. J Indian Aca Oral Med Radiol 2013;25:196–199.

9. Khan AA, Morrison A, Hanley DA, Felsenberg D, McCauley LK, O'Ryan F, et al.: Diagnosis and management of osteonecrosis of the jaw: a systematic review and international consensus. J Bone Miner Res 2015;30:3–23.

10. Kolokythas A, Olech E, Miloro M: Alveolar osteitis: A comprehensive review of concepts and controversies. Int J Dent 2010;2010:249073.

11. Nicolatou-Galitis O, Schiodt M, Mendes RA, Ripamonti C, Hope S, Drudge-Coates L, et al.: Medication-related osteonecrosis of the jaw: definition and best practice for prevention, diagnosis, and treatment. Oral Surg Oral Med Oral Pathol Oral Radiol 2019;127:117–135.

12. Notani K, Yamazaki Y, Kitada H, Sakakibara N, Fukuda H, Omori K, et al.: Management of mandibular osteoradionecrosis corresponding to the severity of osteoradionecrosis and the method of radiotherapy. Head Neck 2003;25:181–186.

13. Rugani P, Acham S, Kirnbauer B, et al.: Stage-related treatment concept of medication-related osteonecrosis of the jaw—a case series. Clin Oral Investig 2015;19:1329–1338.

14. Ruggiero SL, Dodson TB, Fantasia J, Goodday R, Aghaloo T, Mehrotra B, et al.: American Association of Oral and Maxillofacial Surgeons position paper on medication-related osteonecrosis of the jaw – 2014 update. J Oral Maxillofac Surg 2014;72:1938–1956.

15. Sultan A, Hanna GJ, Margalit DN, Chau N, Goguen LA, Marty FM, et al.: The Use of Hyperbaric Oxygen for the Prevention and Management of Osteoradionecrosis of the Jaw: A Dana-Farber/Brigham and Women's Cancer Center Multidisciplinary Guideline. Oncologist 2017;22:343–350.

16. Topazian RG, Goldberg MH, Hupp JR: Osteomyelitis of the jaws. Oral and maxillofacial infections, ed 4. Philadelphia: WB Saunders, 2002:214–242.

Orthodontic mini-implants

21

Sebastian Kühl, Georgios Kanavakis,
Carlalberta Verna, Fabio Saccardin

Indications

Orthodontic mini-implants or miniscrews together with anchorage plates (e.g. Bollard anchors) and palatal implants (see Section 22) are among the available temporary skeletal anchorage devices. Mini-implants have wide-ranging uses in both the maxilla and mandible because of their much smaller dimensions compared with palatal implants. As a stable anchorage point that absorbs all the counterforces, mini-implants are mainly used for the movement of individual teeth or groups of teeth, overbites, retraction of anterior teeth, intrusion of molars in an open bite or to control the vertical dimension of occlusion (Fig 21-1). Mini-implants can be inserted into interradicular bone septa but also into supra-apical, retromolar, and palatal positions or in the area of the zygomaticoalveolar crest. The advantage of insertion on the palatal side is that more and better quality (more compact) bone is available, and, in addition, the implants are constantly surrounded by keratinized gingiva.

The selection of mini-implant systems available on the market is wide and making a choice can be very confusing, especially for novice users. For instance, there are considerable differences in length, diameter, and design of screw head as well as a wide choice of possible retention components that can be secured to them. The choice of screw head depends on the position that was stipulated for the implant by the orthodontist when planning tooth movement.

Mini-implants are typically made of a titanium alloy, are self-cutting, and have a machined surface. Therefore, only limited osseointegration will take place. Nevertheless, the average success rate is 86%[8]. Compared with palatal implants (see Section 22), mini-implants are less invasive, less expensive, and quicker to use; also, due to their widely variable dimensions, they have a greater diversity of uses in orthodontics (Figs 21-2 to 21-6). In contrast to mini-implants, anchorage plates (e.g. Bollard anchors) are fixed with more than just one screw, so that primary mechanical stability is increased, especially against rotational forces (Fig 21-7). Here again, there is a wide selection of different forms (quadrant-dependent), possible orientations of the retention devices, and orthodontic applications.

Contraindications

The insertion of a mini-implant is an elective surgical procedure. Younger patients, in particular, whose compliance cannot be guaranteed ahead of the minor surgical procedure should not be fitted with mini-implants. In the mixed dentition, tooth germs of permanent teeth are an interfering factor, and the surrounding bone tends to be irregular, which increases the risk of making a mistake. Paramedian positioning is possible in these circumstances. Furthermore, such an elective surgical procedure is contraindicated in patients who are classified as inoperable because of their current general medical status (due to, e.g. chemotherapy, HIV infection, untreated or poorly controlled diabetes mellitus, antiresorptive medication, long-term steroid treatment or radiotherapy in the head and neck region).

Specific risks

The most common complication is injury to the adjacent tooth root resulting from contact with the mini-implant[1] (Fig 21-8). If contact with the root is not noticed intraoperatively or postoperatively (although it should be apparent intraoperatively from reduced stability), and hence the mini-implant is left in place, resorptions at the affected tooth root may occur at a later stage. However, if the mini-implant is removed immediately once root contact is detected, complete regeneration of the periodontium is

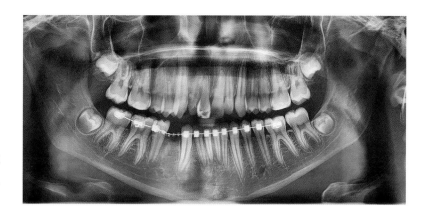

Fig 21-1 Typical indication for skeletal anchorage devices: Mesial shift of the tooth group in the mandibular right second premolar to second molar region.

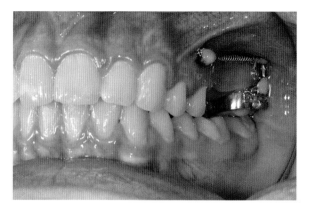

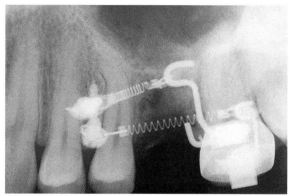

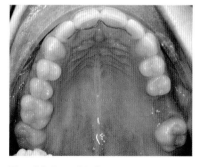

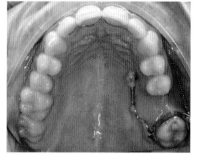

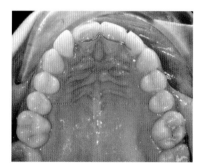

Figs 21-2 to 21-6 Mini-implants positioned buccally and palatally in order to mesialize a maxillary molar (without banding the entire maxillary arch). The force passes through the center of resistance of the tooth and provides maximal control over unwanted tipping movements (images courtesy of Prof C. Verna and Dr Lienert).

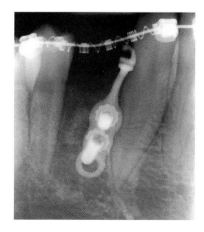

Fig 21-7 Skeletal anchorage with a Bollard anchor, which provides great stability due to the use of several screws but is operatively far more complex than a mini-implant (the same patient as in Fig 21-1 and Video 21-2).

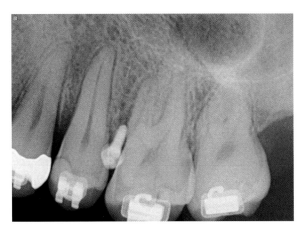

Fig 21-8 A mini-implant in close proximity to the tooth root is one of the most common complications.

usually observed within 6 to 12 weeks, provided only the cementum and dentin are affected. The prognosis is much worse if the pulp was injured during the insertion of the mini-implant. In this instance, secondary damage can range from inflammatory infiltrate and lack of bone regeneration to ankylosis or pulp necrosis. Another common complication is the loss of retention of a mini-implant. Possible reasons for this are contact between the mini-implant and the tooth root, localization of the mini-implant (Table 21-1), and insertion into unattached mucosa or into nonkeratinized gingiva. Fracture of mini-implants, clinical signs of inflammation with hyperplasia of the peri-implant mucosa or mechanically induced ulcerations of the mucosa are further complications. The specific risks also apply to a Bollard anchor with plates.

Step-by-step clinical procedure

Infiltration anesthesia in the area of the future insertion site is generally sufficient. Depending on localization, nerve blocks can also be used as an option. Contralateral local anesthesia is not necessary in most cases. Pain-free palatal placement of mini-implants is possible after a nerve block at the greater palatine nerve and the nasopalatine nerve.

The insertion site is decided from an orthodontic perspective and involves determining the position in the vestibular-oral direction and identifying the precise localization between the roots (Figs 21-9 and 21-10). After local anesthesia, the mini-implant can be inserted directly without pre-drilling. The mini-implant is self-cutting and can be screwed in by hand (with a screwdriver) but also by machine, depending on the specific manufacturer and access possibilities. Pre-drilling may be necessary in rare cases (if the bone structure is very compact). Battery operated handpieces or motors offer maximal flexibility and comfort for the surgeon because they are cordless, but they have less torque compared with classic surgical motors (Video 21-1). The expected bony supply at the particular insertion site is well documented in the literature[3,6,9,10].

However, the length of the mini-implant should be individually determined, for example, based on the preoperative radiograph and/or by probing the mucosa (known as bone sounding). The length is dictated by the type of anchorage because longer mini-implants (10 to 12 mm) are indicated for bicortical insertion. Mini-implants that are 8 to 10 mm in length are preferred for very thick mucosa. If a cortical bone thickness of more than 1 mm is anticipated, shorter mini-implants need to be chosen because primary stability is guaranteed by the cortical bone. It has been shown that oblique insertion between 45 and 70 degrees additionally increases contact with the cortical bone, and hence stability[4]. Longer mini-implants are recommended for thinner cortical bone of less than 1 mm because more bone contact is required. The presence of neighboring anatomical structures such as teeth or the maxillary sinuses also dictates the choice of mini-implant length.

Table 21-1 Frequency of loss of mini-implants with respect to localization[5].

Maxilla			
Buccal		**Palatal**	
Interradicular between first molar and second premolar	9.2%	Central or midline	1.3%
Interradicular between canine and lateral incisor	9.7%	Paramedian	4.8%
Zygomaticoalveolar crest	16.4%	Parapalatal	5.5%
Mandible			
Buccal		**Lingual**	
Interradicular between first molar and second premolar	13.5%	No mini-implants should be inserted lingually	
Interradicular between first premolar and canine	9.9%		

The diameter of the mini-implant is determined by the limited bone supply between two tooth roots, especially for interradicular insertion. In order for the mini-implant to be used successfully later, it is imperative to achieve primary stability (in the same way as for prosthetic implantology). This requires not only adequate bone quality but also a mini-implant with the correct dimensions as well as a straight insertion. A mini-implant diameter of less than 1.2 mm is not recommended because it increases the risk of fracture[2]. The lowest fracture risk is for diameters between 1.2 and 2 mm. The insertion site is also relevant to the choice of diameter size. In the retromolar areas of the mandible or generally, provided the cortical bone is thicker than 2 mm, the recommended diameter is 2 mm. Pre-drilling is advisable for thick cortical bone, even with self-cutting and self-drilling mini-implants, in order to avoid fracture of the mini-implant as a result of excessive torque. In the retromolar region of the maxilla, where thin trabecular bone is present, a diameter of 1.3 mm may be used.

As for all elective surgical procedures, any injury to vital structures must be ruled out. Three-dimensional (3D) imaging is necessary in cases where two-dimensional radiographs

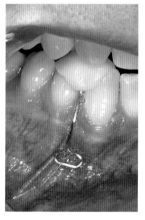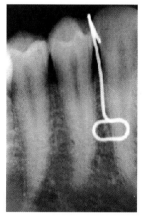

Figs 21-9 and 21-10 During preoperative planning, a metallic marker is used to radiographically check the risk of intraoperative root contact with the mini-implant. The metallic marking (curved wire), previously custom-made by the orthodontist, is secured to the teeth with composite. On the single-tooth radiograph, vertical positioning of the x-ray source is decisive when assessing the correct position.

Video 21-1 Insertion of two mini-implants with the aid of a mobile, battery operated contra-angle handpiece or a motor-driven contra-angle handpiece.

Video 21-2 Fixation of a Bollard anchor in order to move the entire posterior tooth group mesially (to distal to the mandibular right canine).

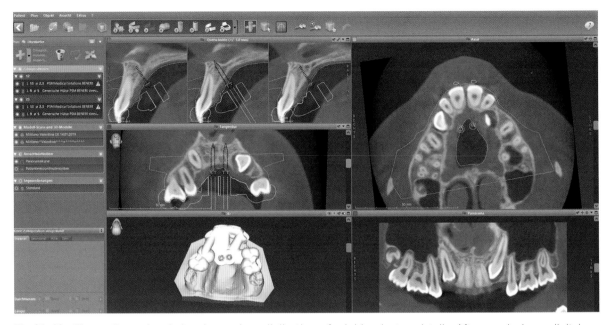

Fig 21-11 Three-dimensional planning and parallelization of mini-implants palatally. After overlaying a digital intraoral scan, a virtual template is designed and fabricated for the procedure using a 3D printer.

combined with clinical examination do not provide clarity regarding anatomical positional relationships (Fig 21-11).

CBCT is the standard technique in this situation. If CBCT is available, it can be used for 3D planning and positioning of mini-implants, in the same way as dental implants, with the aid of a special drilling template (Figs 21-11 to 21-13).

Wound care and closure

Mini-implants do not require any special wound care. However, patients should be instructed to carry out regular oral hygiene measures at home to avoid any accumulation of plaque. For Bollard anchors, sutures should be removed 1 week after insertion because, in contrast to mini-implants, this system requires flap reflection.

Postoperative controls and course

For documentation purposes and to rule out contact between the mini-implant and tooth root, a single-tooth radiograph can be taken postoperatively. Furthermore, an analgesic (ibuprofen or paracetamol) is prescribed as required, depending on the patient's medical history and body weight.

A mini-implant can be immediately loaded, unlike palatal implants. With respect to intervention-related complaints affecting the mucosa, however, it is advisable to allow 2 weeks of healing time before the laboratory fabrication of orthodontic appliances and loading of the mini-implant (Fig 21-13). This coincides with the period during which wound follow-ups can be carried out, if required.

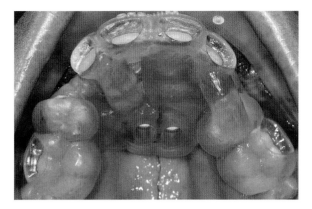

Fig 21-12 Printed template in situ for the procedure. The mini-implants can be inserted with suitable systems guided by the template (image courtesy of Dr Max Rohde).

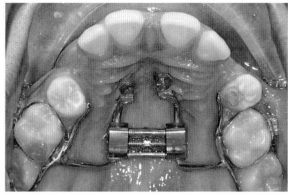

Fig 21-13 Appliance fixed to the mini-implants in situ (image courtesy of Dr Max Rohde).

When the mini-implant is loaded, a condensation of the bone can usually be observed radiographically. In many situations, orthodontic loading and the bone remodeling process can alter the position of the mini-implant. An average deviation of one millimeter (0.1 to 2 mm) and a few degrees (1 to 3 degrees) is described in the literature[7].

After completion of orthodontic treatment, the mini-implant can simply be unscrewed under local anesthesia in the same way as it was inserted. Anchorage plates, on the other hand, can only be removed by flap reflection, which makes the procedure far more complex and time consuming overall.

References

1. Alves M Jr, Baratieri C, Mattos CT, Araújo MT, Maia LC: Root repair after contact with mini-implants: systematic review of the literature. Eur J Orthod 2013;35:491–499.

2. Dalstra M, Cattaneo PM, Melsen B: Load transfer of miniscrews for orthodontic anchorage. Orthodontics 2004;1:53–62.

3. Hourfar J, Kanavakis G, Bister D, Schätzle M, Awad L, Nienkemper M, Goldbecher C, Ludwig B: Three dimensional anatomical exploration of the anterior hard palate at the level of the third ruga for the placement of mini-implants – a cone-beam CT study. Eur J Orthod 2015;37:589–595.

4. Laursen MG, Melsen B, Cattaneo PM: An evaluation of insertion sites for mini-implants: a micro - CT study of human autopsy material. Angle Orthod 2013;83:222–229.

5. Mohammed H, Wafaie K, Rizk MZ, Almuzian M, Sosly R, Bearn DR: Role of anatomical sites and correlated risk factors on the survival of orthodontic miniscrew implants: a systematic review and meta-analysis. Prog Orthod 2018;19:36.

6. Monnerat C, Restle L, Mucha JN: Tomographic mapping of mandibular interradicular spaces for placement of orthodontic mini-implants. Am J Orthod Dentofacial Orthop 2009;135:428–429.

7. Nienkemper M, Handschel J, Drescher D: Systematic review of mini-implant displacement under orthodontic loading. Int J Oral Sci 2014;6:1–6.

8. Papageorgiou SN, Zogakis IP, Papadopoulos MA: Failure rates and associated risk factors of orthodontic miniscrew implants: A meta-analysis. Am J Orthod Dentofacial Orthop 2012;142:577–595.

9. Park J, Cho HJ: Three-dimensional evaluation of interradicular spaces and cortical bone thickness for the placement and initial stability of micro-implants in adults. Am J Orthod Dentofacial Orthop 2009;136:314–315.

10. Winsauer H, Vlachojannis C, Bumann A, Vlachojannis J, Chrubasik S: Paramedian vertical palatal bone height for mini-implant insertion: a systematic review. Eur J Orthod 2014;36:541–549.

Recommended literature

Hourfar J, Lisson JA: Wissenschaftliche Stellungnahme zur Verankerung mit Gaumenimplantaten und Kortikalisschrauben in der Kieferorthopädie. DGKFO, 2017.

Palatal implants

22

Sebastian Kühl, Fabio Saccardin, Andreas Filippi

Palatal implants together with orthodontic mini-implants (see Section 21) and anchorage plates are among the available temporary skeletal anchorage devices.

Insertion of palatal implants

Indications

The purpose of a palatal implant is stable anchorage, allowing reciprocal absorption of orthodontic forces. Despite being locally restricted to the maxilla, palatal implants have a wide diversity of uses (although a palatal implant is not recommended until after the age of 12 years):

■ Intrusion and extrusion of anterior and posterior teeth,
■ Mesialization and distalization of posterior teeth,
■ Molar uprighting,
■ Orthodontic space closure,
■ Treatment of an anterior open bite,
■ Treatment of crowding in the maxilla,
■ Poor compliance for planned extraoral anchorage (e.g. headgear).

Palatal implants are usually made of a titanium alloy. The surface of the endosteal part of palatal implants, unlike mini-implants, is macro- and micro-rough in order to promote osseointegration. Prosthetic implants of similar dimensions, i.e. very short tissue-level implants, are also currently used as palatal implants[3]. This can be advantageous because most dental practices already have a complete set of instruments for dental implants, and hence there is already some familiarity with a specific implant system. Furthermore, this would make a digital workflow (CAD/CAM) possible, although at the expense of higher radiation exposure (especially in the case of CBCT) and cost. A classic palatal implant system (Orthosystem, Straumann) is used in the following case studies (Figs 22-1 and 22-2).

Palatal implants can be regarded as a reliable form of skeletal anchorage, with a success rate of > 95%, and are superior to tooth-supported anchorage and other forms of skeletal anchorage such as mini-implants.

Contraindications

Palatal implants should not be inserted in patients with poor compliance. Furthermore, palatal implants are at least temporarily contraindicated in at-risk patients (due to, e.g. chemotherapy, HIV infection, hemorrhagic diatheses, untreated or uncontrolled diabetes mellitus, antiresorptive medication, long-term steroid treatment or radiotherapy in the head and neck region). The insertion of a palatal implant is an elective surgical procedure. Consequently, possible alternative orthodontic treatment options need to be discussed.

The most common complications reported in the literature in relation to the insertion of palatal implants are lack of primary stability (6.7%) and prolonged pain (6.7%), followed by secondary bleeding (5.8%), perforation of the nasal floor (1.9%), mucosal necrosis (1.9%), and sensory impairment in the anterior palate (1%)[1].

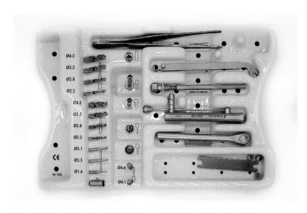

Fig 22-1 Surgical kit of a palatal implant system (Orthosystem).

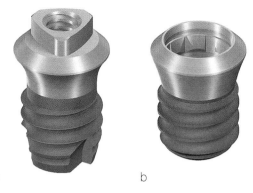

a   b

Fig 22-2 Comparison of (a) a palatal implant (Palatal Implant, SLA, endosteal diameter 4.1 mm, length 4.2 mm, Straumann) with (b) a very short conventional tissue-level implant (Standard Plus, SLActive, endosteal diameter 4.1 mm, length 4 mm, regular neck with shoulder diameter 4.8 mm, Straumann)[3] (©Institut Straumann AG, 2020. All rights reserved. Images courtesy of Institut Straumann AG).

Step-by-step clinical procedure

Infiltration anesthesia administered three times in the area of the future implant position is generally sufficient. A bilateral nerve block in the greater palatine nerve and an additional nerve block in the nasopalatine nerve have been considered as alternatives.

The minor surgical procedure is preceded by comprehensive orthodontic diagnostic assessment and treatment planning. If skeletal growth is completed (recognizable from a radiograph of the hand), the implant is inserted in the area of the median palatine suture, level with the maxillary premolars. If skeletal growth is not yet complete, insertion should be in a paramedian position in the palate. The expected bone supply at the particular insertion site is well documented in the literature[2,4-6]. The exact bone thickness and implant axis can also be determined by means of a lateral cephalogram (Fig 22-3). A vacuum-formed splint with an integrated pin, which initially serves as a radiographic template

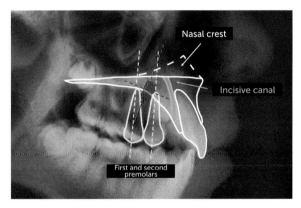

Fig 22-3 Preoperative lateral cephalogram with schematic diagram of the implant position and surrounding anatomical structures.

and later as a surgical template, can be fabricated to provide orientation, if necessary.

After local anesthesia, the thickness of the palatal mucosa is measured using a periodontal probe (known as bone sounding) to establish the preparation depth (Figs 22-4 and 22-5). Insertion takes place entirely without an access flap (flapless), in contrast to dental implants. Therefore, the depth marking on the twist drill during preparation of the implant bed cannot be checked

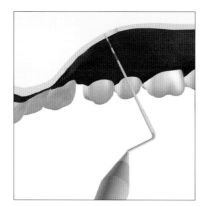
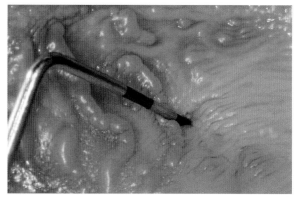

Figs 22-4 and 22-5   Measuring the thickness of the palatal mucosa with a periodontal probe perpendicular to the bone surface (known as bone sounding). Measuring in the depression of the median palatine suture should be avoided as the thickness of the mucosal measurement will be too large (Fig 22-4: ©Institut Straumann AG, 2020. All rights reserved. Image courtesy of Institut Straumann AG).

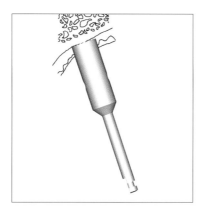
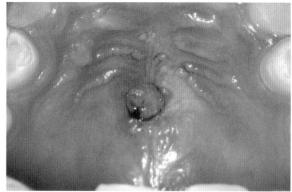

Figs 22-6 and 22-7   The mucosa at the insertion site is removed using a punch corresponding to the diameter of the palatal implant and a fine raspatory (Fig 22-6: ©Institut Straumann AG, 2020. All rights reserved. Image courtesy of Institut Straumann AG).

at the bone level, only at the mucosal level. The preparation depth at the mucosal level is calculated from the sum of the future implant length and the measured mucosal thickness.

After measuring, the mucosa at the insertion site is removed with the aid of a punch corresponding to the diameter of the implant and with a fine raspatory (Figs 22-6 and 22-7). The thickness of the mucosa at this site is checked again.

The bone surface that has been exposed is then smoothed with a rose bur, if necessary.

Irrespective of whether the palatal implant is inserted at the median palatine suture or in a paramedian position, the implant axis should be oriented perpendicularly to the bone surface at the premolar level. The manufacturer of the implant system will stipulate the exact sequence of drills (rose drill, pilot drill, twist drill, etc) and the maximal number of revolutions per minute for each drill for the preparation of the implant bed (Figs 22-8 and 22-9). Drilling should be performed intermittently and always under cooling with sterile isotonic saline. Insertion of a

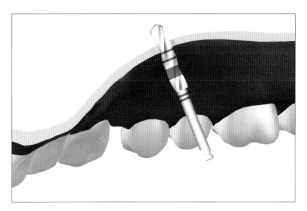

Fig 22-8 The implant bed is prepared according to the manufacturer's instructions (©Institut Straumann AG, 2020. All rights reserved. Image courtesy of Institut Straumann AG).

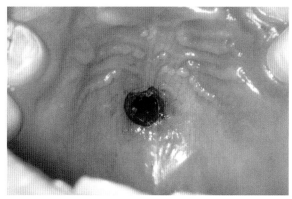

Fig 22-9 Intraoperative situation after preparation of the implant bed.

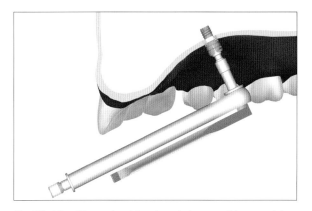

Fig 22-10 The palatal implant is inserted by machine or by hand with a torque ratchet (©Institut Straumann AG, 2020. All rights reserved. Image courtesy of Institut Straumann AG).

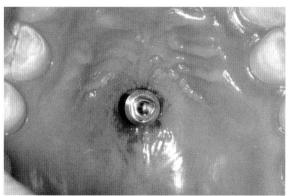

Fig 22-11 Intraoperative situation after implant insertion.

very short tissue-level implant then takes place. A thread cutter might be required, but palatal implants are usually self-cutting.

After preparation of the implant bed, the palatal implant can be inserted with slow clockwise turns using a torque ratchet (maximum 15 rpm) at a maximum tightening torque of 25 Ncm (Fig 22-10). Adequate primary stability is a basic prerequisite for successful osseointegration (Fig 22-11).

Implant insertion is flapless and therefore no wound closure is necessary. However, a healing cap is fitted to the implant and hand-tightened during the healing phase. In terms of hygiene measures, patients should be advised to clean around the implant with a soft toothbrush twice a day from the first day as part of their general cleaning routine. Patients should receive an antiseptic and an analgesic (paracetamol or a nonsteroidal anti-inflammatory drug [NSAID], preferably ibuprofen) after surgery. Dose and dosage need to be adjusted to the patient's body weight and age.

Postoperative controls and course

The first wound check-up is carried out on the second day postoperatively. During this check-up, the wound site is disinfected with an antiseptic. Follow-up can then take place after 1 week and 1 month. Unlike mini-implants, the palatal implant is not loaded with the orthodontic appliance until osseointegration has occurred. The healing phase usually lasts for 8 to 12 weeks. There has been some discussion in the literature of the possibility of earlier loading. At the University Center for Dental Medicine Basel, orthodontic loading normally starts 3 months after implant insertion.

After the healing phase, the orthodontic appliance can be fixed to the rotation-secured palatal implant directly or indirectly with secondary parts. To prevent loss of anchorage of the palatal implant due to deflection, it is important to ensure that the dimensions of the connectors between the implant and the orthodontic appliance are large enough (e.g. transpalatal arch).

Radiographs may subsequently show condensation of the bone as a result of mechanical loading of the palatal implant. If peri-implant mucositis should arise due to poor oral hygiene, short-term application of a chlorhexidine gel (one to two times per day) should be carried out.

Explantation of palatal implants

Indications

Palatal implants as well as other osseous anchorage devices are usually not removed until orthodontic treatment is completed (Figs 22-12 and 22-13).

Contraindications

Premature removal of a palatal implant during ongoing orthodontic treatment is inadvisable. If it becomes apparent afterward that skeletal anchorage was actually still required, it would be very troublesome for everyone involved if it had been removed prematurely.

Specific risks

The most common complications related to palatal implant explantation that are mentioned in the literature are wound-healing complications (6.8%), followed by nasal floor perforations (2.3%) and secondary bleeding (2.3%)[1].

Step-by-step clinical procedure

Local infiltration anesthesia administered three times around the palatal implant generally suffices. A possible alternative is a bilateral nerve block of the greater palatine nerve and the nasopalatine nerve.

Next, a minimally invasive or selective osteotomy in a circle around the palatal implant is

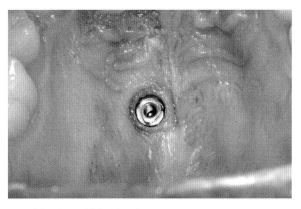
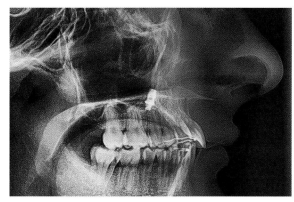

Figs 22-12 and 22-13 Clinical and radiographic situation after completion of orthodontic treatment (situation pre-explantation).

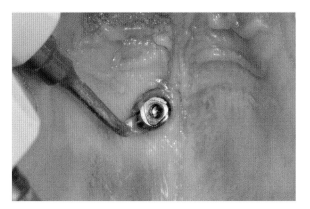
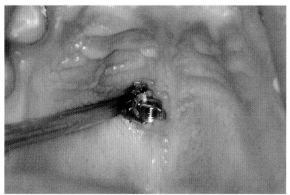

Fig 22-14 A minimal, circular osteotomy is performed around the palatal implant being removed using special piezoelectric surgical attachments. The piezoelectric surgical instrument is kept in constant motion, and little pressure is applied to the bone.

Fig 22-15 The palatal implant is then loosened with an elevator. If the palatal implant still does not move, another osteotomy is performed with the piezoelectric surgical instrument.

performed with specially designed piezoelectric surgical attachments (see Section 4; Fig 22-14). The palatal implant can then be loosened with an elevator (Fig 22-15) and removed with a grasping instrument such as extraction forceps or a Luer bone rongeur (Figs 22-16 to 22-19).

As an alternative, a specially developed explantation set (Bussmann Orthodontie-Labor) can be used for Orthosystem palatal implants. This set comprises a torque ratchet, a screwdriver, and a special adapter (Figs 22-20 to 22-23). The special adapter is made of hard steel

and has a triangular internal profile (Fig 22-24) so that it fits the triangular connector on the Orthosystem palatal implant (Fig 22-25). This means that minimally invasive removal of palatal implants requires minimal technical outlay.

The initial step is to remove the protective cap from the palatal implant and secure the adapter with the occlusal screw and long screwdriver (Figs 22-26 to 22-29). After the correct positioning and secure hold have been carefully checked, a short turn in a clockwise and then a counterclockwise direction is made with the

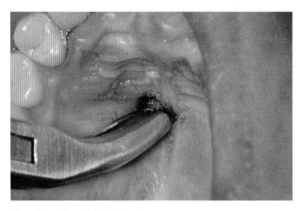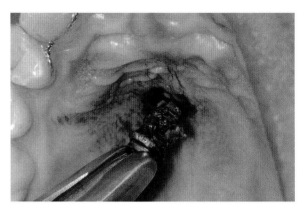

Figs 22-16 and 22-17   Once the palatal implant is loosened, it can be safely removed with a grasping instrument (here, a Luer bone rongeur).

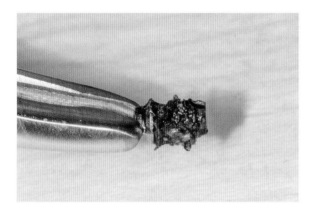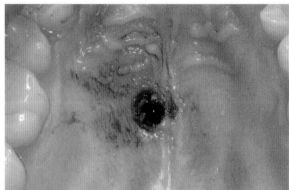

Fig 22-18   Palatal implant ex vivo: Bone fragments can still be seen on the rough implant surface.

Fig 22-19   Wound condition after explantation.

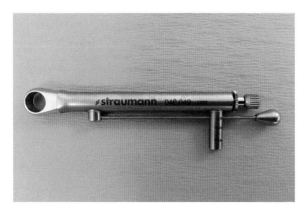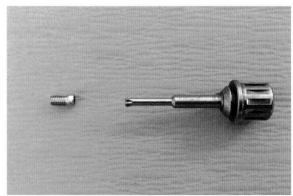

Fig 22-20   Torque ratchet (Straumann).

Fig 22-21   Long SCS screwdriver with SCS occlusal screw (Straumann) for fixation of the screw removal tool.

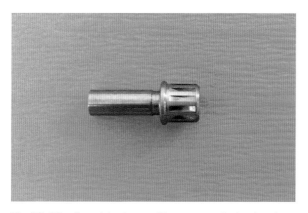

Fig 22-22 Special adapter (Bussmann Orthodontie-Labor).

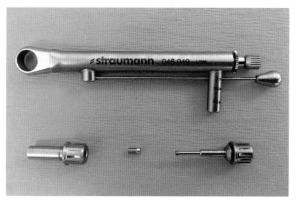

Fig 22-23 All the components of the explantation set together.

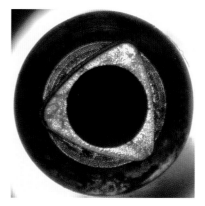

Fig 22-24 Internal triangular profile of the adapter.

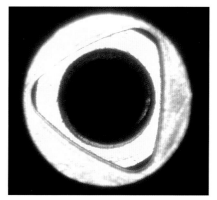

Fig 22-25 Triangular connector on the head of the Orthosystem palatal implant.

attached torque ratchet to loosen the palatal implant from its bony anchorage. It can easily be unscrewed in one further step (Fig 22-30).

Explantation with a trephine drill should be avoided because it is more invasive. Due to the larger diameter of its hollow cylinder, drilling around the palatal implant will create an extensive wound. Complications such as perforation of the nasal floor or injury to adjacent tooth roots are mentioned in the literature in connection with a trephine drill. In a few case reports, maxillary anterior teeth have also been devitalized.

The risk arises primarily when there has been pronounced palatal movement of the anterior tooth roots during orthodontic treatment, e.g. when treating an Angle Class II, division 2 malocclusion after extraction of two premolars, followed by space closure and axial alignment of the anterior teeth.

The patient should perform the nose-blowing test immediately after explantation in order to exclude perforation of the nasal floor. If the test is negative, the wound, which might still be bleeding slightly (Fig 22-31), is compressed for a

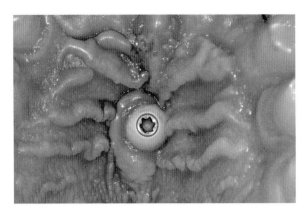

Fig 22-26 Preoperative clinical situation: The protective cap is still located on the palatal implant.

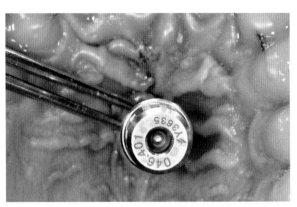

Fig 22-27 The screwdriver is used to remove the protective cap.

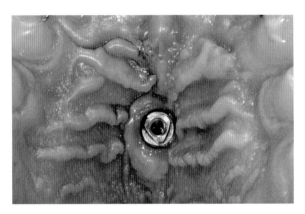

Fig 22-28 Situation after removal of the protective cap: The triangular connector is visible.

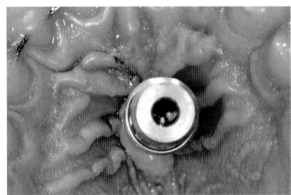

Fig 22-29 The adapter on the palatal implant is secured with an SCS occlusal screw.

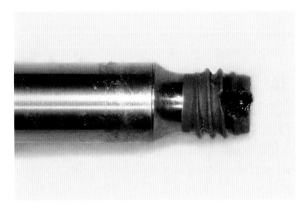

Fig 22-30 Palatal implant ex vivo.

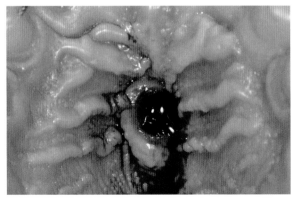

Fig 22-31 Situation after explantation using the explantation set.

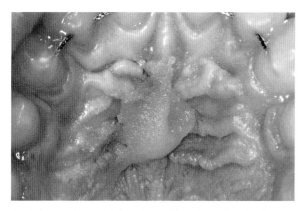

Fig 22-32 Wound dressing with a dental adhesive paste (Solcoseryl).

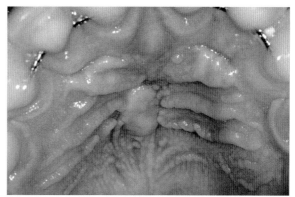

Fig 22-33 Non-irritated wound conditions 2 weeks postoperatively.

few minutes with a sterile swab. A dental adhesive paste (e.g. Solcoseryl, MEDA Pharmaceuticals) can then be applied to the wound area (Fig 22-32). If the nose-blowing test is positive, the oroantral communication can be covered with a vacuum-formed splint. Recall should then follow at short intervals. If conservative treatment of the oroantral communication remains unsuccessful, soft tissue closure is indicated, e.g. with a palatal rotational flap.

The patient should be given a few sterile swabs to take home in case there is more bleeding after the local anesthetic has worn off. The patient should also receive an antiseptic and analgesic in the event that they are required (paracetamol or an NSAID, preferably ibuprofen). Dose and dosage need to be adjusted to the patient's body weight and age.

Postoperative controls and course

The first check-up takes place on the second day postoperatively. During this recall, the wound is disinfected with an antiseptic. The second and final wound check-up can be carried out after 1 to 2 weeks (Fig 22-33).

References

1. Fäh R, Schätzle M: Complications and adverse patient reactions associated with the surgical insertion and removal of palatal implants: a retrospective study. Clin Oral Implants Res 2014;25:653–658.

2. Kawa D, Kunkel M, Heuser L, Jung BA: What is the best position for palatal implants? A CBCT study on bone volume in the growing maxilla. Clin Oral Investig 2017;21:541–549.

3. Schätzle M, Mühlemann S, Hersberger-Zurfluh M, Bussmann T, Näf P, Patcas R: Prosthetic implants used as orthodontic anchor-age – Introducing a complete digital workflow for clinical use. Swiss Dent J 2020;130:887–892.

4. Schlegel KA, Kinner F, Schlegel KD: The anatomic basis for palatal implants in orthodontics. Int J Adult Orthodon Orthognath Surg 2002;17:133–139.

5. Stockmann P, Schlegel KA, Srour S, Neukam FW, Fenner M, Felszeghy E: Which region of the median palate is a suitable location of temporary orthodontic anchorage devices? A histomorphometric study on human cadavers aged 15-20 years. Clin Oral Implants Res 2009;20:306–312.

6. Wehrbein H, Merz BR, Diedrich P: Palatal bone support for orthodontic implant anchorage – a clinical and radiological study. Eur J Orthod 1999;21:65–70.

Recommended literature

Hourfar J, Lisson JA: Wissenschaftliche Stellungnahme zur Verankerung mit Gaumenimplantaten und Kortikalisschrauben in der Kieferorthopädie. DGKFO, 2017.

Züger M, Hänggi M, Kühl S, Filippi A: Ein neues Explantationsverfahren für Gaumenimplantate. Quintessenz 2015;66:197–202.

Evidence-based aspects

23

Frank Peter Strietzel, Henrik Dommisch

The purpose of quality assurance measures in diagnostics and therapy is ultimately to optimize patient treatment safety. It is important that we critically reflect on our own knowledge, experience, and internal evidence while taking into account the existing external evidence. The latter includes considering the latest published results from clinical trials as well as **systematic literature review articles** and **meta-analyses**. These results will have been obtained following specific scientifically accepted processes focusing on particular issues. Literature reviews and meta-analyses can prove a particularly useful source of information. However, we should critically question the results of meta-analyses in terms of their transferability to clinical practice and their possible limitations[20]. **External evidence** can complement, filter or refine individual clinical experience but is no substitute for it[78]. **Internal evidence** denotes "all knowledge about our individual [patients] themselves, which can often only be clarified in a meeting between each unique [patient] and the therapist[18]." Other important factors are additional knowledge and experience obtained from our daily clinical activity, i.e. our **individual clinical expertise**[97]. If we take into account the additional element of patient wishes or preferences, an initially traditional (patriarchal) approach can evolve into a **participatory decision-making process** when developing a therapeutic approach[96].

More and more frequently, decision making by clinicians also incorporates **guidelines**. These are statements regarding the current state of knowledge about a certain disease or specific treatment method and are systematically and increasingly developed on the basis of systematic literature reviews[21,80,105]. The latter are based on findings updated at regular intervals (usually every 3 to 5 years) that are discussed by experienced professionals or experts; these discussions increasingly also involve professional policymakers as well as patients, interest groups or representatives, and include the best scientifically published evidence. Nevertheless, guidelines still require critical appraisal with regard to their implementability under everyday clinical conditions and under the particular circumstances of the type of intervention as they relate to the patient's individual requirements or characteristics[87].

Selected aspects of external evidence relating to some of the areas of focus in the previous sections of this book are examined below.

Interventions to preserve alveolar process dimensions

After tooth extraction, the alveolar process undergoes dimensional changes in terms of a reduction in width and height, which can be significant and can influence the subsequent treatment options regarding prosthetic or implant-prosthetic rehabilitation after tooth loss[19,90]. Measures to stabilize the alveolar process in order to maintain the dimensions of the bony alveolar ridge and the soft tissue (especially the peri-implant soft tissue) are becoming increasingly important. The measures used in this context are described earlier in this book (see Section 6).

Stabilization of alveolar process dimensions

Systematic literature review articles have generally reported a positive effect of ridge-stabilizing measures following tooth extraction in favor of a smaller reduction of the alveolar process in terms of its buccolingual width and height compared with dimensional changes in untreated extraction sockets[34,90]. However, it is clearly not possible to prevent dimensional changes to the alveolar ridge generally by measures to stabilize the alveolar process[90].

It is generally acknowledged that measures to stabilize the alveolar process create better initial conditions for eventual implant placement. However, no recommendations have been made in favor of one specific material or technical approach over another, not least because of the interrelations of numerous variables and the lack of long-term studies. The long-term effects on implant success or peri-implant tissue resulting from measures to stabilize the alveolar ridge also have not been established[10].

Quantitative analyses of data from various studies for the purposes of meta-analyses have selectively provided some clarification. For instance, a significant reduction of the horizontal as well as the vertical mesial, distal, and buccal dimensions of the alveolar process in the socket area has been demonstrated as a result of measures to stabilize the alveolar ridge[12,17,45,59,106]. In approximately 90% of areas where the alveolar ridge was thus treated, implants could later be placed without additional augmentation measures, whereas this was possible for only 79% of untreated sockets[106].

Some meta-analyses[10,59] regarding the nature of the intervention to stabilize the alveolar process do not provide recommendations about alternative interventions in the absence of usable data. Meanwhile, other meta-analyses regarding the type of intervention and the bone substitute materials used do offer a few focused statements. For instance, primary wound closure had a significant, positive effect on the preservation of the horizontal dimension of the alveolar ridge[11,12,17]; however, a reduced width of keratinized gingiva was identified in this context[16].

Ridge-stabilizing measures had a significantly greater effect when used in sockets with defects in the socket walls compared with sockets with intact walls[17].

The type of bone replacement material used had a significant influence on the outcome of the ridge-stabilizing measure[17,44]. In particular, xenogeneic bone substitutes (as the most commonly tested materials) seem to result in short-term

success regarding ridge-stabilizing measures. Furthermore, xenogeneic or allogeneic bone replacement materials were shown to have advantages over alloplastic materials[11,12,17]. Allogeneic bone substitute material had the best stabilizing effects on the height of the alveolar process and autologous bone on its width compared with untreated sockets[45]. However, most of these studies were found to show a strong bias[10].

The use of a barrier membrane had a significant positive effect on the outcome of alveolar ridge-stabilizing measures[11,12,17]. When a combination of xenogeneic or allogeneic bone substitute material and a resorbable membrane was used in the context of tooth extraction, significant stabilization of ridge dimensions postextraction was achieved[45,95].

In a few systematic literature review articles and meta-analyses, the sole use of autologous platelet concentrates has not shown any advantages or effects to date in terms of the dimensional stability of the alveolar process or osteoblastic activity postextraction. With regard to bone density, a wide and partly contradictory range of results has been reported, from a lack of influence on bone density[56] in the area of the former socket to significantly higher bone density after 1, 3, and 6 months[31]. However, evidence of accelerated soft tissue wound healing and the reduction of postoperative symptoms such as swelling and trismus was consistently found[5,31].

Histologic and histomorphometric analyses overall show that, when allogeneic bone replacement material was used, the proportion of newly formed bone was highest and the proportion of remnants of biomaterial was lowest after 3 months compared with xenogeneic bone substitute (in which case, the proportion of newly formed bone was lowest after 5 months). However, the difference was not significant. At the same time, it did not seem necessary to wait more than 3 to 4 months after alveolar ridge-stabilizing measures before carrying out implant placement[33].

Implants inserted in the area of a former ridge-stabilizing intervention had similar retention and success rates and a comparable marginal bone contour to implants inserted in the area of formerly untreated sockets[61].

Some meta-analyses favor certain methods or materials while others do not. This may be an indicator of structural and methodologic variations between the systematic literature review articles or meta-analyses, which, in fact, has been confirmed[64]. Hence, it should be noted that the quality or informative value of a systematic literature review article or meta-analysis depends on the quality of the published evidence available or on their critical selection as well as on their methodologic quality.

Stabilization of peri-implant soft tissue

For the most part, published articles on the importance of peri-implant soft tissue do not make a distinction between attached or keratinized peri-implant soft tissue, even though they are separate characteristics. Thus, the importance of one or the other of these components for peri-implant health cannot be clearly defined[50]. However, the existence of attached and keratinized peri-implant mucosa does seem to be significant in the prevention of peri-implant disease.

A lack of adequate **keratinized peri-implant mucosa**[57] as well as soft tissue deficiencies such as insufficient vestibular depth, scar tissue or the pull of labial or buccal frenula on the peri-implant mucosa are significantly associated with increased plaque accumulation, inflammation, mucosal recession, and attachment loss[41,73]. However, metric details for the minimal required width of attached or keratinized peri-implant mucosa are not given in review articles. In a cross-sectional study on 37 patients, a width of < 2 mm of keratinized peri-implant mucosa

was shown to have a significant correlation with diseases of the peri-implant tissue[63]. Without giving details of the required width of keratinized peri-implant mucosa, a prospective study involving 89 patients showed that implants not surrounded by keratinized mucosa had a higher accumulation of plaque and soft tissue recessions after 10 years[75]. The use of a free mucosal graft in this situation led to markedly improved plaque control[75].

During the course of a consensus conference, it was noted that achieving an adequate width of keratinized peri-implant soft tissue had significant advantages in terms of reducing plaque and gingivitis indices and probing depths[38].

Regarding **soft tissue thickness**, a noticeably thick phenotype has a positive influence on the esthetic outcome due to higher resistance to mechanical injury or surgical manipulations and mucosal recessions of the peri-implant soft tissue, and not least because the tissue volume is beneficial for prosthetic restorations[36].

There appears to be some controversy at present about the required crestal peri-implant soft tissue thickness. In a systematic literature review article, Akcalı et al[1] concluded, based on the wide heterogeneity of the available studies, that there was insufficient evidence of more pronounced crestal bone resorption when the soft tissue thickness initially present was < 2 mm as well as a lack of evidence of less crestal bone resorption for a soft tissue thickness of 2 mm or more. In a meta-analysis, Thoma et al[91] showed advantages for soft tissue augmentation in terms of the health of the peri-implant tissue, especially when using autogenous grafts for widening the keratinized peri-implant mucosa (thereby improving the bleeding indices and maintaining the marginal bone level) and for thickening the mucosa (providing significantly less marginal bone resorption over time).

The use of autologous connective tissue grafts led to a widening of the keratinized peri-implant mucosa and a thickening of the soft tissue after an observation period of up to 48 months. However, a volume decrease is to be expected within the first 3 months[72]. Furthermore, soft tissue augmentation with free connective tissue grafts to thicken the peri-implant mucosa in esthetically demanding areas led to significantly less marginal bone resorption over time, but did have significant repercussions for bleeding on probing, probing depths, and plaque indices compared with nonaugmented regions[38].

The results of soft tissue augmentation to increase the thickness of peri-implant buccal and crestal mucosa and to widen the keratinized mucosa do not differ significantly in relation to the use of a xenogeneic collagen matrix compared with an autologous connective tissue graft, nor when considering postoperative morbidity. Only the treatment time was significantly shorter when a xenogeneic collagen matrix was used[37].

Tooth-preserving surgery

A distinction is generally made between the **retention or survival rate** and the **success rate** of a tooth in assessments of treatment outcome following apicoectomy, intentional replantation or autologous tooth transplantation. Evaluation of the success rate includes the criteria of tooth retention in situ, the condition of the tooth and the periodontal tissue (including the periapical region – clinical and radiographic evaluation), checks of tooth loosening and percussion sound, and the presence or absence of clinical symptoms[86].

Apicoectomy

Apicoectomy (see Section 10) may be used as the last resort for preserving an endodontically treated tooth, bearing in mind the indication and certain prevailing conditions[54,86]. A recent meta-analysis reported post-apicoectomy tooth retention rates of 94% (95% confidence interval [CI]: 91% to 97%) after 2 to 4 years and 88% (95% CI: 84% to 92%) after 4 to 6 years[94]. The success rates are slightly lower at 90% (95% CI: 86% to 94%) after 2 to 4 years and 84% (95% CI: 67% to 96%) after 4 to 6 years[94]. The microsurgical approach was studied in this instance.

If alternative treatment methods are also considered for comparative purposes – always assuming the correct indication exists – the success rates after endodontic revision differ significantly in an observation period of 2 to 4 years, according to a systematic literature review article. A higher success rate (77.8%) was found after apicoectomy compared with endodontic revision treatments (70.9%). A success rate of 83% was found 4 to 6 years postintervention after endodontic revision compared with apicoectomy (71.8%)[92]. Similar results were published in a more recent review article: endodontic revision treatments led to a tooth retention rate of 84% to 89% after 4 to 10 years, while a rate of 59% to 93% was reported for apicoectomy after 1 to 10 years[22]. After a short observation period, Kang et al[49] found a success rate of 84% for endodontic revision versus 95% for apicoectomy. After 2 to 4 years of observation, there were still significant differences in the results (71% for endodontic revision and 90% for apicoectomy), whereas the differences no longer existed after 4 years (82% for both groups).

These results show that apicoectomy evidently leads to higher success rates than endodontic revision treatments in the short term, but this effect seems to level out in the longer term[53]. In view of this uncertainty, it is worth asking critically to what extent the studies included dropouts after longer treatment periods. Furthermore, to some extent, the studies considered are very heterogenous. Repetition of apicoectomy seems to be associated with a significantly lower prospect of success than results following the first apicoectomy. Von Arx et al[98,102] partly attribute this to negative selection in compromised initial conditions.

Various **influencing factors** are crucial to the success of apicoectomy. These include factors that should be considered in advance of the intervention such as establishing the correct indication[54]. Furthermore, one of the fundamental requirements for a successful post-apicoectomy treatment outcome is the exclusion of a persistent root canal infection by endodontic treatment after tight root canal filling and after tight crown restoration[29,54,65]. The accompanying topographic, anatomical, and pathologic circumstances also influence the outcome of apicoectomy. For instance, the condition of the marginal periodontium with associated apicomarginal defects[84] has an adverse effect on apicoectomy outcome, as does marginal bone resorption of > 3 mm[101].

The preoperative size of the lesion influences the success rate, at least tendentially. The larger the lesion, the lower the postoperative success rate[15,71,100,102]. In this context, diabetes mellitus also appears to affect the incidence and progression of **apical periodontitis** and the size of the apical lesion[81].

The location of the tooth has an impact on the treatment outcome post-apicoectomy. Incisors show the highest success rate (100% to 84.5%), followed by premolars (81.4% to 69%) and molars (78% to 68.1%)[30,102,103]. The success rates are higher in the maxilla than in the mandible[71,102,103], while the results can definitely vary after a longer period of time[101].

General surgical conditions also have an influence on outcome. Retrograde cavity preparation with ultrasonic tips produces significantly better results than conventional preparation with a rotary instrument[30,51,102].

Hydraulic silicate cements (e.g. mineral trioxide aggregate [MTA]) as a filling material for a retrograde cavity compared with an intermediate restorative material (IRM), aluminum-reinforced zinc oxide eugenol cement modified by the addition of ethoxybenzoic acid (SuperEBA, Bosworth) as well as thermoplastically processed gutta-percha showed success rates of 84% to 90% after at least 1 year, with no significant difference between MTA and IRM. Both materials had the best results[26,79,88,103], while other studies showed significantly better results for MTA than for SuperEBA[100,101].

Optical magnifying aids (e.g. loupes, microscopes, endoscopes; see Section 2) seem to help clinicians achieve better success rates. The difference compared with results after conventional methods were not significant in some studies[32,35,89,99,102]. In a recent meta-analysis, however, the use of powerful magnifying aids (operating microscope or endoscope) in the molar region showed a significant advantage in relation to success rates compared with a traditional method[82] and working with loupe magnification[83].

With regard to age (distinguishing between patients under or over 40 to 45 years of age) and gender, a meta-analysis revealed no significant difference in the success rate after apicoectomy with retrograde root canal filling[102]. However, a more recent epidemiologic study did show a difference, with a significantly higher success rate in males (84%) than in females (81%)[74].

Intentional replantation

Assessment of treatment outcomes after intentional replantation (see Section 12) is based on the above-mentioned criteria, in the same way as for apicoectomy. However, there are fewer clinical studies on intentional replantation with a smaller number of patients, widely varying observation periods (but tending to rather shorter follow-up periods), and relatively nonhomogenous retention rates. Current publications from the past 10 years report retention rates of 72% to 100% after 3 months to 11 years[8,14,23-25,46,58,67].

A recent systematic literature review reports retention rates of 88% (95% CI: 81% to 94%, N = 838, 11% root resorptions) for intentionally replanted teeth[93]. Intentional replantation was most commonly performed on maxillary and mandibular second molars. The reasons for this, apart from the root topography being suitable, were difficulty of access for endodontic surgical procedures, the proximity of anatomical structures such as the maxillary sinus or mandibular canal, and the lower treatment costs compared with alternative therapies (e.g. implant-prosthetic single-tooth replacement)[60]. On the other hand, the results are also influenced by the learning curve and the organization of processes (e.g. the tooth should be extracted with minimal trauma and the shortest possible extraoral treatment time in order to avoid damage to the periodontal ligament; in a systematic literature review, it was 11 to 12 minutes on average[60]). Possible postoperative complications include root resorption and ankylosis[93,104].

Tooth transplantation

Calculation of the success rate takes into account retention of the transplanted tooth (see Section 11) in its recipient site (calculation of the **retention and survival rate**), the absence of ankylosis or inflammatory root resorption, the presence of normal physiologic tooth mobility, and continued root growth[76].

In the process, the following factors influence the success rates after autologous tooth transplantation: the patient's age and the associated developmental stage of the autotransplanted tooth, its location, an atraumatic surgical procedure while keeping the periodontal tissue of the graft and recipient region vital, absence of inflammation and favorable bone supply in the recipient region, and the duration of extra-alveolar storage of the tooth for transplantation; other factors include the motivation and cooperation of the patient and good oral hygiene[7,9,42,43,47,55,76,77].

The prognosis is better for autotransplanted teeth at the stage of one-third to three-quarters root formation (but also up to fully formed root length with an open apical foramen), autotransplanted premolars, and maxillary recipient sites[9,76]. For third molars as transplanted teeth, the ideal stage is reportedly two-thirds of root length development[7]. The open apical aspect of the autotransplanted teeth was identified as a significant prognostic factor in meta-analyses[9,76].

Rohof et al[76] reported the retention rates for autotransplanted teeth (premolars showed a better prognosis than molars) as 97.4% (95% CI: 96.2% to 98.2%) after 1 year, 97.8% (95% CI: 95% to 99%) after 5 years, and 96.3% (95% CI: 89.8% to 98.7%) after 10 years; the weighted success rate was calculated to be 96.6% (95% CI: 94.8% to 97.8%) per year, and the weighted complication rates were given as 2% (95% CI: 1.1% to 3.7%) for ankylosis, 2.9% (95% CI: 1.1% to 5.5%) for root resorption, and 3.3% (95% CI: 1.9% to 5.6%) for pulp necrosis, per year[76]. If ankylosis occurs, a higher risk of the loss of the autotransplanted tooth is to be expected[9].

Based on retrospective studies, autotransplanted teeth with completed root growth and a closed apical foramen after endodontic treatment reportedly showed success rates of 71% after an average of 5.8 years[52], and 53.3% (≥ 55-year-olds), 76.7% (25- to 39-year-olds), and 83.8% (40- to 54-year-olds) after up to 10 years[108]. Autotransplanted canines exhibited success rates of 83% after an average of 14.5 years[70], molars had success rates of 84% after 15 months[13], and third molars showed success rates of 88% after 6 months[85].

Temporary implants for orthodontic anchorage

The introduction of mini-implants to aid skeletal anchorage for orthodontic movement (see

Section 21) has expanded treatment options in orthodontics. Unlike conventional implants for attachment or support of dentures, these are temporary implants that are usually removed after the completion of orthodontic treatment. Mini-implants facilitate orthodontic movement of individual teeth or groups of teeth in a significantly shorter treatment time than conventional methods[6,68].

The **success rates** of orthodontic mini-implants are reported to be 86%[27], 87.7%[68], and between 79% and 96%[28]; the mean rates of loss are reported to be between 6%[48] and 13.5%[69]. The **risk of loss** of orthodontic mini-implants correlates significantly with patient age under 20 years, peri-implant mucositis, poor oral hygiene, smoking, implantation in the mandible[28,62], and contact with adjacent roots[40,62]. The **loss rates** for orthodontic mini-implants also differ with respect to the individual jaw regions or the area of use. For instance, in terms of palatally inserted implants, loss rates of 1.3% were calculated for the median position, 4.8% for the paramedian position, and 5.5% for parapalatal insertion of implants[62]. For buccal insertion sites, loss rates of 9.2% and 9.7% were found for the regions between the second premolar and first molar or canine and lateral incisor, respectively, while a loss rate of 16.4% was found for insertion in the area of the zygomaticoalveolar crest[62]. In the mandible, loss rates of 13.5% were reported for buccally inserted mini-implants between the second premolar and first molar, and 9.9% when insertion was between the canines and first premolars[62].

Penetration of mini-implants into the integrity of the roots is regarded as a **complication**. If the periodontal space, cementum or dentin in the marginal areas of the tooth root are affected, regeneration is possible. However, if the integrity of the pulp is damaged, regeneration is unlikely, even in the periodontal space[4,39]. Gradual dislocation of mini-implants during the course of orthodontic treatment is also a possibility and can lead to the penetration of the periodontal ligament space. Therefore, when positioned in interradicular areas, mini-implants should be inserted as far away as possible from the direction of force[66].

In addition to the **anatomical aspects** of positioning outlined above, insertion sites 3 mm posterior to the incisive foramen and 3 to 9 mm paramedian as well as 12 mm posterior to the incisive foramen and 9 to 12 mm paramedian were identified as suitable for **palatal** paramedian anchorage of mini-implants with respect to vertical bone supply[107]. AlSamak et al[2] ascertained that the optimal palatal implantation sites were positions 3 to 6 mm posterior to the incisive foramen and 2 to 9 mm lateral thereof. AlSamak et al[3] highlighted the region between the canine and the first premolar as being the most favorable insertion sites for orthodontic mini-implants in the **anterior region** of the maxilla and mandible. The regions between the canine and lateral incisor are given as alternative implant placement sites for both jaws. However, the distances between the roots must be respected as a limiting factor[3]. In the **posterior regions** of the maxilla and mandible, the region between the first and second molars offers the best anchorage possibilities, with the region between the second premolar and first molar being an alternative possibility[2].

References

1. Akcalı A, Trullenque-Eriksson A, Sun C, Petrie A, Nibali L, Donos N: What is the effect of soft tissue thickness on crestal bone loss around dental implants? A systematic review. Clin Oral Implants Res 2016;28:1046–1053.

2. AlSamak S, Gkantidis N, Bitsanis E, Christou P: Assessment of potential orthodontic mini-implant insertion sites based on anatomical hard tissue parameters: a systematic review. Int J Oral Maxillofac Implants 2012;27:875–887.

3. AlSamak S, Psomiadis S, Gkantidis N: Positional guidelines for orthodontic mini-implant placement in the anterior alveolar region: a systematic review. Int J Oral Maxillofac Implants 2013;28:470–479.

4. Alves Jr M, Baratieri C, Mattos CT, de Souza Araujo MT, Maia LC: Root repair after contact with mini-implants: a systematic review of the literature. Eur J Orthodont 2013;35:491–499.

5. Annunziata M, Guida L, Piccirillo A, Sommese L, Napoli C: The role of autologous platelet concentrates in alveolar socket preservation: a systematic review. Transfus Med Hemother 2018;45:195–203.

6. Antoszewska-Smith J, Sarul M, Lyczek J, Konopka T, Kawala B: Effectiveness of orthodontic miniscrew implants in anchorage reinforcement during en-masse retraction: a systematic review and meta-analysis. Am J Orthod Dentofacial Orthop 2017;151:440–455.

7. Armstronq L, O'Reilly C, Ahmed B: Autotransplantation of third molars: a literature review and preliminary protocols. Br Dent J 2020;228:247–251.

8. Asgary S, Marvasti LA, Kolahdouzan A: Indications and case series of intentional replantation of teeth. Iran Endod J 2014;9:71–78.

9. Atala-Acevedo C, Abarca J, Martínez-Zapata MJ, Díaz J, Olate S, Zaror C: Success rate of autotransplantation of teeth with open apex: systematic review and meta-analysis. J Oral Maxillofac Surg 2017;75:35–50.

10. Atieh MA, Alsabeeha NHM, Payne AGT, Duncan W, Faggion CM, Esposito M: Interventions for replacing missing teeth: alveolar ridge preservation techniques for dental implant site development. Cochrane Database Syst Rev 2015. CD010176.

11. Avila-Ortiz G, Chambrone L, Vignoletti F: Effect of alveolar ridge preservation interventions following tooth extraction: A systematic review and meta-analysis. J Clin Periodontol 2019;46(Suppl 21):195–223.

12. Avila-Ortiz G, Elangovan S, Kramer KWO, Blanchette D, Dawson DV: Effect of alveolar ridge preservation after tooth extraction: a systematic review and meta-analysis. J Dent Res 2014;93:950–958.

13. Bae JH, Choi YH, Cho BH, Kim YK, Kim SG: Autotransplantation of teeth with complete root formation: a case series. J Endod 2010;36:1422–1426.

14. Baltacioglu E, Tasdemir T, Yuva P, Celik D, Sukuroglu E: Intentional replantation of periodontallly hopeless teeth using a combination of enamel matrix derivative and demineralized freeze-dried bone allograft. Int J Periodontics Restorative Dent 2011;31:75–81.

15. Barone C, Dao TT, Basrani BB, Wang N, Friedman S: Treatment outcome in endodontics: the Toronto study – phases 3, 4, and 5: apical surgery. J Endod 2010;36:28–35.

16. Barone A, Toti P, Piattelli A, Iezzi G, Derchi G, Covani U: Extraction socket healing in humans after ridge preservation techniques: comparison between flapless and flapped procedures in a randomized clinical trial. J Periodontol 2014;85:14–23.

17. Bassir SH, Alhareky M, Wangsrimongkol B, Jia Y, Karimbux N: Systematic review and meta-analysis of hard tissue outcomes of alveolar ridge preservation. Int J Oral Maxillofac Implants 2018;33:979–994.

18. Behrens J: EbM ist die aktuelle Selbstreflexion der individualisierten Medizin als Handlungswissenschaft. (Zum wissenschaftstheoretischen Verständnis von EbM). Z Evid Fortbild Qual Gesundh wesen (ZEFQ) 2010;104:617–624.

19. Chappuis V, Araujo MG, Buser D: Clinical relevance of dimensional bone and soft tissue alterations post-extraction in esthetic sites. Periodontol 2000 2017;73:73–83.

20. Chenot J-F, Reber KC: Metaanalysen lesen und interpretieren: eine praktische Anleitung. Zeitschrift für Allgemeinmedizin 2015;11:1–8.

21. Chenot R, Schmidt J, Jordan AR: Informationsbedürfnisse und Stellenwert von Leitlinien im Praxisalltag: eine qualitative Studie. Dtsch Zahnärztl Z 2017;72:390–397.

22. Chércoles-Ruiz A, Sánchez-Torres A, Gay-Escoda C: Endodontics, endodontic retreatment and apical surgery versus tooth extraction and implant placement: a systematic review. J Endod 2017;4:679–686.

23.   Cho SY, Lee Y, Shin SJ, Kim E, Jung IY, Friedman S, Lee SJ: Retention and healing outcomes after intentional replantation. J Endod 2016;42: 909–915.

24.   Cho SY, Lee Y, Kim E: Clinical outcomes after intentional replantation of periodontally involved teeth. J Endod 2017;43:550–555.

25.   Choi Y, Bae J, Kim Y, Kim HY, Kim SK, Cho BH: Clinical outcome of intentional replantation with preoperative orthodontic extrusion: a retrospective study. Int Endod J 2014;47:1168–1176.

26.   Chong BS, Pitt Ford TR, Hudson MB: A prospective clinical study of mineral trioxide aggregate and IRM when used as root-end filling materials in endodontic surgery. Int Endod J 2003;36:520–526.

27.   Cunha AC, da Veiga AMA, Masterson D, Mattos CT, Nojima LI, Nojima MCG, Maia LC: How do geometry-related parameters influence the clinical performance of orthodontic mini-implants? A systematic review and meta-analysis. Int J Oral Maxillofac Surg 2017;46:1539–1551.

28.   Dalessandri D, Salgarello S, Dalessandri M, Lazzaroni E, Piancino M, Paganelli C, Maiorana C, Santoro F: Determinants for success rates of temporary anchorage devices in orthodontics: a meta-analysis (n>50). Eur J Orthodont 2014;36:303–313.

29.   Danin J, Linder LE, Lundqvist G, Ohlsson L, Ramsköld LO, Strömberg T: Outcomes of periradicular surgery in cases with apical pathosis and untreated canals. Oral Surg Oral Med Oral Pathol Oral Radiol Endod 1999;87:227–232.

30.   De Lange J, Putters T, Baas EM, van Ingen JM: Ultrasonic root-end preparation in apical surgery: a prospective randomized study. Oral Surg Oral Med Oral Pathol Oral Radiol Endod 2007;104:841–845.

31.   Del Fabbro M, Bucchi C, Lolato A, Corbella S, Testori T, Taschieri S: Healing of postextraction sockets preserved with autologous platelet concentrates. A systematic review and meta-analysis. J Oral Maxillofac Surg 2017;75:1601–1615.

32.   Del Fabbro M, Taschieri S: Endodontic therapy using magnification devices: a systematic review. J Dent 2010;38:269–275.

33.   De Risi V, Clementini M, Vittorini G, Mannocci A, de Sanctis M: Alveolar ridge preservation techniques: a systematic review and meta-analysis of histological and histomorphometrical data. Clin Oral Impl Res 2013;26:50–68.

34.   Faria-Almeida R, Astramskaite-Januseviciene I, Puisys A, Correia F: Extraction socket preservation with or without membranes, soft tissue influence on post extraction alveolar ridge preservation: a systematic review. J Oral Maxillofac Res 2019;10:e5.

35.   Filippi A, Lüthi Meier M, Lambrecht JT: Endoskopische Wurzelspitzenresektion – eine klinisch-prospektive Studie. Schweiz Monatsschr Zahnmed 2006;116:12–17.

36.   Fu JH, Lee A, Wang HL: Influence of tissue biotype on implant esthetics. Int J Oral Maxillofac Implants 2011;26:499–508.

37.   Gargallo-Albiol J, Barootchi S, Tavelli L, Wang HL: Efficacy of xenogenic collagen matrix to augment peri-implant soft tissue thickness compared with autogenous connective tissue graft: a systematic review and meta-analysis. Int J Oral Maxillofac Implants 2019;34:1059–1069.

38.   Giannobile WV, Jung RE, Schwarz F: Evidence-based knowledge on the aesthetics and maintenance of peri-implant soft tissues: Osteology Foundation Consensus report part 1 – effects of soft tissue augmentation procedures on the maintenance of peri-implant soft tissue health. Clin Oral Impl Res 2018;29(Suppl 15):7–10.

39.   Gintautaite G, Gaidyte A: Surgery-related factors affecting the stability of orthodontic mini-implants screwed in alveolar process interdental spaces: a systematic literature review. Stomatologija 2018;19:73–81.

40.   Gintautaite G, Kenstavicius G, Gaidyte A: Dental roots' and surrounding structures' response after contact with orthodontic mini implants: a systematic review. Stomatologija 2017;20:10–18.

41.   Giovannoli JL, Roccuzzo M, Albouy JP, Duffau F, Lin GH, Serino G: Local risk indicators – consensus report of working group 2. Int Dent J 2019;69(Suppl):7–11.

42.   Gonissen H, Politis C, Schepers S, Lambrichts I, Vrielinck L, Sun Y, Schuermans J: Long-term success and survival rates of autogenously transplanted canines. Oral Surg Oral med Oral Pathol Oral Radiol Endod 2010;110:570–578.

43.   Grisar K, Nys M, The V, Vrielinck L, Schepers S, Jacobs R, Politis C: Long-term outcome of autogenously transplanted maxillary canines. Clin Exp Dent Res 2019;5:67–75.

44.   Haugen HJ, Lyngstadaas SP, Rossi F, Perale G: Bone grafts: which is the ideal biomaterial? J Clin Periodontol 2019;46(Suppl 21):92–102.

45. Iocca O, Farcomeni A, Pardinas-Lopez S, Talib HS: Alveolar ridge preservation after tooth extraction: a Bayesian network meta-analysis of grafting materials efficacy on prevention of bone height and width reduction. J Clin Periodontol 2016;44:104–114.

46. Jang Y, Lee SJ, Yoon TC, Roh BD, Kim E: Survival rate of teeth with a C-shaped canal after intentional replantation: a study of 41 cases for up to 11 years. J Endod 2016;42:1320–1325.

47. Kafourou V, Tong HJ, Day P, Houghton N, Spencer RJ, Duggal M: Outcomes and prognostic factors that influence the success of tooth autotransplantation in children and adolescents. Dent Traumatol 2017;33:393–399.

48. Kakali L, Alharbi M, Pandis N, Gkantidis N, Kloukos D: Success of palatal implants or mini-screws placed median or paramedian for the reinforcement of anchorage during orthodontic treatment: a systematic review. Eur J Orthodont 2019;41:9–20.

49. Kang M, In Jung H, Song M, Kim SY, Kim HC, Kim E: Outcome of nonsurgical retreatment and endodontic microsurgery: a meta-analysis. Clin Oral Investig 2015;19:569–582.

50. Kleinheinz J: Kap. 12. Hot topic: Weichgewebs-management. In: Grötz KA, Haßfeld S, Schmidt-Westhausen AM (Hrsg): Handbuch MKG. MKG-Update 2020. Wiesbaden: Med Public, 2020.

51. Kohli MR, Berenji H, Setzer FC, Lee SM, Karabucak B: Outcome of endodontic surgery: a meta-analysis of the literature – part 3: comparison of endodontic microsurgical techniques with two different root-end filling materials. J Endod 2018;44:923–931.

52. Kokai S, Kanno Z, Koike S, Uesugi S, Takahashi Y, Ono T, Soma K: Retrospective study of 100 autotransplanted teeth with complete root formation and subsequent orthodontic treatment. Am J Orthod Dentofacial Orthop 2015;148:982–989.

53. Kreisler M: Kap. 14 Orale Chirurgie: Wurzel-spitzenresektion. MKG Update. Handbuch MKG. Wiesbaden, Med Update, 2020.

54. Kühl S: Wurzelspitzenresektion. In: Filippi A, Kühl S (Hrsg): Atlas der modernen zahnerhaltenden Chirurgie. Berlin: Quintessenz, 2018:51–68.

55. Kvint S, Lindsten R, Magnusson A, Nilsson P, Bjerklin K: Autotransplantation of teeth in 215 patients. A follow-up study. Angle Orthod 2010;80:446–451.

56. Lin CY, Chen Z, Pan WL, Wang HL: Effect of platelet-rich fibrin on ridge preservation in perspective of bone healing: a systematic review and meta-analysis. Int J Oral Maxillofac Implants 2019;34:845–854.

57. Lin GH, Chan HL, Wang HL: The significance of keratinized mucosa on implant health: a systematic review. J Periodontol 2013;84:1755–1767.

58. Lee EU, Lim HC, Lee JS, Jung UW, Kim US, Lee SJ, Choi SH: Delayed intentional replantation of periodontally hopeless teeth: a retrospective study. J Periodontal Implant Sci 2014;44:13–19.

59. MacBeth N, Trullenque-Eriksson A, Donos N, Mardas N: Hard and soft tissue changes following alveolar ridge preservation: a systematic review. Clin Oral Impl Res 2017;28:982–1004.

60. Mainkar A: A systematic review of the survival of teeth intentionally replanted with a modern technique and cost-effectiveness compared with single-tooth implants. J Endod 2017;43:1963–1968.

61. Mardas N, Trullenque-Eriksson A, MacBeth N, Petrie A, Donos N: Does ridge preservation following tooth extraction improve implant treatment outcomes: a systematic review. Clin Oral Impl Res 2015;26(Suppl 11):180–201.

62. Mohammed H, Wafaie K, Rizk MZ, Almuzian M, Sosly R, Bearn DR: Role of anatomical sites and correlated risk factors on the survival of orthodontic miniscrew implants: a systematic review and meta-analysis. Progr Orthod 2018;19:36.

63. Monje A, Blasi G: Significance of keratinized mucosa/gingiva on peri-implant and adjacent periodontal conditions in erratic maintenance compliers. J Periodontol 2019;90:445–453.

64. Moraschini V, dos SP Barbosa E: Quality assessment of systematic reviews on alveolar socket preservation. Int J Oral Maxillofac Surg 2016;45:1126–1134.

65. Nair PNR, Sjögren U, Figdor D, Sundqvist G: Persistent periapical radiolucencies of root-end filled human teeth, failed enodontic treatments, and periapical scars. Oral Surg Oral Med Oral Pathol Oral Radiol Endod 1999;87:617–627.

66. Nienkemper M, Handschel J, Drescher D: Systematic review of mini-implant displacement under orthodontic loading. Int J Oral Sci 2014;6:1–6.

67. Nizam N, Kaval ME, Gürlek Ö, Atila A, Caliskan MK: Intentional replantation of adhesively reattached vertically fractured maxillary single-rooted teeth. J Endod 2016;49:227–236.

68. Papadopoulos MA, Papageorgiou SN, Zogakis IP: Clinical effectiveness of orthodontic mini-screw implants: a meta-analysis. J Dent Res 2011;90:969–976.

69. Papageorgiou SN, Zogakis IP, Papadopoulos MA: Failure rates and associated risk factors of orthodontic miniscrew implants: a meta-analysis. Am J Orthodont Dentofacial Orthop 2012;142: 577–595.

70. Patel S, Fanshawe T, Bister D, Cobourne MT. Survival and success of maxillary canine autotransplantation: a retrospective investigation. Eur J Orthodont 2011;33:289–304.

71. Peñarrocha M, Martí E, García B, Gay C: Relationship of periapical radiologic lesion size, apical resection, and retrograde filling with the prognosis of periapical surgery. J Oral Maxillofac Surg 2007;65:1526–1529.

72. Poskevicius L, Sidlauskas A, Galindo-Moreno P, Juodzbalys G: Dimensional soft tissue changes following soft tissue grafting in conjunction with implant placement or around present dental implants: a systematic review. Clin Oral Implants Res 2017;28:1–8.

73. Pranskunas M, Poskevicius L, Juodzbalys G, Kubilius R, Jimbo R: Influence of peri-implant soft tissue condition and plaque accumulation on peri-implantitis: a systematic review. J Oral Maxillofac Res 2016;7:e2.

74. Raedel M, Hartmann A, Bohm S, Walther MH: Three-year outcome of apicectomy (apicoectomy): mining an insurance database. J Dent 2015;43:1218–1222.

75. Roccuzzo M, Grasso G, Dalmasso P: Keratinized mucosa around implants in partially edentulous posterior mandible: 10-year results of a prospective comparative study. Clin Oral Implants Res 2016;27:491–496.

76. Rohof EC, Kerdijk W, Jansma J, Livas C, Ren Y: Autotransplantation of teeth with incomplete root formation: a systematic review and meta-analysis. Clin Oral Investig 2018;22:1613–1624.

77. Ronchetti MF, Valdec S, Pandis N, Locher M, van Waes H: A retrospective analysis of factors influencing the success of autotransplanted posterior teeth. Progr Orthod 2015;16:42.

78. Sackett DL, Rosenberg WMC, Gray JAM, Haynes RB, Richardson WS: Evidence based medicine: what it is and what it isn't. BMJ 1996;312:71–72.

79. Saunders WP: A prospective clinical study of periradicular surgery using mineral trioxide aggregate as root-end filling. J Endod 2008;34: 660–665.

80. Schütte U, Weber A, Stratmann R: Leitlinien in der Zahn-, Mund- und Kieferheilkunde. Dtsch Zahnärztl Z 2010;65:278–280.

81. Segura-Egea JJ, Castellanos-Cosano L, Machuca G, López-López J, Martín-González J, velasco-Ortega E, Sánchez-Domínguez B, López-Frías FJ: Diabetes mellitus, periapical inflammation and endodontic treatment outcome. Med Oral Patol Oral Cir Bucal 2012;17:356–361.

82. Setzer FC, Shah SB, Kohli MR, Karabucak B, Kim S: Outcome of endodontic surgery: a meta-analysis of the literature – part 1: comparison of traditional root-end surgery and endodontic microsurgery. J Endod 2010;36: 1757–1765.

83. Setzer FC, Kohli MR, Shah SB, Karabucak B, Kim S: Outcome of endodontic surgery: a meta-analysis of the literature – part 2: comparison of endodontic microsurgical techniques with and without the use of higher magnification. J Endod 2012;38:1–10.

84. Skoglund A, Persson G: A follow-up study of apicoectomized teeth with total loss of the buccal bone plate. Oral Surg Oral Med Oral Pathol 1985;59:78–81.

85. Sobhi MB, Rana MJ, Manzoor MA, Ibrahim M, Tasleem-ul-Hudda: Autotransplantation of endodontically treated third molars. J Coll Physicians Surg Pak 2003;13:372–374.

86. Strietzel FP: Erfolgsraten. In: Filippi A, Kühl S (Hrsg): Atlas der modernen zahnerhaltenden Chirurgie. Berlin: Quintessenz, 2018:151–163.

87. Strietzel FP: Evidenzbasierte Aspekte in der Oralchirurgie. In: Filippi A, Saccardin F, Kühl S (Hrsg.): Das kleine 1 x 1 der Oralchirurgie. Berlin: Quintessenz, 2020.

88. Tang Y, Li X, Yin S: Outcomes of MTA as root-end filling in endodontic surgery: a systematic review. Quintessence Int 2010;41:557–566.

89. Taschieri S, del Fabbro M, Testori T, Francetti L, Weinstein R: Endodontic surgery using 2 different magnification devices: preliminary results of a randomized controlled study. J Oral Maxillofac Surg 2006;64:235–242.

90. Ten Heggeler JM, Slot DE, Van der Weijden GA: Effect of socket preservation therapies following tooth extraction in non-molar regions in humans: a systematic review. Clin Oral Implants Res 2020;22:779–788.

91. Thoma D, Naenni N, Figuero E, Hämmerle CHF, Schwarz F, Jung RE, Sanz-Sanchez I: Effects of soft tissue augmentation procedures on peri-implant health or disease: a systematic review and meta-analysis. Clin Oral Impl Res 2018;29(Suppl 15):32–49.

92. Torabinejad M, Corr R, Handysides R, Shabahang S: Outcomes of nonsurgical retreatment and endodontic surgery: a systematic review. J Endod 2009;35:930–937.

93. Torabinejad M, Dinsbach NA, Turman M, Handysides R, Bahjri K, White SN: Survival of intentionally replanted teeth and implant-supported single crowns: a systematic review. J Endod 2015;41:992–998.

94. Torabinejad M, Landaez M, Milan M, Sun CX, Henkin J, Al-Ardah A, Kattadiyil M, Bahjri K, Dehom S, Cortez E, White SN: Tooth retention through endodontic microsurgery or tooth replacement using single implants: a systematic review of treatment outcomes. J Endod 2015;41:1–10.

95. Troiano G, Zhurakivska K, Lo Muzio L, Laino L, Cicciù M, Lo Russo L: Combination of bone graft and resorbable membrane for alveolar ridge preservation: a systematic review, meta-analysis, and trial sequential analysis. J Periodontol 2018;89:46–57.

96. Türp JC, Antes G: Evidenzbasierte Medizin – aktueller Stand. Dtsch Zahnärztl Z 2013;68: 72–75.

97. Vollmuth R, Groß D: Zwischen Gütesiegel und Scheinargument: Der Diskurs um die Evidenzbasierte Zahnmedizin am Beispiel der professionellen Zahnreinigung. Dtsch Zahnärztl Z 2015;72:382–388.

98. von Arx T: Apical surgery: a review of current techniques and outcome. Saudi Dent J 2011;23:9–15.

99. von Arx T, Frei C, Bornstein M: Periradikuläre Chirurgie mit und ohne Endoskopie. Eine klinisch-prospektive Vergleichsstudie. Schweiz Monatsschr Zahnmed 2003;113:860–865.

100. von Arx T, Jensen SS, Hänni S: Clinical and radiographic assessment of various predictors for healing outcome 1 year after periapical surgery. J Endod 2007;33:123–128.

101. Von Arx T, Jensen S, Hänni S, Friedman S: Five-year longitudinal assessment of the prognosis of apical microsurgery. J Endod 2012;38:570–579.

102. von Arx T, Peñarrocha M, Jensen S: Prognostic factors in apical surgery with root-end filling: a meta-analysis. J Endod 2010;36:957–973.

103. Wälivaara DÅ, Abrahamsson P, Isaksson S, Blomqvist JE, Sämfors KA: Prospective study of periapically infected teeth treated with periapical surgery including ultrasonic preparation and retrograde intermediate restorative material root-end fillings. J Oral Maxillofac Surg 2007;65:931–935.

104. Wang L, Jiang H, Bai Y, Luo Q, Wu H, Liu H: Clinical outcomes after intentional replantation of permanent teeth: a systematic review. Bosn J Basic Med Sci 2020;20:13–20.

105. Weber A: Leitlinien sind enorm wichtige Entscheidungshilfen für den Zahnarzt. Interview. Dtsch Zahnärztl Z 2019;74:152–153.

106. Willenbacher M, Al-Nawas B, Berres M, Kämmerer PW, Schiegnitz E: The effects of alveolar ridge preservation: a meta-analysis. Clin Implant Dent Relat Res 2016;18:1248–1268.

107. Winsauer H, Vlachojannis C, Bumann A, Vlachojannis J, Chrubasik S: Paramedian vertical palatal bone height for mini-implant insertion: a systematic review. Eur J Orthodont 2014;36:541–549.

108. Yoshino K, Kariya N, Namura D, Noji I, Mitsuhashi K, Kimura H, Fukuda A, Kikukawa I, Hayashi T, Yamazaki N, Kimura M, Tsukiyama K, Yamamoto K, Fukuyama A, Hidaka D, Shinoda J, Mibu H, Shimakura Y, Saito A, Ikumi S, Umehara K, Kamei F, Fukuda H, Toake T, Takahashi Y, Miyata Y, Shioji S, Toyoda M, Hattori N, Nishihara H, Matsushima R, Nishibori M, Hokkedo O, Nojima M, Kimura T, Fujiseki M, Okudaira S, Tanabe K, Nakano M, Ito K, Kuroda M, Takiguchi T, Fukai K, Matsukubo T: Influence of age on tooth autotransplantation with complete root formation. J Oral Rehab 2013;40:112–118.